INFUSING COMPASSIONATE PRESENCE
INTO YOUR DAILY LIFE

Dearest Tara + Greg!
Thank you so much for your endless
love and support!
I love you both so much!
Love you forever ♡ *Love,*
Kelly

365

DAYS OF
COMPASSION

BOOK COVER DESIGN: Nicole O'Keefe
CREATIVE DIRECTOR & TYPESET: Devon Adamson

First Printing, December 2023
Published by Ho'ola Publishing

pursuit365.com
onecaringhuman.org

instagram.com/**kellygrahamtick**
linktr.ee/**kellygrahamtick**

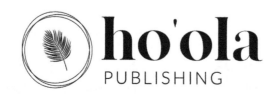

Dedicated to my Mama, Joyce Graham, from whom this journey began and continues, for willfully choosing your path, creating community with each person you met, loving with your whole heart, and being my biggest fan.

Also dedicated to Thom Hansen, for sharing your vulnerability and smiles with me through the last year of your life, and for teaching me so much.

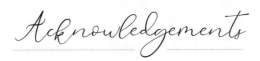

Acknowledgements

My sincerest gratitude to:

Shelly Lynn Hughes and Ho'ola Publishing, for helping me get this project off the ground.

Bif Naked, for all the love, generosity, and open heartedness.

Lyndsay Barrett, editor extraordinaire, for teaching me about authentic writing.

Devon Adamson, for making this book work and look stunning in the process.

Nicole O'Keefe, for gorgeous cover artistry.

Ashley Ramer and Cedar & Ocean Photography, for heart-opening experiences and photos.

Writers, mentors, and creative muses; Clarissa Pinkola Estes, Robin Wall Kimmerer, Richard Wagamese, Elizabeth Gilbert, Brene Brown, Gabor Mate, Glennon Doyle, Martha Beck, Renee Magnusson – OG girl gang creatress, instigator, and muse, Rhian Lockard – magical moon mama, Chris Zydel – creative inspirator, and Simone Grace Seol – #garbagepostchallenge creator and joyful marketing coach.

And I am eternally grateful for:

Highlands United Community, cast, crew, and support team, especially Ken Irwin, Gillian Irwin, Doug Irwin, Joy Dancey, Geordie Roberts, Carolyn Bergstrand, and Joanne Lacroix Doldon, for carrying me through grief and my mama's celebration of life, and for allowing fun and joy to seep back in.

Callan Rush and my Female Strong cohort, for sharing love and whooshes, and for inspiring my creativity and confidence. My Wayfinder Life Coaching cohort, for constantly having my back, loving honestly and transparently, sharing vulnerability, supporting so fully and thoughtfully, and being such a rad group of beautiful humans.

My fiercely loving and brilliant wolf pack babies, Kirni Gill and Rachel McClelland, and our One Caring Human Initiative peeps. My brave and beautiful patients, for sharing their stories and vulnerability with me.

My soul sisters, Kassie Kolins, Stephanie Chenoll, and Danica Hansen-Hughes, for your endless love, hugs, and support. Thank you for holding me for so many years, at my best and my worst.

My sister, Cari Michelle Broyles, for your sensitive heart, and for everything you did to care for Mum.

My family of siblings, aunts, uncles, cousins, nieces, nephews, all our fur babies, for an interwoven connection of the best and beautiful quirky support and generosity, especially thankful for Nicole, Alex, Denver, Gavin, Shane, Holly, Christopher, Taylor, Cari, Rob, Ginger, and Rush, for joining to spread Nana and Papa's ashes.

My kind-hearted and soulful children, Gavin, and Shane, for your love, your generous spirit, endless hugs, and so many cups of tea. I love you both forever.

My heart and love of my life, Ginger, for your limitless faith in me, continuous support, laughter, cuddles, adventures, and honesty. Thank you for lifting me up with your love, knowing when I need a break to hug a tree, for cooking all the time – it truly saves my life, for seeing me for everything I am and loving me anyway, and for holding me through all our days together.

Foreword

by Bif Naked, Canadian Punk Rock Legend

I may be known for being a bold, punk rock 'n' roll singer, but the truth is, I'm soft as a puppy. I love love, and I want to encourage the feeling in others. I've been this way as long as I can remember. And folks may be surprised to learn I found my true calling off the stage, as a hospital volunteer in healthcare when I was a cancer patient.

Oh, I survived breast cancer, and eventually graduated from the chemo and radiation wards with flying colors, but I couldn't shake off the desire to be in the hospital and the palliative care wards. I kept getting asked to visit patients and I just couldn't say no. I loved being there, loved the people, and not only do I love entertaining them, I love loving them.

I want everybody to feel better.
Living in gratitude is something I like to do, it's a habit, and it feels good. Not just because of my crazy life experience but because of the cool people that I get to sit with, be with, work with, or meet all over the world. For example, Kelly Graham Tick, a living angel.

Kelly was introduced to me by my dear friend, Shelly Lynn Hughes, famous for her thoughtfully curated book series Pursuit 365. It is motivational and inspirational, and I was blessed to be a part of it… not just once, but twice!

I definitely expected to be moved and inspired by this book, but I never expected to have my life completely changed, and that's exactly what Kelly did. Her writing broke my heart wide open and made my brain explode. She changed me for the better.

That may sound kind of insane but it's true. During my first conversation with Kelly,
I quickly discovered a human being so unyieldingly lovely and boundlessly compassionate, that I kind of fell in love with her.

Kelly has always been a force of loving nature, her background being a Registered Massage Therapist, working with people in Hospice and care homes, and teaching students of massage therapy to be exceptional caregivers themselves.
She is an extraordinary healer and light worker. She brings compassionate presence and safe touch to humans who need it.

And if that wasn't enough, she is a living soul doula, coaching others to find their truth, integrity, and alignment with their own paths.
Not only is she a soul doula - I believe she is mine.

I feel so utterly aligned with Kelly, so enamored - like a little kid who can't stop staring. I had to catch my breath. Can she be real? I thought, is she actually a living angel on earth?
It's possible.

She actually lives in this world, providing loving kindness, understanding, love, and healing touch to seriously ill and dying patients.
I look up to her. She is a mentor, a teacher, a living example of what we could and should all be. She inspires me to open my own compassion further, and to offer my own love more deeply.

Kelly inspires a more tender-hearted connection to all beings. She helps me discover true peace with my own spacious heart.
When I was asked to write the forward for Kelly's book, I almost had to turn it down. I simply didn't feel worthy.

Her writing is spectacular, open like the sky, as vast as the ocean, and unforgettable.
It hit me hard, every page.
It moved me.
It changed me.
Her words let me breathe and trust.

I needed it.
And so will you.

This body of work is perfect. It's a reflection of her heart and the memorable moments she has discovered through her work. Kelly heals through her words, and offers positivity, love, and this unbelievable radiant hope that we can feel the freedom to surrender to.

I humbly accepted to write the forward and as I write, it is my earnest effort to convey how I truly feel about this work, these words, and about Kelly's powerful message.

Kelly can help us, and heal us, through her words and the delicate energy behind them, because her words are from her ginormous, honorable, endlessly loving heart. As she generously shares her astonishing experiences from her life and work, and deeply private glimpses into her beloved mother's journey, she sensitively shows us the art of true, loving kindness.

She receives lessons to keep honoring herself during her darkest, lowest times, her humility shining during reflections with quotes like, "Sending love to all those wandering humbly toward holiness, may you soon find peace". I will always carry these words with me.

Her truth is beautiful.
It's meaningful, and Kelly's writing aims to help everyone acknowledge their own beauty and worthiness and let go of the rest. Kelly says purpose can grow within us like a sunrise, and I feel it…and so will you.

I felt love grow, and become brighter than any sun, from reading every page that she lovingly wrote, and because she has a tremendous calling for helping others, she lives for it.

Kelly helps us slide across the spectrum of vulnerability with grace and love. This book is a rare treasure, a gift to the world as the unparalleled living love that is the unparalleled Kelly Graham Tick.seeing me for everything I am and loving me anyway, and for holding me through all our days together.

- Bif Naked, 2023

365 Days of Compassion

Infusing compassionate presence into your daily life
By Kelly Graham Tick

365 Days of Compassion is a cathartic day-to-day journey through the illness and death of my mama and getting through the grief that followed.

Daily writing helped me wipe the sand off the messages that were bottled up and express the thoughts that arose with every gentle tide and crashing wave of emotion, throughout a challenging year.

I learned more than any other year how to speak the language of my soul and translate the simultaneous pain and bliss into a sense of wholeness.

Everyone has experienced or will face the death of a loved one, and ultimately will move through the transition themselves.

Though it is not a new situation, each person holds a unique perspective on how to face the challenges of aging, dying, and living.

Every part of our lives may be affected when viewed through the eyes of compassion.

These pages are the emotions of my daily thoughts, questions, reflections, insights, sadness, grief, joy, love notes, and calls for compassionate presence that I hope will take you on an intimate journey of your own.

Epiphany can arrive in unexpected moments and understanding can arise through the words of others.
My sincerest wish for you is to see yourself reflected in the vulnerable expressions I share here.

Kelly is a Canadian Registered Massage Therapist, a teacher, a writer, and founder of One Caring Human Initiative, an organization that offers compassionate presence and therapeutic touch to the elderly and the dying in care homes, hospice, and palliative hospitals.

Everybody deserves exceptional care

You are an exceptional being.

You deserve no less than exceptional kindness,
honour, love, care, connection, and compassion.

Every human and non-human requires care,
nurturing, and to be known, **in order to thrive.**

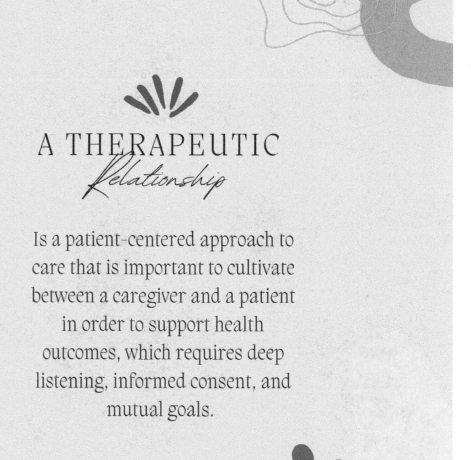

A THERAPEUTIC
Relationship

Is a patient-centered approach to care that is important to cultivate between a caregiver and a patient in order to support health outcomes, which requires deep listening, informed consent, and mutual goals.

A relationship with a caregiver is significant enough to expect thoughtful, intentional presence, focused on what you need to feel supported.

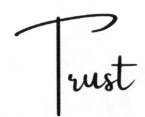

IN THERAPEUTIC RELATIONSHIP BEGINS WITH:

Physical Safety
Emotional Safety
Psychological Safety
Confidentiality

Feeling safe in vulnerable situations,
especially in a healthcare setting, is needed
for healing and relief to be possible
outcomes.

**Do you have deep trust for your healthcare
providers?**

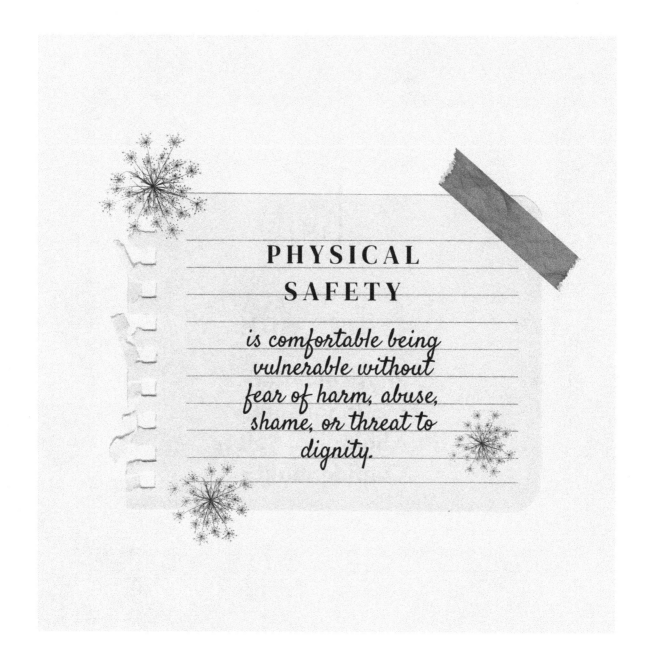

PHYSICAL SAFETY

is comfortable being vulnerable without fear of harm, abuse, shame, or threat to dignity.

Priorities in a caregiver/patient relationship.

Psychological safety is feeling comfortable expressing concerns without fear of rejection, humiliation, or ridicule.

Do you trust your healthcare practitioners and caregivers to treat you with dignity and respect in regard to your mental and emotional health?

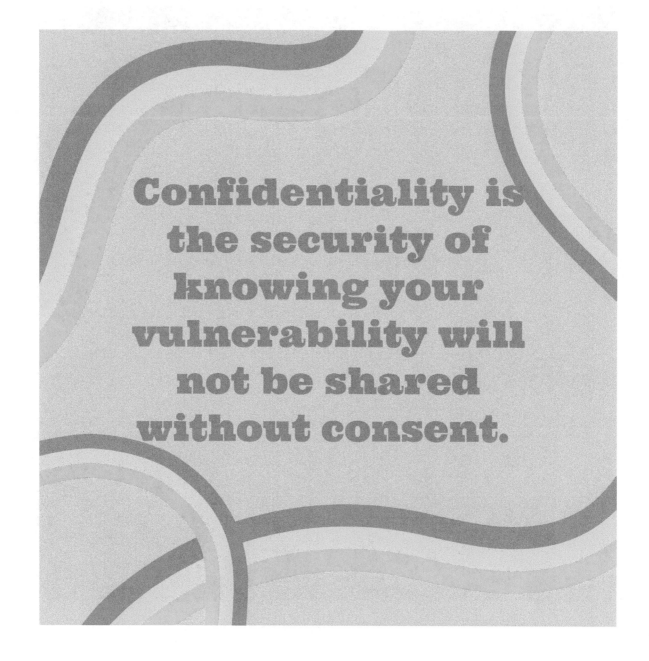

Confidentiality is the security of knowing your vulnerability will not be shared without consent.

Confidence in healthcare must include confidentiality to feel safe.

Did you know that confidentiality is part of the Code of Ethics in every regulated health profession in Canada?

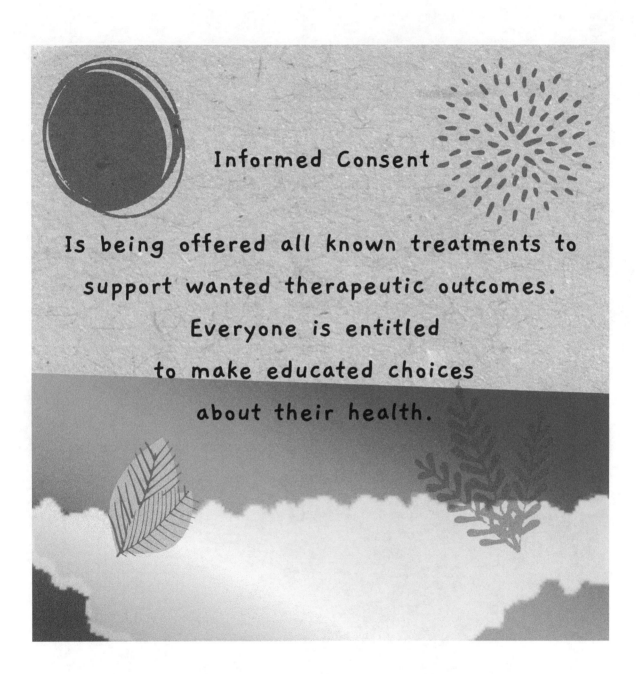

Informed Consent

Is being offered all known treatments to support wanted therapeutic outcomes. Everyone is entitled to make educated choices about their health.

Sovereignty allows our hearts to be aligned with our actions and decisions.

Taking the time to understand and ask questions is vital to giving consent.

You have the right to direct your own care.

SHOWING LOVE IN A HEALTHCARE SETTING LOOKS LIKE

Compassionate Presence

Dignity

Safety

You deserve this kind of care.

We need our caregivers to be present with us, to offer dignity, and ensure every layer of safety.

If one of these is missing, the other two are invalidated.

You Deserve to be
Trusted
To Make Healthcare
Decisions

Our systems can make it challenging to feel honoured and
trusted to make the choices that are right for us.

Slow down enough to ask for time to make decisions that
honour your path, rather than the directive of a caregiver,
even if it ends up being the same outcome.

Autonomy. Nothing less.

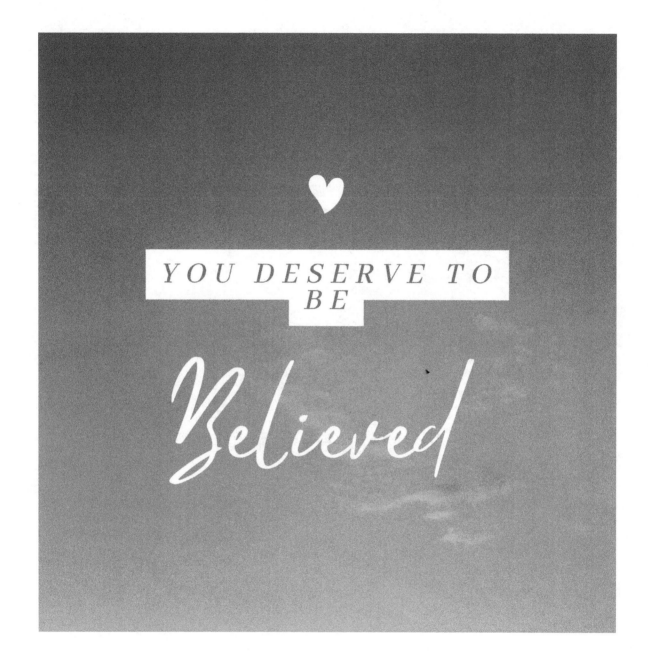

You know your truth better than anyone else in this world.

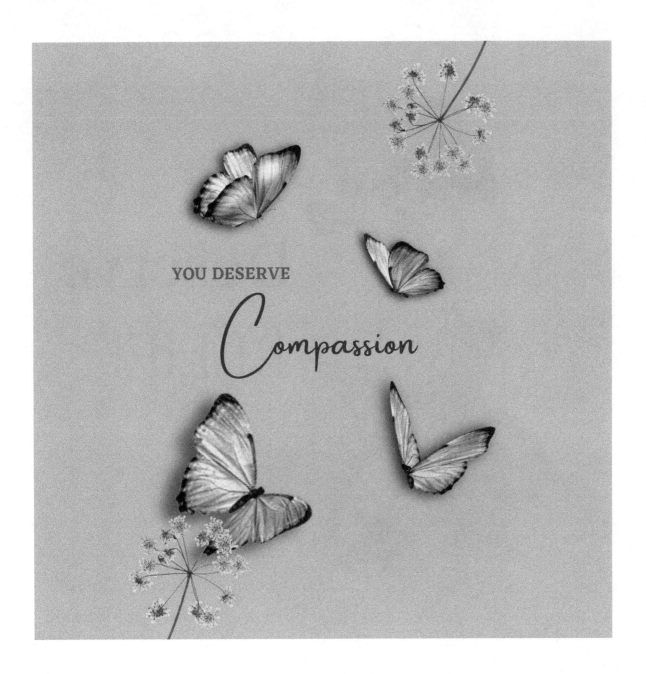

YOU DESERVE

Compassion

Compassion creates connection.

It allows a space between the tender heart and its exposure
to the outside elements, a cushion to keep us warm during
the hardest moments in life.

Compassion in the healthcare system can easily be
forgotten.

Reminders of humanity are so so important.

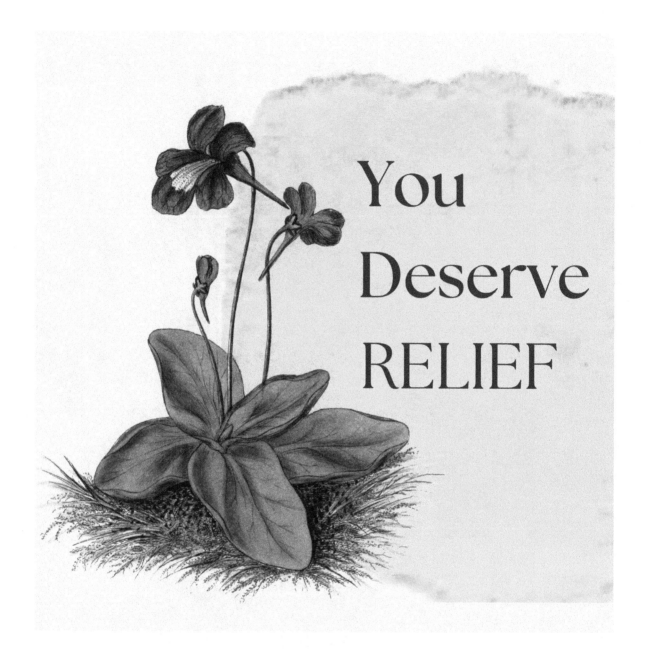

You
Deserve
RELIEF

Relief doesn't need to be big to be impactful.

Just a tiny shift in perception can create tremendous comfort, whether physical, emotional, psychological, or spiritual.

It's been a tough day. Many people I know are in the hospital tonight. I'm sending anyone who is struggling and in pain some sweet relief and love.

Take care of you.

You Deserve Compassionate Caregivers

You deserve to feel seen, heard, valued, and cared for.

We often get used to being treated poorly, even if it feels wrong somewhere in our bodies.

Noticing when compassion is absent is the first step to recognizing something that needs to change, and then move toward asking for it.

Everyone has pressures that can distract us from being present, including caregivers.

It is a gift to yourself and them to ask for presence and compassion.

Therapeutic relationships with caregivers in healthcare and other realms of your life that feel safe, loving, kind, and thorough, promote healing, self-compassion, and authenticity.

YOU DESERVE SUPPORT

When we feel supported, our nervous system responds by opening and relaxing.

Your body is a great indicator of tension and relief, check in with your muscles and your breath to feel where support could make a difference.

We are not meant to do this alone.

Any of it.

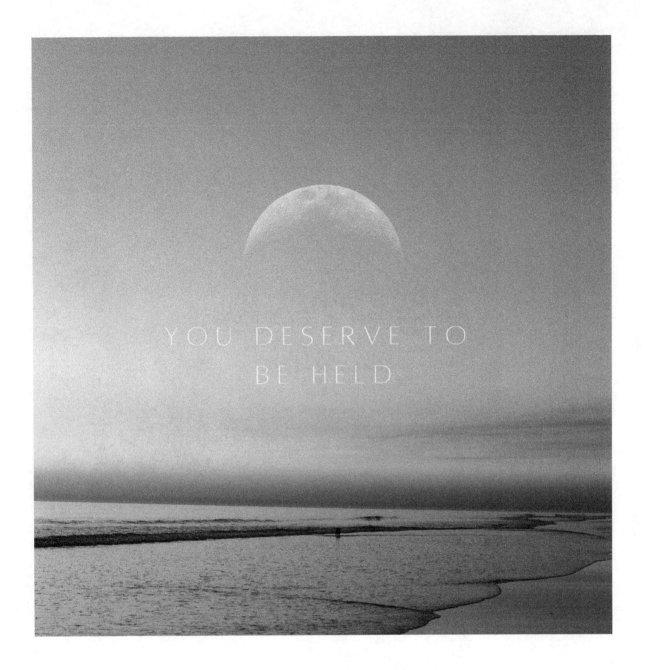

YOU DESERVE TO
BE HELD

Pain and shame changes when we are held in compassion
and non-judgement.

Notice what parts of you need to be held.

How can you hold yourself in your own compassion, joy,
love, and integrity?

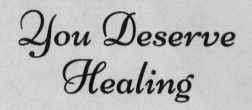

You Deserve Healing

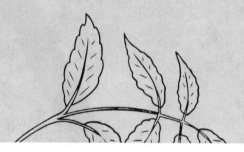

You deserve profound healing, multi-layered healing, in
your wholeness, by your own definition.

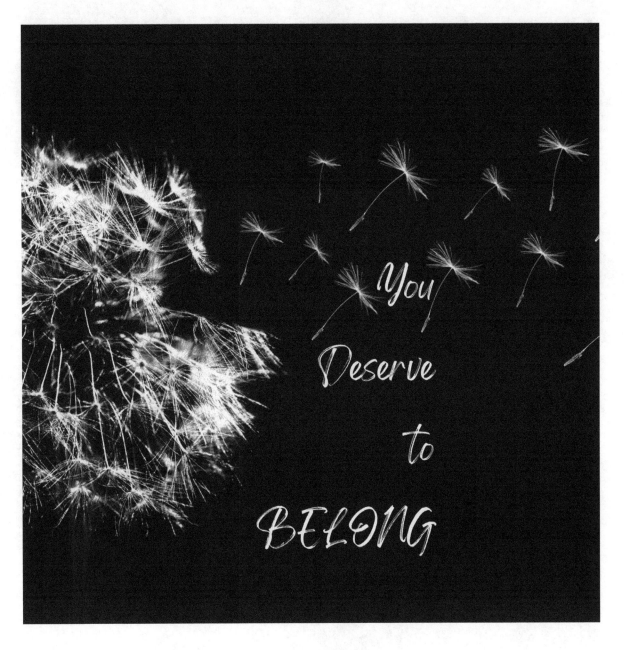

You
Deserve
to
BELONG

Belonging is a core need for all humans.

Without it, our sense of self suffers and can become
hypervigilant in self-protection.

Feeling truly part of a community allows us to explore
our truths, shadows, and desires, and find peace within,
through the cultivation of reciprocal relationship.

Authentic belonging creates a unique sense of security that
promotes a relaxed joy in being yourself.

Inclusion is for everyone.

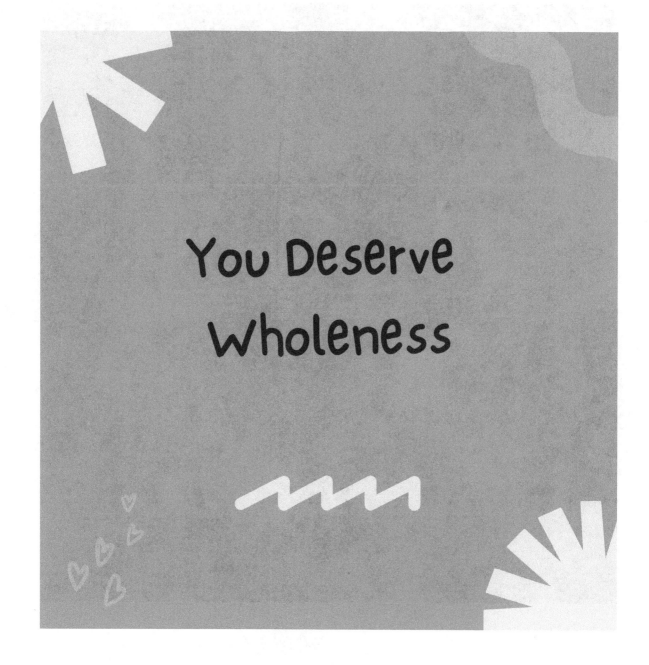

You Deserve Wholeness

You deserve your whole self; your mind, body, spirit, soul, emotions, needs, desires, concerns, and goals to be addressed, engaged, held, respected, and honoured... together, as one whole being.

You Deserve to Know what Peace Feels Like

Peace... in mind, in body, in your environment.

Cultivate peace within yourself and ask for it from your personal and professional relationships. This does not mean you must be calm all the time, or even ever, it means you understand what peace feels like, and hold boundaries in those moments, or relationships that try to move you away from that knowing.

Allowing yourself to sink to your core and discover the constant support that is always there, deep under social conditioning, is fundamental to your joy. Normalize supporting others in this endeavor and asking for adequate support for yourself.

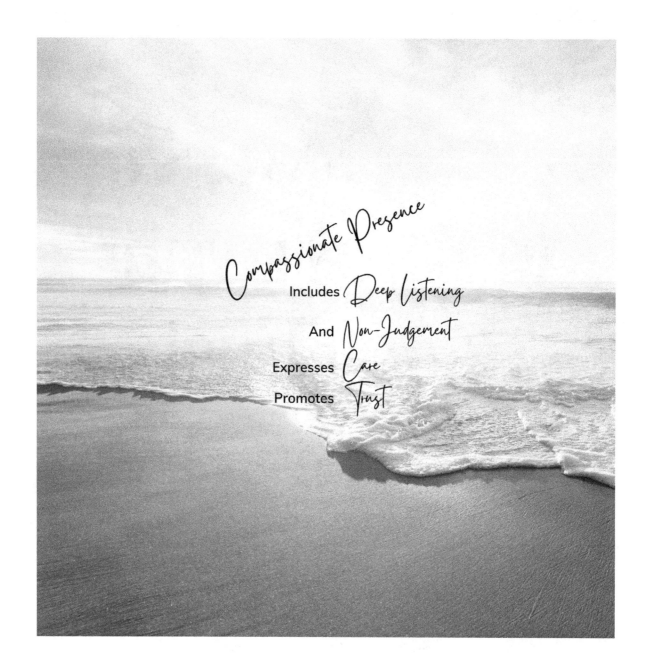

Compassionate Presence

Includes Deep Listening

And Non-Judgement

Expresses Care

Promotes Trust

Do you experience this with your healthcare team?

You Deserve a Society that values generosity and cooperation over greed and power.

Poverty should not exist in a world with thousands of billionaires.

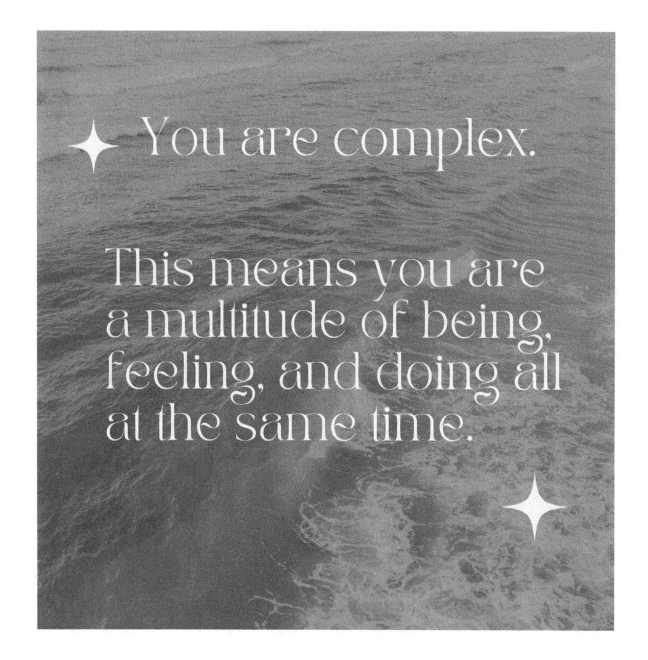

You are complex.

This means you are a multitude of being, feeling, and doing all at the same time.

Some days, it feels like we can experience a million feelings at once, other days we notice barely one. We are complex containers with capacity for expansive thoughts and emotions.

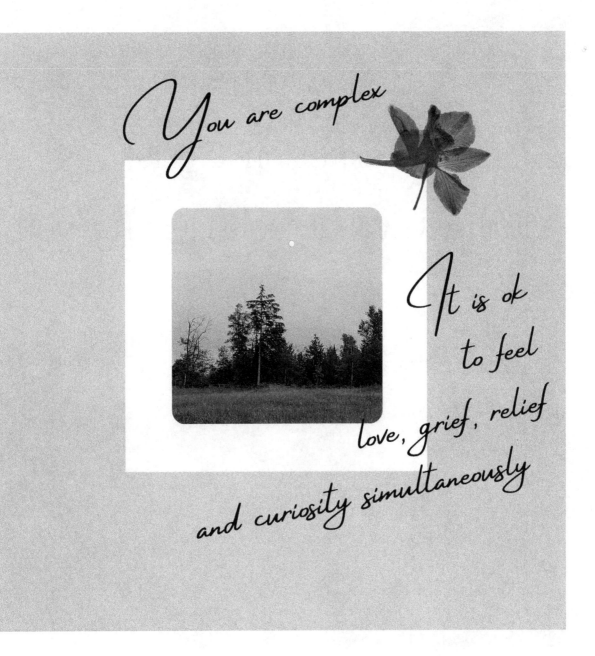

You are complex

It is ok
to feel
love, grief, relief
and curiosity simultaneously

Allow yourself

to experience grief

in the way that feels right for you.

"Grief is just love with no place to go."
-Alyson Noel

Please find an outlet for your unconditional love and
grieving heart.

I'm sending love to all of you who are grieving.

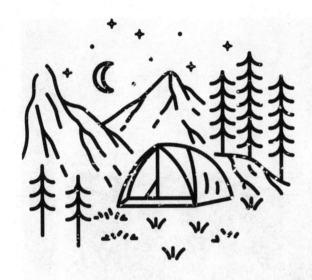

THE NATURE OF BELONGING WILL GROW
NEW NEURAL PATHWAYS IN THE BRAIN THAT HAVE
THE POWER TO CONNECT US WITH PERSPECTIVES WE HAVEN'T
CONSIDERED, CHANGE OUR INNER DYNAMIC AND
PATTERNS OF BEHAVIOR.

Belonging changes your brain.

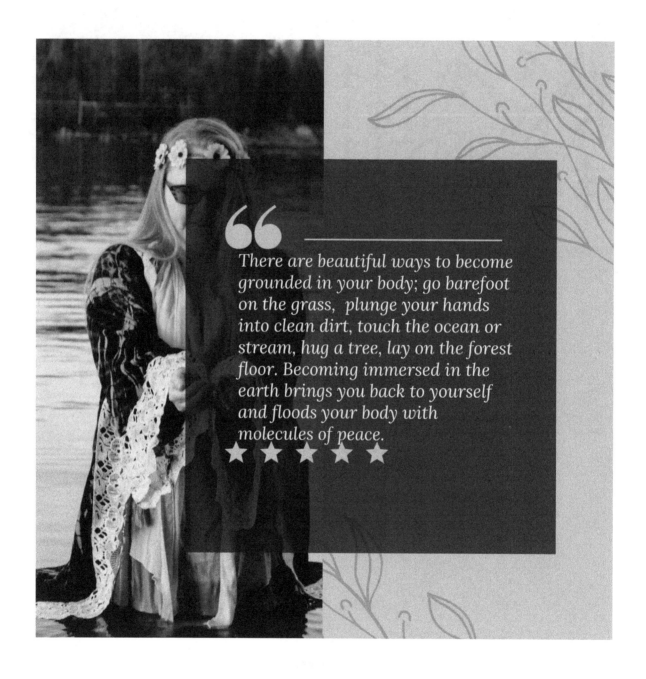

" There are beautiful ways to become grounded in your body; go barefoot on the grass, plunge your hands into clean dirt, touch the ocean or stream, hug a tree, lay on the forest floor. Becoming immersed in the earth brings you back to yourself and floods your body with molecules of peace.

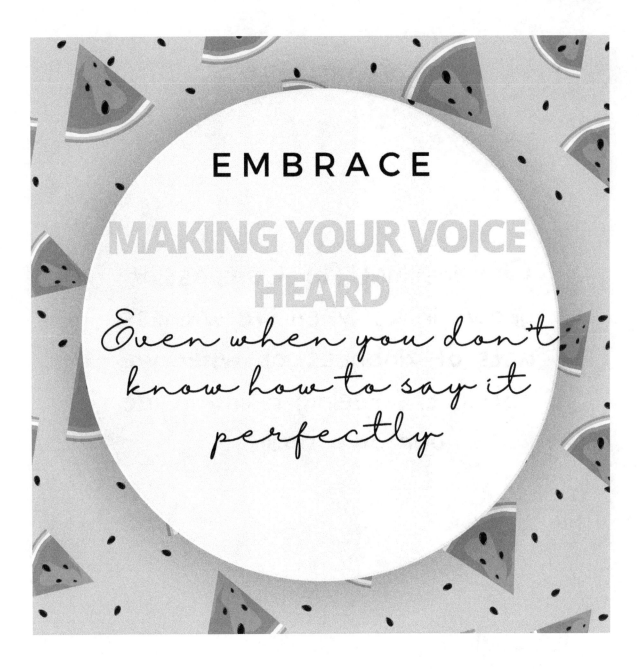

EMBRACE

MAKING YOUR VOICE HEARD

Even when you don't know how to say it perfectly

Nobody knows what they're doing 100% of the time, or likely even 50 % of the time. Life is a lot of choices and chances, winging it and hoping for the best. Putting yourself out there give others permission to do it too and gives them a chance to support you as well.

That's what these posts are for me, just flinging my thoughts and heart out there, and finding out what will stick, what will resonate with others who may need to hear my words. It is vulnerable and scary, but you know I'm not perfect.

So, I know you can do it too, and I'll support the heck out of it!

Our instinct for Compassion grows in us when we witness acts of kindness, or when we notice the feeling rising inside our own bodies.

"In some recent studies I've conducted, we have found that when people perform behaviors associated with compassionate love – warm smiles, friendly hand gestures, affirmative forward leans – their bodies produce more oxytocin. This suggests compassion may be self-perpetuating: Being compassionate causes a chemical reaction in the body that motivates us to be even more compassionate."

- Dacher Keltner, The Compassionate Instinct, Greater Good Magazine

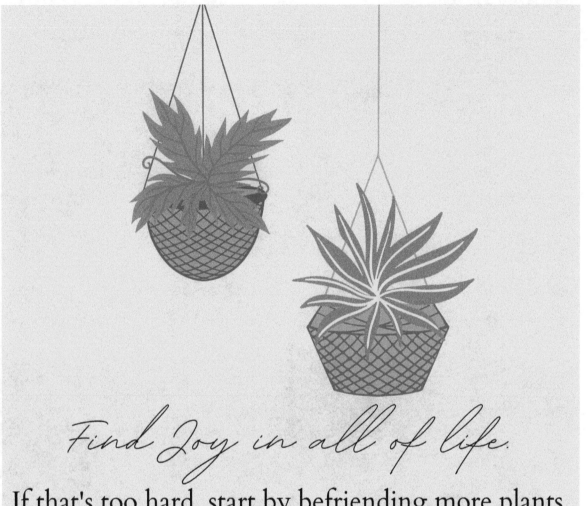

Find Joy in all of life.

If that's too hard, start by befriending more plants.

Plants are non-human friends. They uplift your spirit, give you oxygen, and shows you how to offer beauty without expectation of something in return. Talking to and taking care of plants when everything else seems too hard, is a non-threatening way to connect with another being.

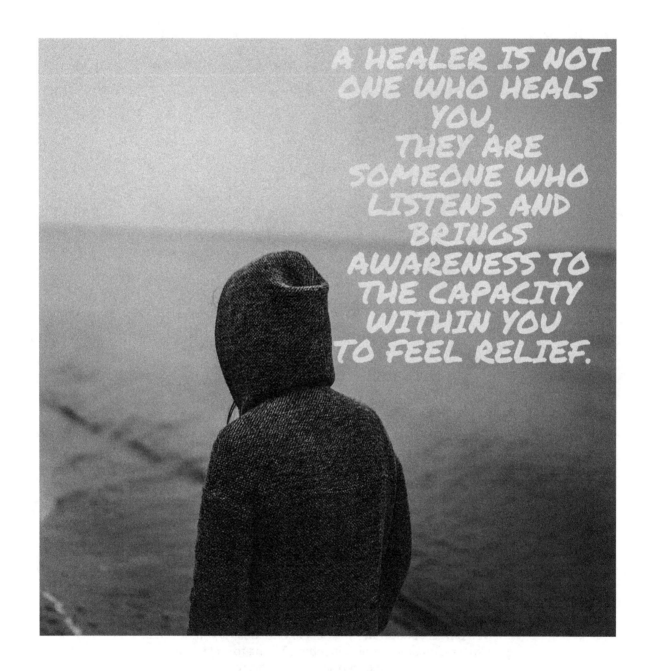

A HEALER IS NOT ONE WHO HEALS YOU, THEY ARE SOMEONE WHO LISTENS AND BRINGS AWARENESS TO THE CAPACITY WITHIN YOU TO FEEL RELIEF.

Create spaces for
you to feel safe in,
and then build them
for others.

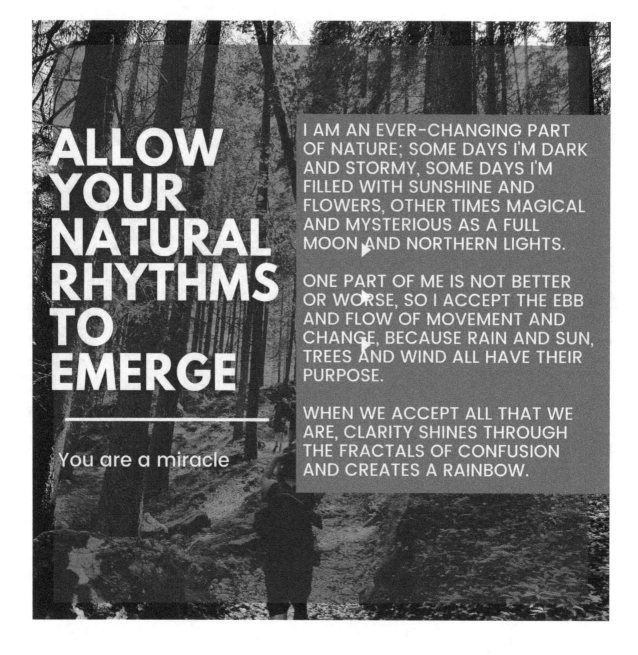

ALLOW YOUR NATURAL RHYTHMS TO EMERGE

You are a miracle

I AM AN EVER-CHANGING PART OF NATURE; SOME DAYS I'M DARK AND STORMY, SOME DAYS I'M FILLED WITH SUNSHINE AND FLOWERS, OTHER TIMES MAGICAL AND MYSTERIOUS AS A FULL MOON AND NORTHERN LIGHTS.

ONE PART OF ME IS NOT BETTER OR WORSE, SO I ACCEPT THE EBB AND FLOW OF MOVEMENT AND CHANGE, BECAUSE RAIN AND SUN, TREES AND WIND ALL HAVE THEIR PURPOSE.

WHEN WE ACCEPT ALL THAT WE ARE, CLARITY SHINES THROUGH THE FRACTALS OF CONFUSION AND CREATES A RAINBOW.

COMPASSIONATE PRESENCE IS
FOCUSED INTENTIONAL ENERGY THAT
CAN BE PERCEIVED ON EVERY LEVEL
BY THE ONE RECEIVING IT

THERAPEUTIC INTENTION IS THE DESIRE TO AFFECT THE

Well-Being of others

A therapeutic relationship is created between a medical practitioner and a patient, or a caregiver and the one they care for. Anyone can have therapeutic intention, if they simply have the desire to see another have relief, healing, or a better quality of life.

You may not think you have the ability to affect another's well-being, but it is possible to give a smile, a hug, a hand to hold, a safe, nurturing touch, a listening ear, compassionate presence. These gifts and more, can absolutely have a therapeutic effect.

Everyone deserves more love and attention.

It's beautiful to

Be someone's rock

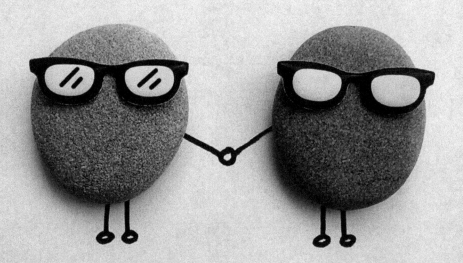

And to let them be yours

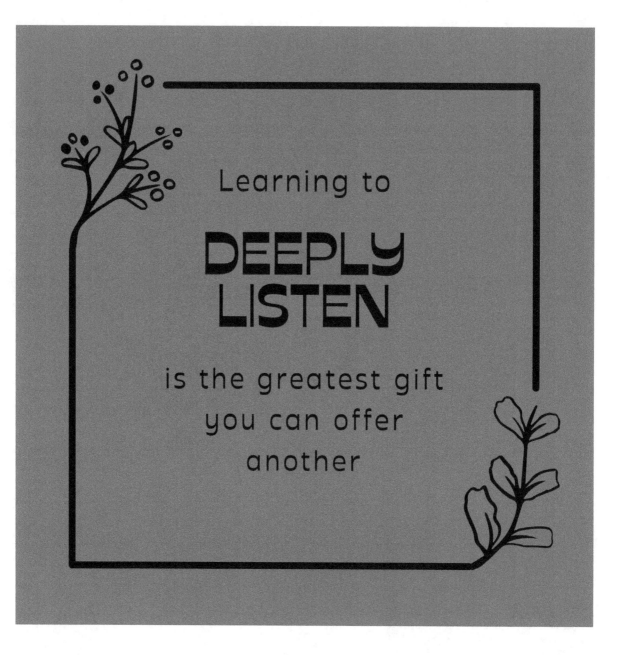

Learning to

DEEPLY
LISTEN

is the greatest gift
you can offer
another

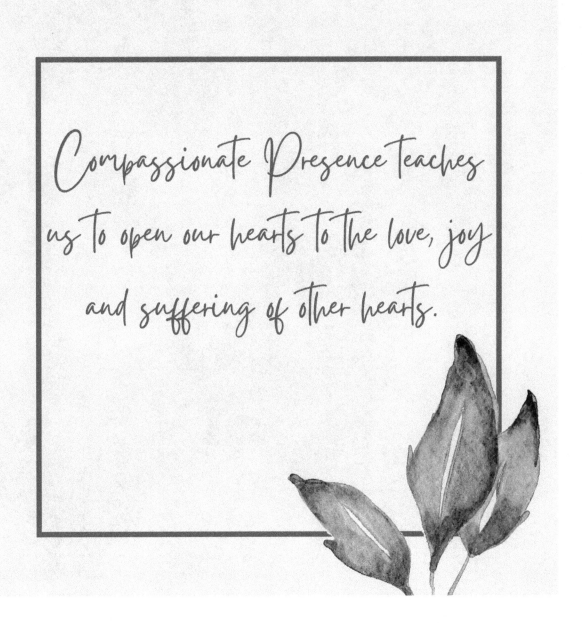

Compassionate Presence teaches us to open our hearts to the love, joy and suffering of other hearts.

When we allow ourselves to slow down enough to truly
hear what others are going through, we are able to become
expanded within, to be changed by the connection that
results from authenticity.

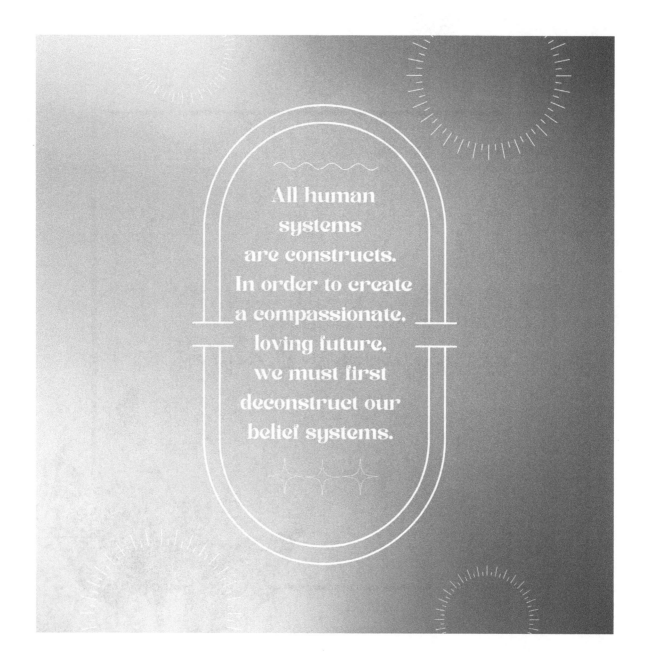

All human
systems
are constructs.
In order to create
a compassionate,
loving future,
we must first
deconstruct our
belief systems.

To create a more compassionate present and future, we
must first be aware of what we believe, and look for paths
toward kinder systems. Change begins within.

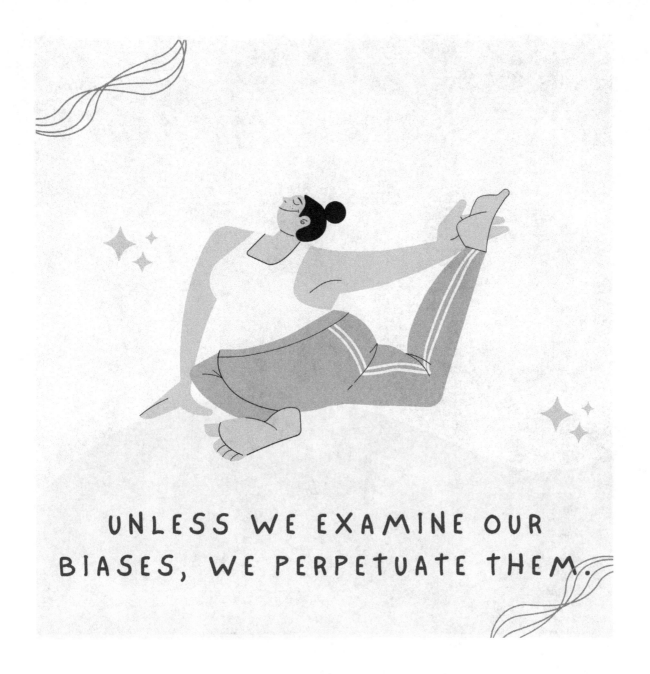

UNLESS WE EXAMINE OUR BIASES, WE PERPETUATE THEM.

"Unless we challenge stigma, we reproduce it."

- Ashton Applewhite, author of "This Chair Rocks, A Manifesto Against Ageism" (a fantastic book by the way!)

Inspired by this quote, I want to articulate that contribute to healthy, compassionate relationships, communities, and organizations, we all need to be aware of our deeply held beliefs and biases, challenge stigma, and embrace opportunities for growth, intuitive wisdom, and thoughtful communication.

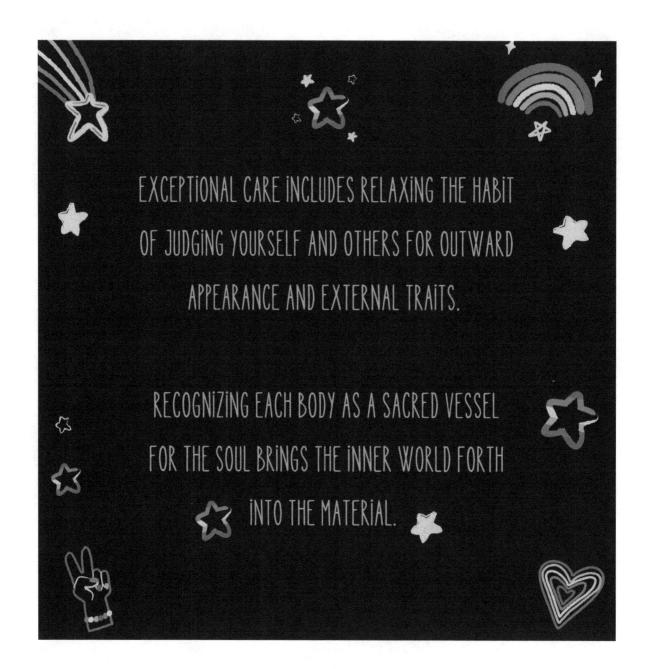

EXCEPTIONAL CARE INCLUDES RELAXING THE HABIT OF JUDGING YOURSELF AND OTHERS FOR OUTWARD APPEARANCE AND EXTERNAL TRAITS.

RECOGNIZING EACH BODY AS A SACRED VESSEL FOR THE SOUL BRINGS THE INNER WORLD FORTH INTO THE MATERIAL.

When we judge less and see each person as the miracle they are, the world becomes infinitely more compassionate and strikingly beautiful.

Dignity must not be reserved only for those with money, power, or status. This weakens society and the health of those within it.

Health and dignity are not meant only for those who have the ability to pay for it.

Interconnectivity and collaboration are the stuff of humanity.

We are connected in ways that haven't even been conceived by the mind yet.

What we do to one, we do to ourselves.

How we treat human and non-human relations grows.

Compassion and community are crucial to our survival.

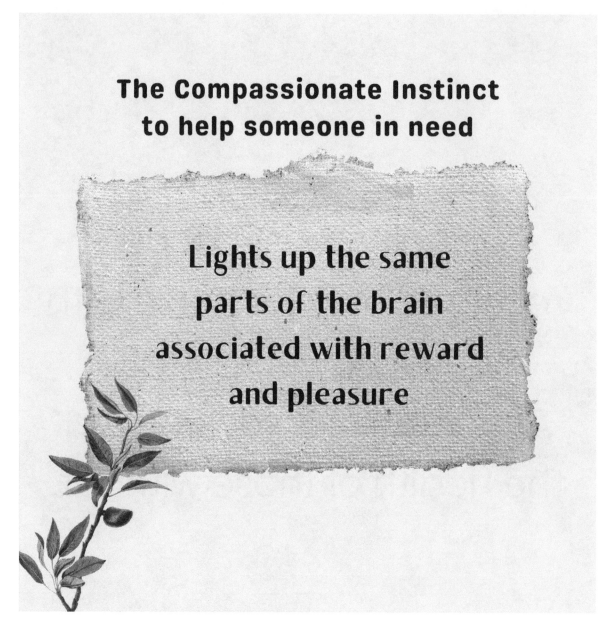

**The Compassionate Instinct
to help someone in need**

Lights up the same
parts of the brain
associated with reward
and pleasure

Isn't this amazing?

We are wired to help others in need.

What happens when we ignore this instinct?

I can only imagine it in the context of "use it or lose it."

I don't believe it goes away completely, but it would make sense that not acting on compassion could feed those neural connections less and create faster responses in the nerves that fear the consequences of compassion.

What we pay attention to becomes habitual.

In essence, being compassionate is healthy for the brain, and helps others at the same time.

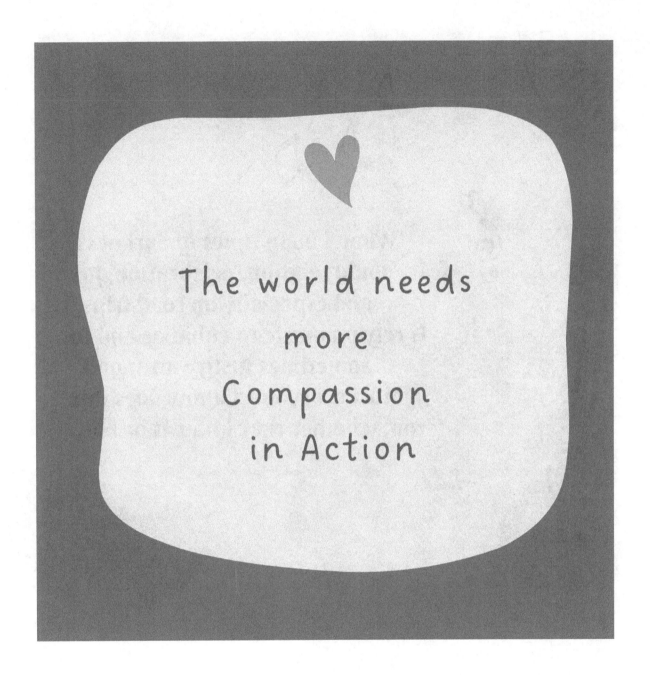

The world needs more Compassion in Action

This kind of love says, 'I see you, let me hold you for a while.'

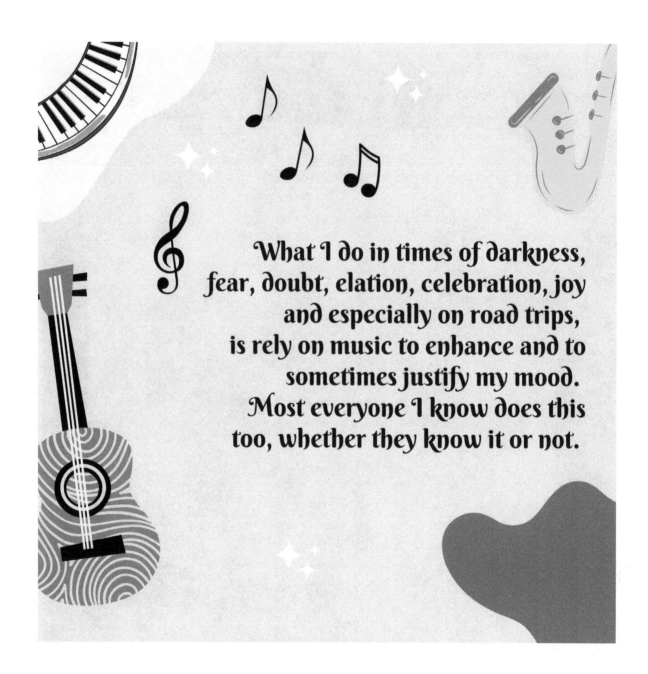

What I do in times of darkness,
fear, doubt, elation, celebration, joy
and especially on road trips,
is rely on music to enhance and to
sometimes justify my mood.
Most everyone I know does this
too, whether they know it or not.

Music infuses my experiences with meaning, comfort,
clarity, protest, awakening, love, grounding, focus, energy,
and hope. I am so grateful for the subversive artists who
continue to share their gifts regardless of the opinions of
others and those who try to control.

Much love!

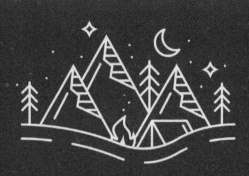

It is breathtaking to imagine the profound impact
Radical support

for self-care

could have on society

In your wildest imaginings, what are all the ways you could feel deeply, radically cared for?

Make a list if it's helpful to see the words in front of you.

And then dream up all the ways you could be in alignment with your values and integrity, do the things that make your heart sing, and have fulfillment, if you had the support to thrive and honour yourself.

Add to your list whenever you can.

Relief can show up as surprise when you realize you CAN ask to be treated better than you have been before.

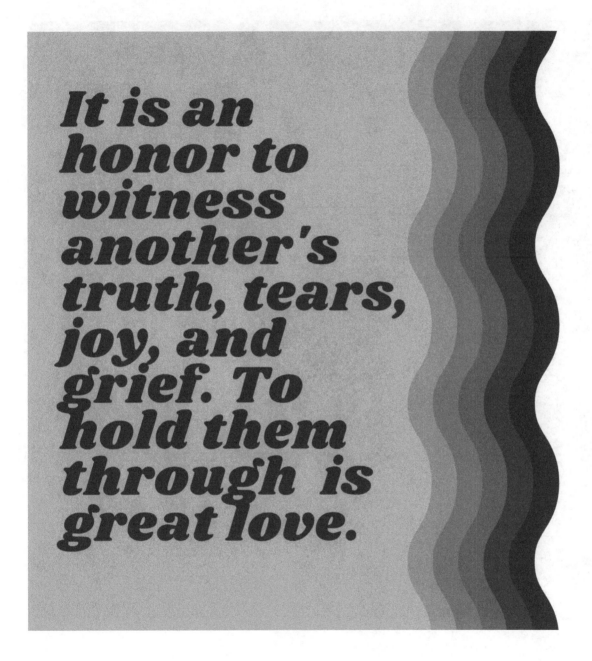

It is an honor to witness another's truth, tears, joy, and grief. To hold them through is great love.

Holding space for another's truest self shows great love for them, and helps grow your own capacity for listening, love, and compassion.

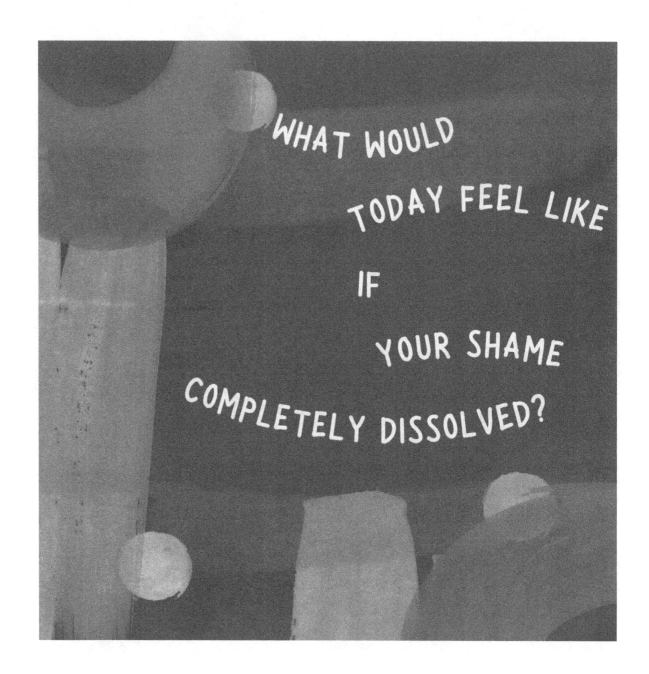

WHAT WOULD TODAY FEEL LIKE IF YOUR SHAME COMPLETELY DISSOLVED?

Shame holds us back from being who we want to be,
because we fear being judged for having shadows. When
we allow light to touch our shadows in safe spaces, those
shadows become indistinguishable from the light.

A universe lives inside you.

NO OTHER HUMAN ON THE
PLANET HAS YOUR UNIQUE
PERSPECTIVE.

YOUR GIFTS ARE BUBBLING
BENEATH THE SURFACE OF
YOUR MUNDANE LIFE, THEY LIVE
IN THE RIVER OF AN EXPANSIVE
INNER WORLD.

YOU HAVE UNEXPLORED
CREATIVITY EXCITEDLY
WAITING TO EMERGE INTO THE
CONSCIOUS, TO JOIN THE SOUL
OF THE WORLD THROUGH
YOU!

You are the muse, a human vessel of creativity.

Share your gifts.

The world needs you.

WHATEVER YOU
THINK OTHERS WILL
JUDGE YOU FOR

*They are already
judging themselves
about*

Feelings of inadequacy, hurt, and self-criticism without consequences can lead to judgement of others without basis. Judgement from another does not necessarily reflect who you are, it is often based on the insecurity of the one who judges you.

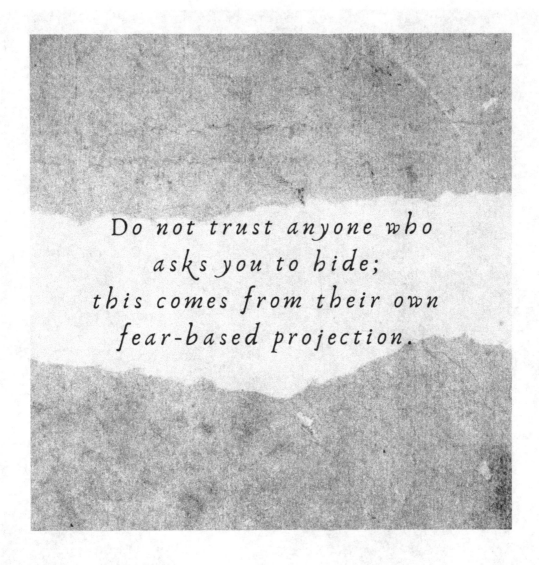

Do not trust anyone who asks you to hide; this comes from their own fear-based projection.

I once had a partner who asked me to hide my hair when we went out walking on his granddad's property because he didn't want the neighbors to tell his grandfather if they happened to spy us. His U.S. granddad didn't approve of his relationship with me because I'm Canadian, as he felt he "lost" his own son (my bf's dad) when he moved to Canada.

Rather than be honest or discuss these fears with his grandparent, he put the burden on me to not be myself, literally, to make himself feel safe.

This felt horrible and wrong in my body and mind, it went against my integrity, I felt like I wasn't good enough being authentic, a whole human. And yet, I compromised myself for him in the moment.

That relationship didn't work out. But it had psychological repercussions.

People and society ask us all the time to compromise ourselves for the sake of fitting in, keeping the status quo. If we do it long enough, an exoskeleton of fear builds thick around us, and becomes difficult to break out of. We feel fear and doubt and insecurity and imposter syndrome. We think, "who am I to have desires or dreams?"

I say f@#* that.

Do whatever it takes, find whatever support you need to discover your true self and start living your precious life!

Being true to YOU is more important than disappointing someone else.

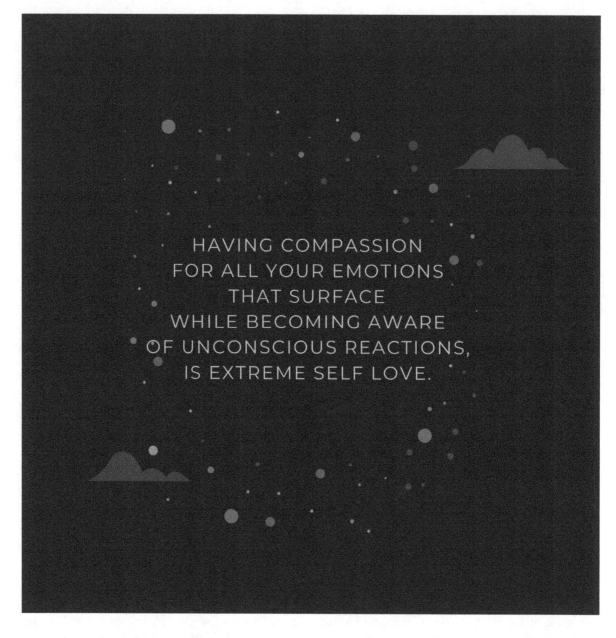

HAVING COMPASSION
FOR ALL YOUR EMOTIONS
THAT SURFACE
WHILE BECOMING AWARE
OF UNCONSCIOUS REACTIONS,
IS EXTREME SELF LOVE.

The first time I remember the feeling of abandonment is when I was 4. My parents divorced, our family dynamic shifted, and I had to create thoughts around those big feelings that kept me connected to safety in the only way I knew how as a child.

This meant I sometimes froze when I thought I might lose connection or affection. Other times it meant I would cut ties with people before they could abandon me. And it also meant that sometimes I would abandon myself, for fear of being judged or left alone.

It has been a common theme in my life, and once

I began to recognize my internal, unconscious reactions to the feeling of fear, I learned to give these feelings space and get curious about where inside me they are coming from. This has led to much revelation, which has grown my self compassion, and my compassion for others.

Holding myself with a different mind than the part of me that is scared is a massive saving grace. I hope that you can learn to hold yourself in grace and love, through the messiness of life and your challenging beliefs, and make known your unconscious reactions.

Love love love. So much love.

YOU HAVE
BOTH
FIRE AND
MAGIC
INSIDE YOU

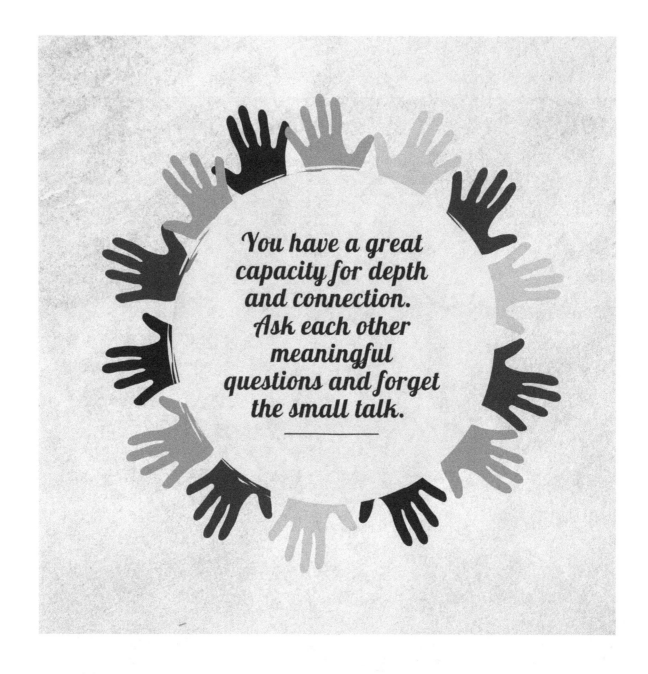

You have a great capacity for depth and connection. Ask each other meaningful questions and forget the small talk.

Relentless small talk causes me to lose interest in the conversation very quickly.

I want to know what you value, what breaks your heart, what brings meaning to your life, and your visions of a better future.

People have become so used to say hello in passing, or not saying hello at all, that we have forgotten the art of conversation, and the shared compassion in deeply listening to one another.

If you are afraid of abandonment or heartbreak, remember you have felt it before. It may at first, feel like an enemy.

You have held it for yourself and for others, because you know they fear it too. Fear has a message, it says, 'do not shut down for me, open instead to dear one's also affected.'
It says, 'you know that love you are afraid to express? Share it!'
For then you will understand the gift of your emotions, even the ones that don't look like friends at first.

Love is to share, as a flower shares its beauty with the world.

THOUGH MY PERSPECTIVE SEEMS OBVIOUS AND ORDINARY TO ME, IT'S ALWAYS A BEAUTIFUL EXPERIENCE WHEN OTHERS REFLECT THE INSIGHT THEY GAIN WHEN I'M BRAVE ENOUGH TO SHARE MY HEART.

Share your heart, I promise you it is worth it.

When I do, I always either find truth, confidence, softness, acceptance, or soul.

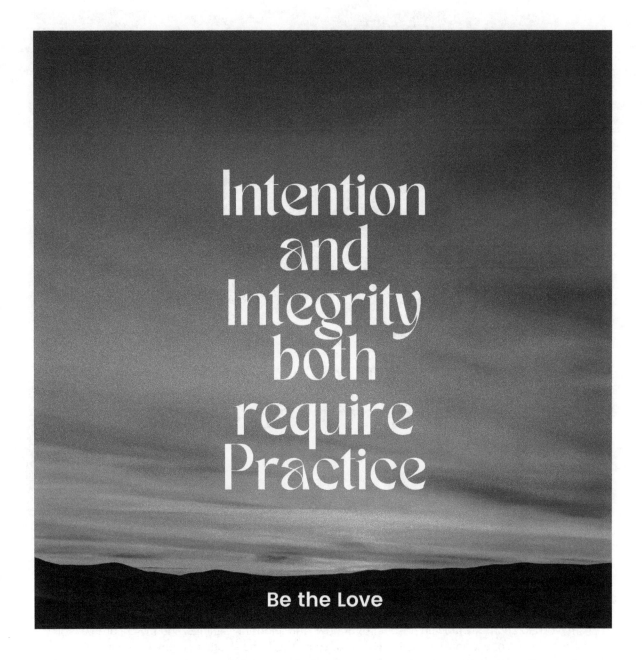

Intention
and
Integrity
both
require
Practice

Be the Love

Having clear intentions and alignment with integrity is more rare than, and as stunning as a gorgeous sunset. We may be fortunate enough to witness both for a short time each day, be it in ourselves or another. The point is to be present enough to stop and notice the beauty when it presents itself to us.

Holding awareness is part of the practice.

Check-in with yourself everyday.

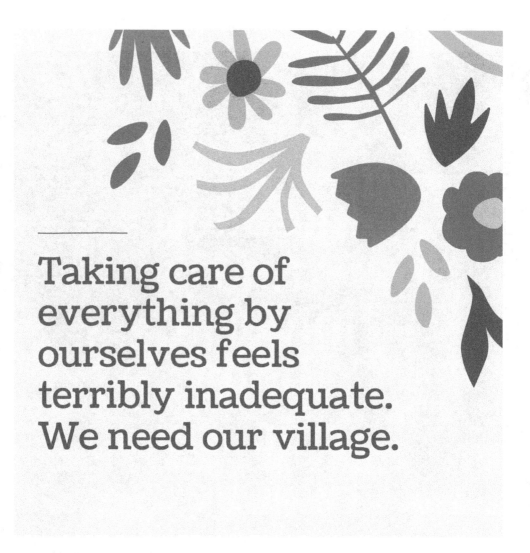

Taking care of everything by ourselves feels terribly inadequate. We need our village.

Even though we aren't actually doing everything alone, it can feel that way in our minds. We are suffering alone. Our hearts and nervous systems need to be in loving, supportive connection with others to feel that our load is shared.

I am worried about my mum in hospital right now, and about my siblings, and my children. I worry about the state of economic hardship rising for so many, in the struggle to pay for essential needs. I worry about our ecosystems and climate in the hands of profiteering systems. I worry about the healthcare and education systems that leave so many people behind.

At times, it is excruciating to feel alone in these worries, even though there are millions with the same struggles.

We have got to reconnect in loving, supportive ways, so we don't feel so alone with the exact same overwhelming thoughts.

I want to do something about it.

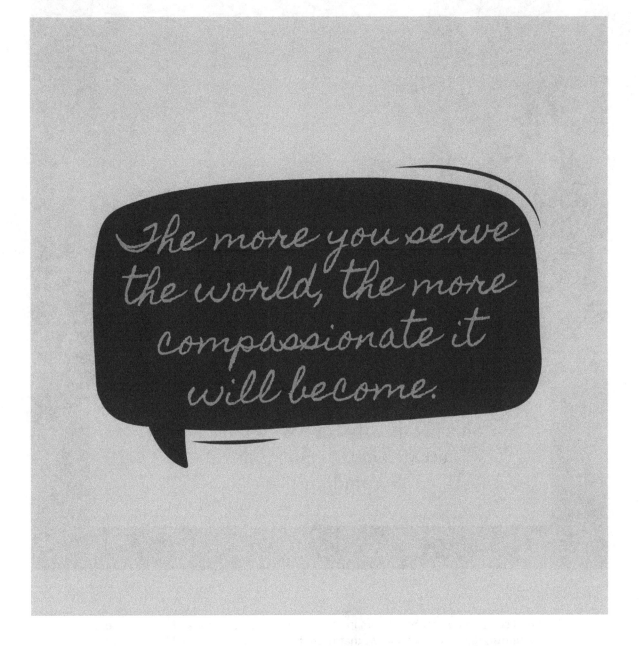

Compassionate presence can witness the world in a way
that brings infinite kindness.

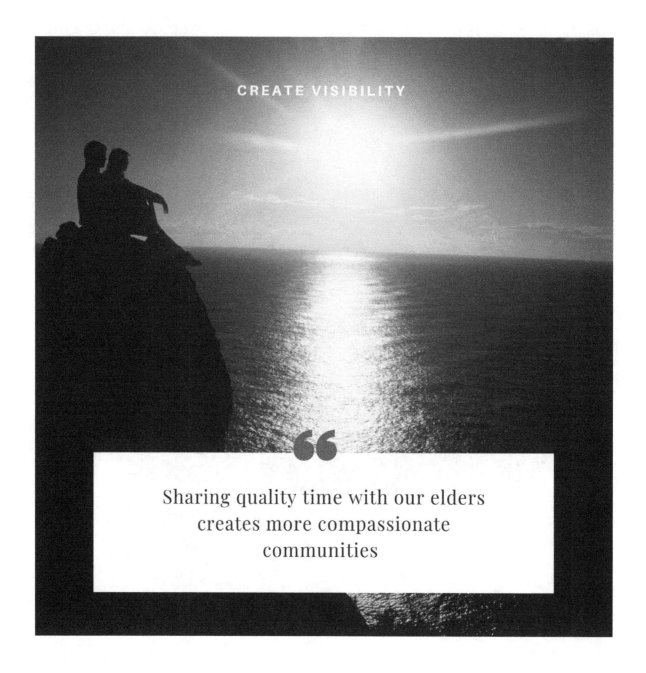

CREATE VISIBILITY

"

Sharing quality time with our elders creates more compassionate communities

When I spend time serving seniors in care homes, offering compassionate presence and nurturing touch, I am shown that there is FAR FROM ENOUGH caring touch and quality time being given to our olders, and not enough visibility of what they go through daily.

It seems that the value of the generations just disappears when they are hidden in tidy, convenient housing, away from the view of the rest of society.

Because of this, we are missing the wisdom and connections that could bring intergenerational relationships, collaboration, and the sharing of knowledge for the benefit of all, and the robust community that would result.

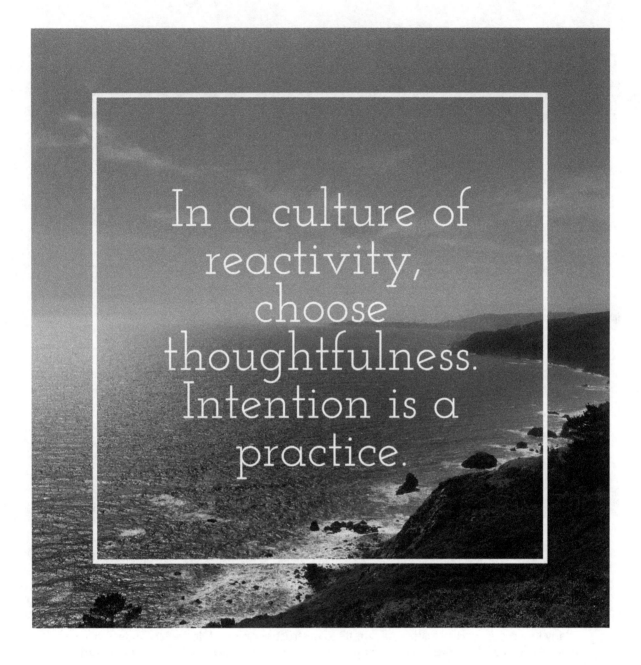

In a culture of reactivity, choose thoughtfulness. Intention is a practice.

How we choose to respond to the circumstances that surround us creates the culture we live within, and which lives within us.

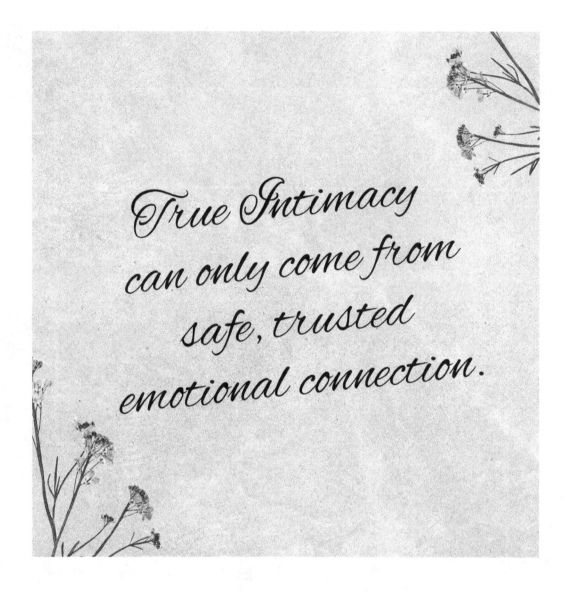

True Intimacy can only come from safe, trusted emotional connection.

Because most of us have lived through adverse childhood events, intimacy can be very scary. Many times, our survival instinct taught us to mistrust our natural desire to connect, because this wasn't safe or available for one reason or another. Our body did what it had to in order to maintain life.

As we grow, small occurrences reinforce this need for protection, making it harder to open to true connection. This is confusing to the primal part of us that needs to be seen, honored, desired, touched, and loved.

When we are able to re-engage in practice of listening to our intuition, our bodies, and hearts, we tap into the skill of discerning what is true for us, and eventually it becomes easier to trust within the framework of our own boundaries. It becomes easier to actually honor our need for boundaries that make us feel safe. In this context, emotional connection can deepen. Fulfillment grows from this place.

Love in Listening

YOU KNOW YOU ARE LISTENING WHEN YOU STOP THINKING OF WHAT YOU WILL SAY NEXT, AND HAVE SOME KIND OF EMOTIONAL AWARENESS ABOUT WHAT A PERSON IS CONVEYING.

Humans have a vital need for connection. Our bodies detect when another is attuned to us and when they are not, even from our earliest moments after we are born. It is a built-in instinct for the purpose of survival.

When someone is intent on giving their full attention to you, they are attuning to you through your nervous system. And when you choose to deeply listen to another, you are doing the same. This is connection. Listening is giving the gift of seeing someone as they are; and that is love.

IN MASSAGE THERAPY, COMPASSIONATE PRESENCE MAKES THE DIFFERENCE BETWEEN A REGULAR TREATMENT AND AN EXCEPTIONAL EXPERIENCE.

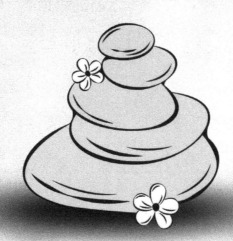

Being present transforms the moment and creates space for connection, no matter what job you're doing, no matter who is in front of you, even if you're simply looking in the mirror.

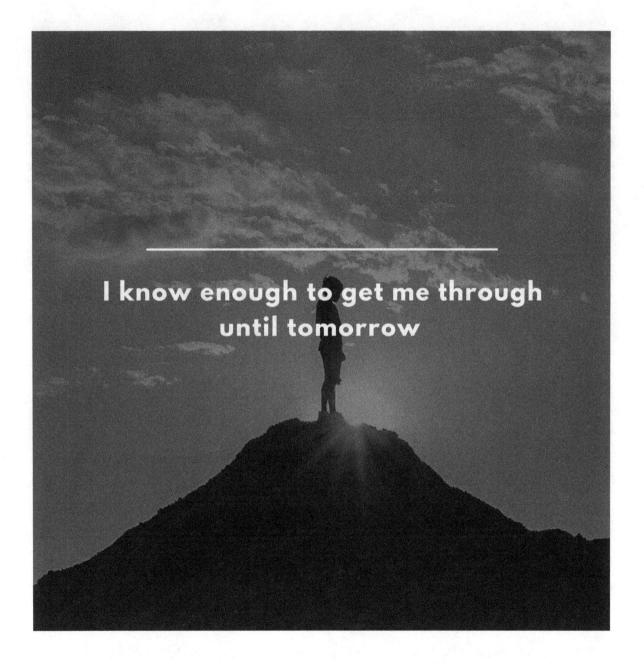

I know enough to get me through
until tomorrow

When you are doubting the next right thing, remember that
you know everything you need for today.

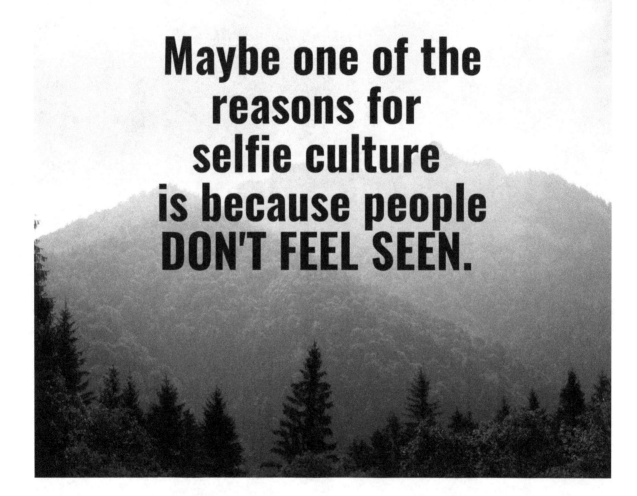

Maybe one of the reasons for selfie culture is because people DON'T FEEL SEEN.

The innate caregivers of the family are so often the memory keepers, and as Amanda Doyle says, they are also the magic makers for their children and others but can feel invisible much of the time. Very rarely do those who care for their loved ones get captured in the magical moments or are honoured and valued for how beautiful they make the mundane feel.

Please let us start including taking snapshots of these beautiful souls during ordinary moments and love them into being the extraordinary moments. This is showing them they are seen, valued, and loved through the eyes of those who adore them.

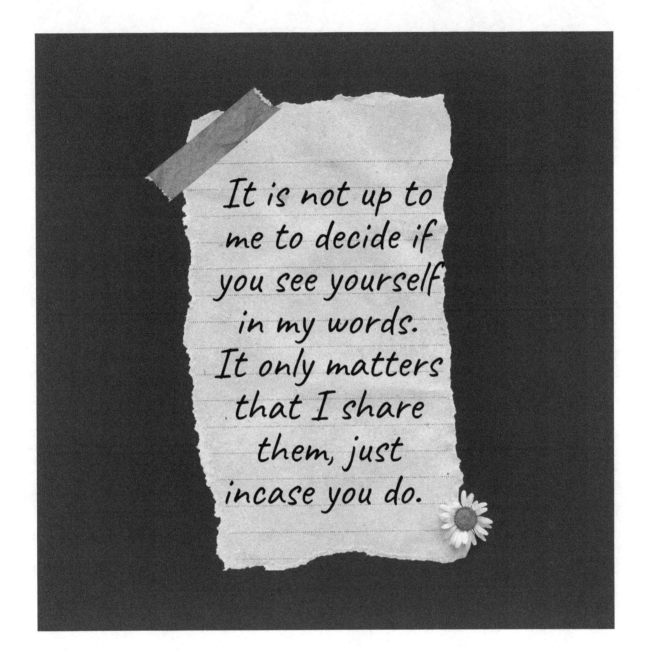

It is not up to me to decide if you see yourself in my words. It only matters that I share them, just incase you do.

Some of my greatest teachers and mentors have been those who have touched me with their words. Books, podcasts, poetry, insights, articles. I am so grateful to them, and they have no idea the impact they have had on my life.

In my quest to find my deepest self, and most fulfilling and meaningful life, I would be truly honored if my words touched another soul in a way that mattered to them. Thank you for reading my words and the hearts of others; may you find your most fulfilling and meaningful life also.

★ ★ ★

Your nervous system craves
Stillness
within the busy

find your peace

Give yourself permission to stop moving your body and your brain for a few
minutes every few hours each day.

The pauses in the middle of busy-ness help you to integrate information
and experiences, gives breath to creativity, and can increase your energy.

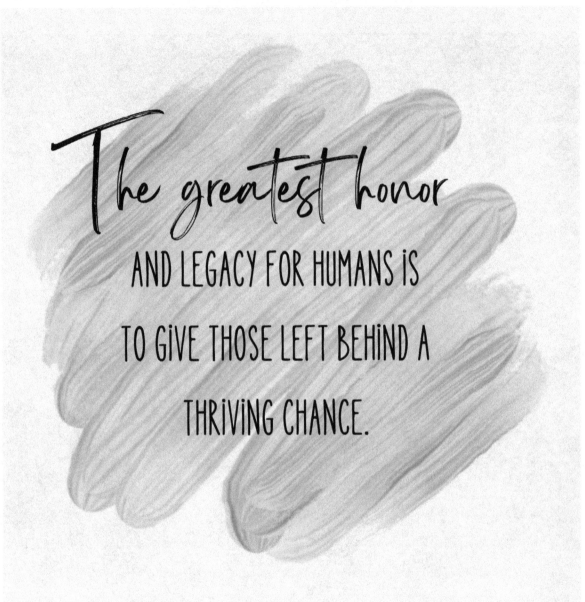

The greatest honor
AND LEGACY FOR HUMANS IS
TO GIVE THOSE LEFT BEHIND A
THRIVING CHANCE.

It is our responsibility to give our children systems that help them love, connect, and thrive in. We have the choice to keep supporting the status quo, or to question our biases, open to other perspectives, continuously learn how to do better, and make life-giving changes.

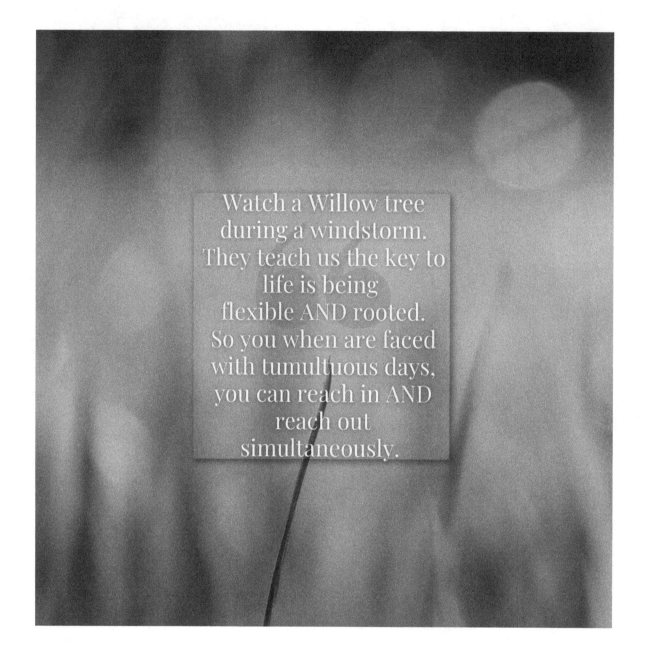

Watch a Willow tree
during a windstorm.
They teach us the key to
life is being
flexible AND rooted.
So you when are faced
with tumultuous days,
you can reach in AND
reach out
simultaneously.

Trees have such insight for us.

They talk to you if you listen.

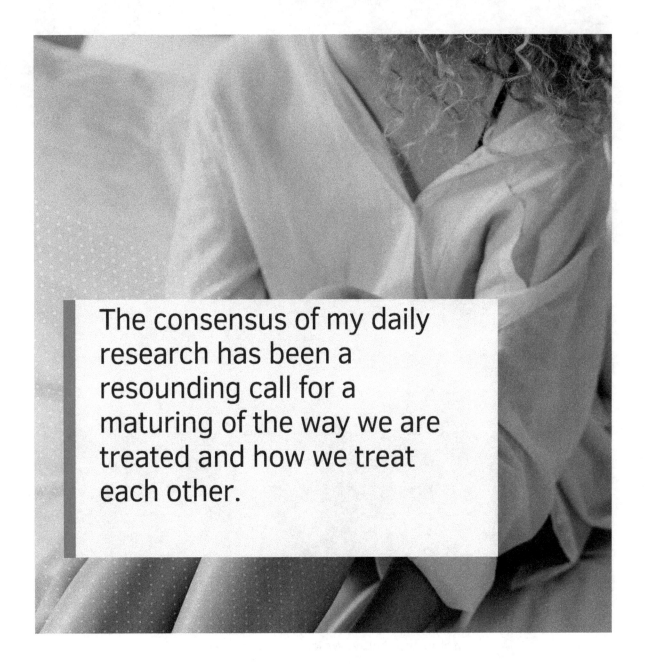

The consensus of my daily research has been a resounding call for a maturing of the way we are treated and how we treat each other.

There is no question that the world needs more love. Patients have told me everyday for the last 10 years how they have been treated unjustly, ignored, felt gaslit, or have been abused by someone in the healthcare industry. These systems truly serve very few, the wealthy, the privileged, those in power. It is not right to expect to have good health ONLY if you can afford to pay for it.

There is a great need for systems that serve everyone equitably, with kindness, by compassionate caregivers. If it does not yet exist, we must create it.

Let it begin with you and me.

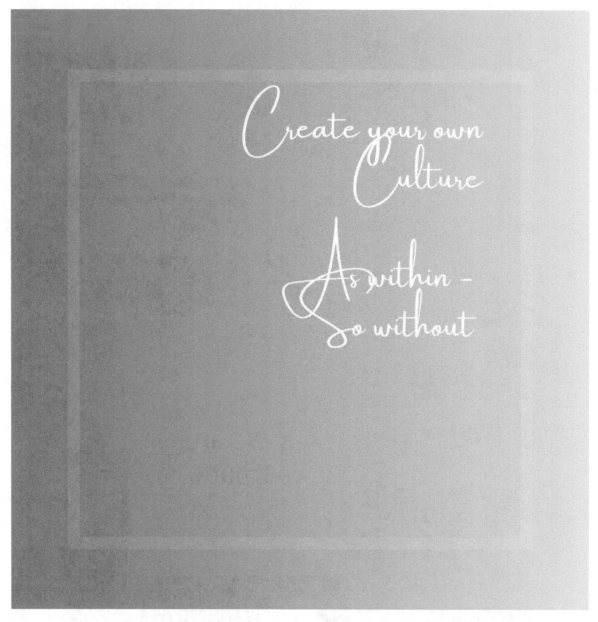

Create your own
Culture

As within –
So without

When a plant, a garden, or a crop fails to thrive, we look to solutions in the culture or environment they are growing in. We don't say the plant is behaving badly or making bad choices. We look for the root cause.

When we blame ourselves for not thriving, we aren't looking at the cause, the environment, or the culture that is contributing to the dis-ease we feel.

Are you aware of the internal culture that you feed inside your mind and body? Try to cultivate that awareness, so that you can add or remove elements that move you away from toxicity and toward relief, ease, and health.

We see in our outer culture what we hold in our inner environment. Once we feed ourselves the nutrients we are missing, we cultivate a rich inner environment, which in turn reflects in our culture.

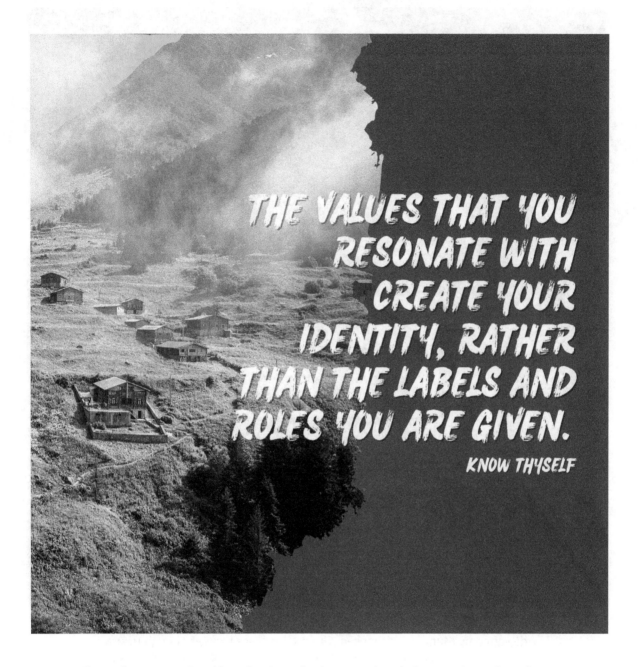

THE VALUES THAT YOU RESONATE WITH CREATE YOUR IDENTITY, RATHER THAN THE LABELS AND ROLES YOU ARE GIVEN.

KNOW THYSELF

Becoming aware of and learning to embody your values helps you determine what roles you accept and roles you don't.

Consider each label or role you have adopted for one reason or another, and literally sit with the word in your mouth, mind, and heart, and ask if you want this title. Feel what your body is telling you. Do you truly align with a full body yes!? If not, get curious about why. Is it a societal expectation, do you not understand the full meaning of the label, is it not exact enough?

You are allowed to find descriptions of you and identities that fit and align more fully and completely with how you truly feel, and how you want to show up in the world. You Deserve the calmness and peace of knowing who you are. You Deserve to feel aligned in your body, mind, heart, and spirit.

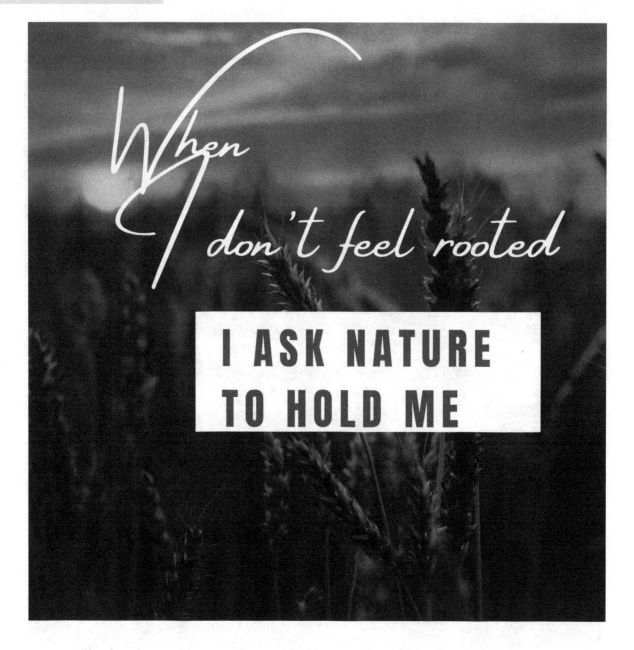

When I don't feel rooted

I ASK NATURE TO HOLD ME

The day after my Mum was diagnosed with cancer, I was blessed enough to stay at a cabin on a lake for a few days with loved ones around me. I did not know how to hold myself then. I was stunned, confused, sad. I felt uprooted.

I walked out into the lake up to my chin, as tears fell into the water.

I felt the gentle rocking of the waves cradling me and accepting my tears, my pain, telling me I would be held for as long as I needed to be.

In that moment of acceptance, I was grounded in nature. My salty emotion blending with the clarity of the lake.

Nature is restorative and unconditional.

May you be held in the same way.

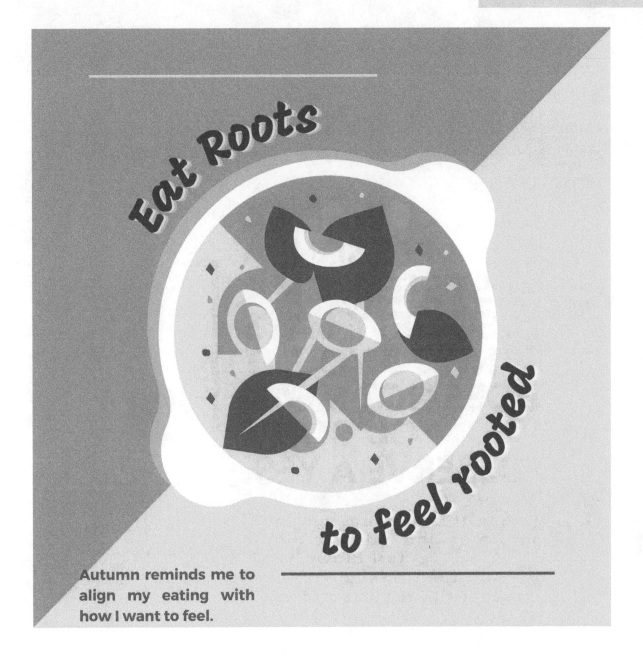

Eat Roots

to feel rooted

Autumn reminds me to align my eating with how I want to feel.

The deeper in or the closer to the ground food grows, the more grounded I feel when I eat it.

Research shows that root vegetables increase the feeling of being grounded, mentally and physically, improves stamina, stability, and endurance.

I made the YUMMIEST veggie Shepard's pie tonight. It feels good to eat healthy.

WHEN A PERSON, A SYSTEM, OR A SOCIETY SAYS NO TO YOU, IT DOES NOT MEAN YOU DON'T DESERVE A YES.

When this happens, go into nature or find a dog to get a full blown YES!
And then re-evaluate the spaces that surround you.

You Deserve to feel safe, seen, and loved. There are many systems that perpetuate the idea that you are not ok, that you need to be perfect, that you don't deserve your needs to be met or you don't deserve rest. These are broken systems; it is not you who is broken. You are enough, you are worthy.

You always have been, and always will be.

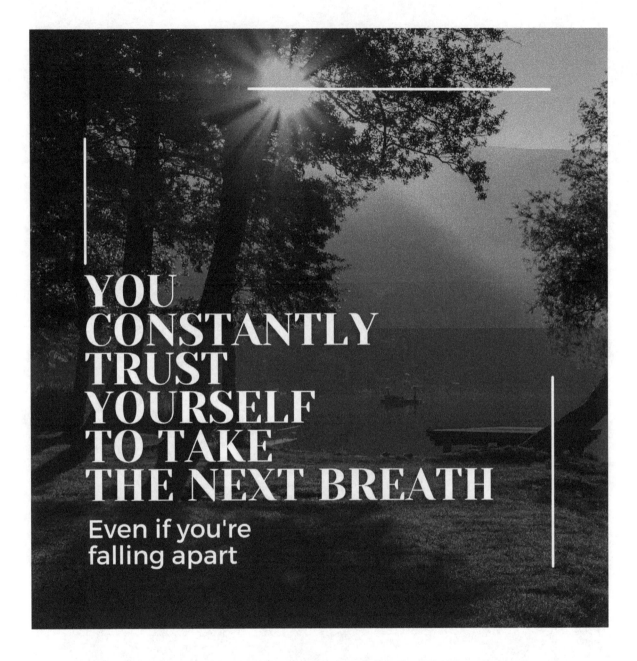

YOU
CONSTANTLY
TRUST
YOURSELF
TO TAKE
THE NEXT BREATH

Even if you're
falling apart

Remember your breath when you are experiencing challenging emotions. Unless there is life-threatening respiratory illness, your body will inhale and exhale for you if you forget. Most people can access the foundation of support that breathing offers, intentionally or subconsciously.

Breathing is literal alchemy, it transforms molecules of oxygen into carbon dioxide, it can be a pathway out of fear and toward calm, it allows us to express ourselves through sound and song, it feeds our cells with life. To inhale means inspiration.

Remember your breath when you need to trust in a process, to trust yourself, your wisdom, or just to make it to the next moment.

My soul talks to me

I see your worry and fear and I whisper to you, you are safe. You feel broken and I say, you are whole. You are sad and lonely and I tell you, you are not alone. You try to ingnore me, block me out, and call me silly, crazy, or woo.

You don't understand why you're even here, and I remind you that you are always wrapped in my love, and you are here to feel joy in the bittersweet and celebration, the profound and the mundane experiences of this life, through the unique gift of your physical senses, guided always by your whispering spirit.
There is magic here. We are here together.

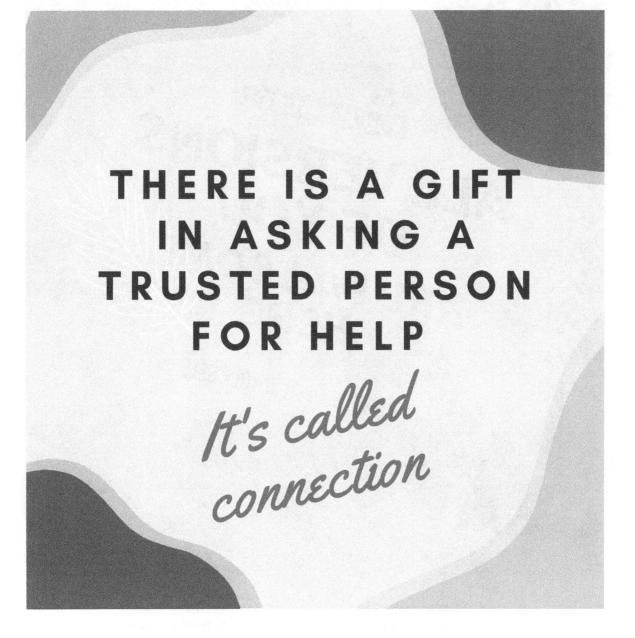

THERE IS A GIFT IN ASKING A TRUSTED PERSON FOR HELP

It's called connection

Many people feel like a burden if they need help when they are struggling with something. Even though it's impossible to do this life independently of others.

When we don't ask for help when we really need it, we are depriving others of the chance to support and feel useful to you. AND we miss the opportunity to connect on a deeper level with those you love and who love you.

Sharing your experience, your vulnerability, though it's difficult and feels bad to be needy (heads up, we ALL have needs!), it is helpful by showing others how to do the same when you'd love the opportunity to help them one day.

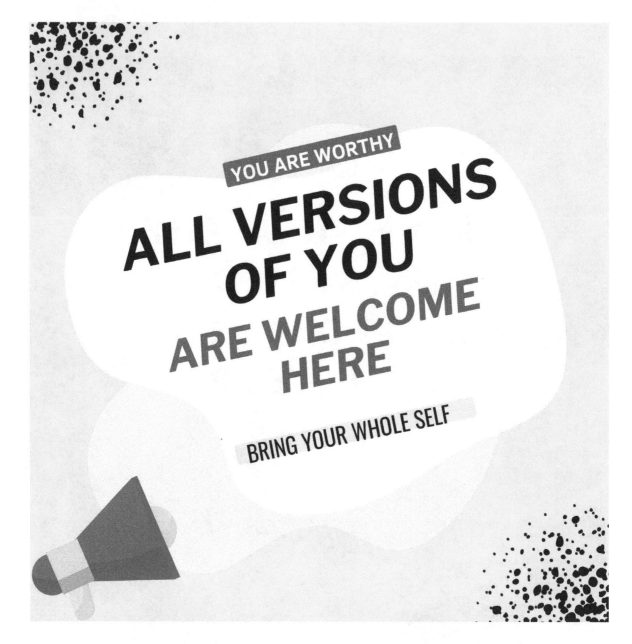

YOU ARE WORTHY

ALL VERSIONS OF YOU

ARE WELCOME HERE

BRING YOUR WHOLE SELF

I used to hide parts of myself, because some people were uncomfortable around certain aspects of my personality. They mistook my friendliness for flirting, my kindness for sucking up, my big heart for weakness, my frustration for being irrational.

This authentic piece of me, she was suffocating. As she learned to recognize her tendency to shrink, and to accept the bits that kept getting suppressed, she was able to start showing her face again. She gained more confidence. She taught me so much about living authentically, to breathe again.

When you only let one or two parts of yourself to be seen or heard, how will you ever feel whole and honoured for the entire complex, messy, beautiful being that your are?

You Deserve to fully know and love every bit of you and be known and loved.

Try out unexplored parts of yourself with safe others and see if they feel good. As you learn more, each day could feel different, more whole.

Feeling a sense of purpose, most often comes from being of service to or connecting with others in a meaningful way.

Imagine the difference between two older persons living in a care home; one sits alone watching TV all day and rarely talks to other people, the other has a little dog and a big plant in their room to care for, and they help out decorating the walls with artwork with the staff and other residents. An extreme but clear example of what occurs all the time. You can likely see how quality of life would differ for these two folks.

Research shows that when you are engaged in activities that help in some way, be it the planet, animals, other people, you feel greater meaning in life.

A sense of purpose leads to better health outcomes and increased longevity, and higher satisfaction overall, regardless of challenges along the way.

Kindness reminder

There are moments, hours, or whole days that are overwhelming for people. At these times, they struggle to connect to any morsel of comfort. If you're able, be a soft place for them to land.

I'm working with patients who are experiencing varying levels of dementia today. My heart explodes all day long supporting their beautiful messiness, and their deep longing for touch and wanting to be heard. Being able to offer acceptance and a soft place for the frustration, the confusion, the overwhelm, the difficult feelings, and the joy is such a huge gift. They are my peeps.

Remember that many whom you encounter on a daily basis struggle with big feelings, even if they keep it well hidden.

If you have the capacity to offer acceptance and a soft place for any version of them they can be today, you are a gift.

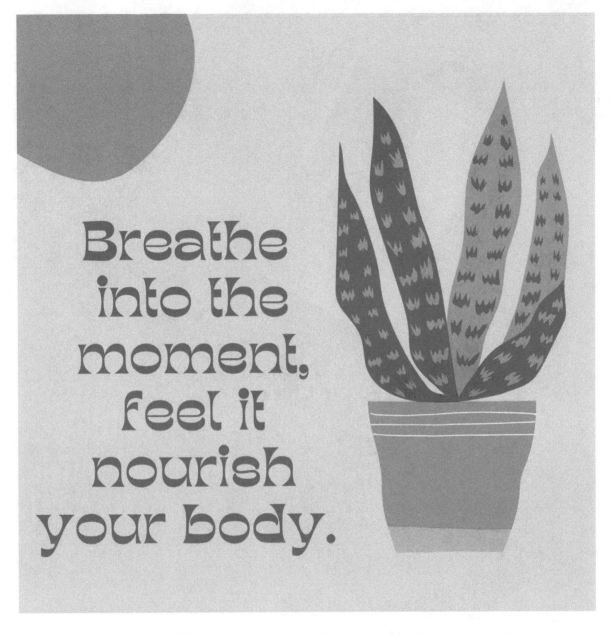

Breathe into the moment, feel it nourish your body.

Have you been breathing today?

This may sound like a silly question.

Sometimes people forget to breathe because of stress, pain, injury, heartache.

I have had patients with aches that have disappeared once they became aware of their breathing habits and allowed themselves to breath again.

Intentionally breathing, in whatever capacity you have available to you is a kind way to nourish your cells. A full breath will stimulate your vagus nerve (a nerve that runs from your cranium to your lungs, heart, and digestive system), and because of this helps regulate your circulatory and digestive systems, among other amazing things.

Notice where your breath goes as you inhale, feel it moving into your lungs and imagine it flowing down your arms and legs and into your brain to touch every cell.

This is a great visualization for focus.

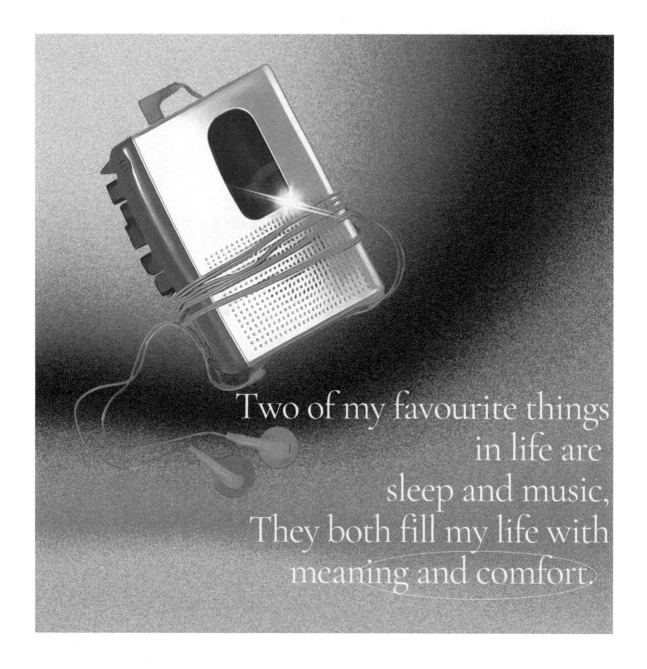

Two of my favourite things
in life are
sleep and music,
They both fill my life with
meaning and comfort.

I've always been in love with sleeping. Getting cozy and comfy in soft blankets and pillows is one of my favorite things. To this day, I can still sleep for 10 hours straight, given the chance. I can identify my top two best naps in my life. **Priorities!**

One of the only things that would get me out of bed when I was younger, was music. I have an early memory of being woken up to ABBA playing loudly in our

house. My sisters knew that I'd come groovin' down the stairs for breakfast, even at 6 years old, when they played Dancing Queen.

Of course, there are many other ways I feel comfort and meaning, but these are among the important.

What are 2 things that sustain you, give you comfort, and connect you to yourself?

Knowing what I value most has been the clarity I needed to find my community.

———

My driving values are love, caring, nurturing, human dignity, and continuous learning. Bring me deep philosophical questions and conversations, tell me stories of what you went through to grow and learn about your own depth, wildness, or acceptance. What vision do you have of the world that brings you to tears? How do you find love and peace inside the chaos, contradictions and messiness?

I long to know who you are and what you value, what scares you, and what makes you feel loved. I desire this connection.

Being honest with myself and others about what fills me, draws us together, it lights a path toward finding my peeps.

Who do you want your community to be?

Are you drawing the people you long for to you, by sharing who you truly are?

YOU are the beacon to light a path for your peeps to find you!

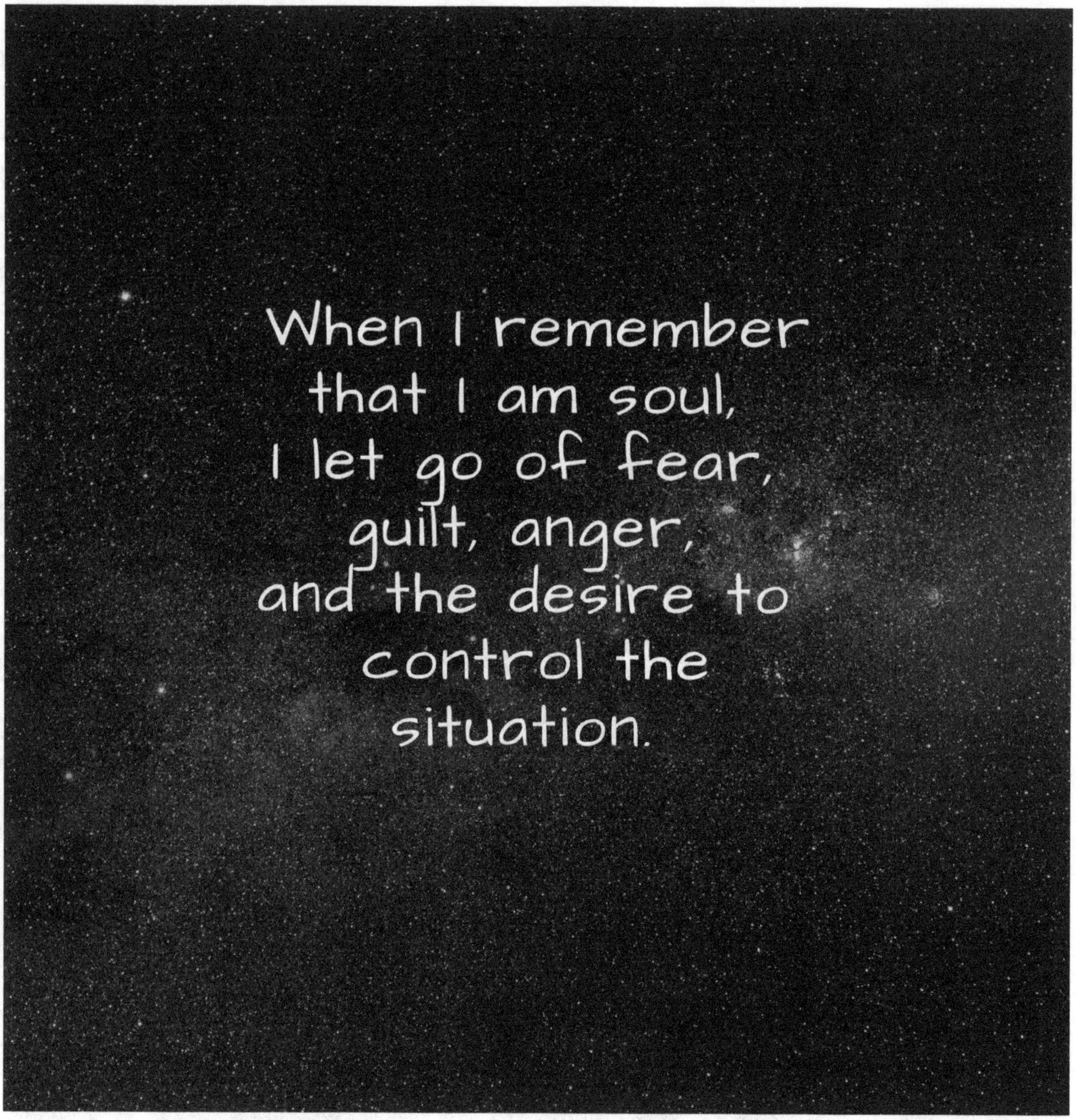

> When I remember
> that I am soul,
> I let go of fear,
> guilt, anger,
> and the desire to
> control the
> situation.

In moments when deep turmoil is activated within me, I first must remove myself from the physical space, vent, turn it over in my mind a few hundred times, and then look within to my connection with all that is.

It is not a straight line from turmoil to connection. It takes awareness, an emptying of toxicity, a willingness to shift energy, and a softening of emotions.

It may not be an instant shift, or even timely at all. But the magic inside us IS the magic inside us. When I open to love, the process of alchemy begins within me. It can be difficult AND so freeing. This is worth every second of my journey through the chrysalis of discovery.

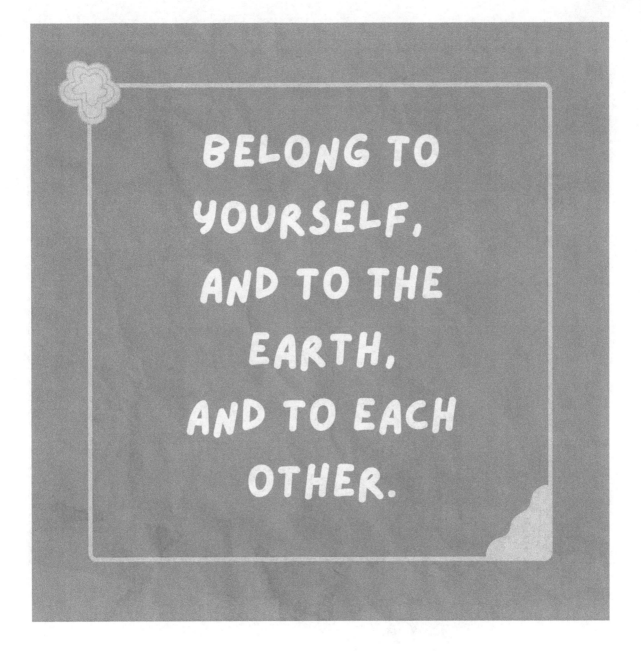

BELONG TO YOURSELF, AND TO THE EARTH, AND TO EACH OTHER.

When you belong to yourself, you inhabit your body with presence and kindness, understanding that you are in it for life.

When you belong to the earth, you tread with presence and love, honouring the life- giving gifts she provides for all.

When you belong to each other, you hold presence and awe in your heart, feeling the magic of interconnectivity, and the living breathing synergy of a connected community.

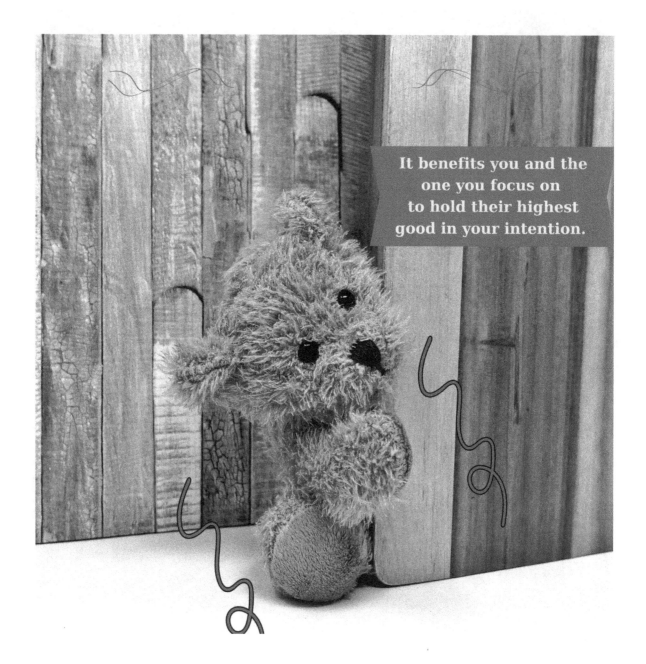

It benefits you and the one you focus on to hold their highest good in your intention.

Intention has powerful effects.

When you hold someone in your thoughts, send them love and peace, and imagine them at their best, your heart and empathy are engaged, and you benefit from your energy being focused on helping another.

You also benefit from the loving energy being sent from you. Love isn't a one-way energy, you get it all over you when you give it to another!

The receiver of your intentions benefits from your compassion and focused attention. (Like sending them a teddy bear hug in your mind!)

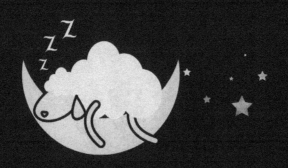

Hustle culture is senseless.

I am so tired of being exhausted.
I'm saddened to witness those
around me affected by it, feeling
there is no option for rest.
I grieve for the harm it causes.
We desperately need respite.
We deeply need this
paradigm to change.

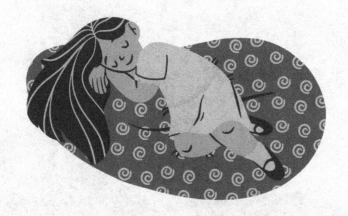

SURRENDER TO DEEP REST

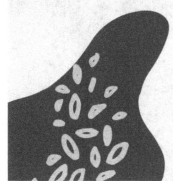
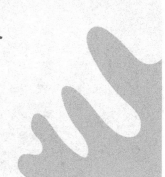

Much of the northern hemisphere of our beautiful, cyclical planet is moving toward a period of deep rest and hibernation.

Nature has the innate wisdom of the birth-death-birth cycle. It knows that times of stillness and times of movement and growth are equally important to life.

Deep rest is regenerative, allows space, and from it our connection and creativity are born. You too deserve and need this inner stillness. We draw strength from the pauses. How will you honor your pause this winter? Yes, there is much to do, and rest is required to gather strength for your journey.

Be a safe space

We face so much that is hard in life.

ALLOWING OTHERS TO HOLD YOU WITH LOVE

gives you
soft places
to land.

Sending love to all who need it today.

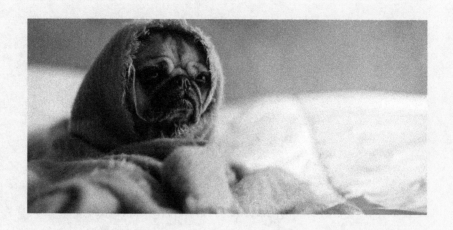

Some days I need to
wrap myself in love and
stay under my blanket.

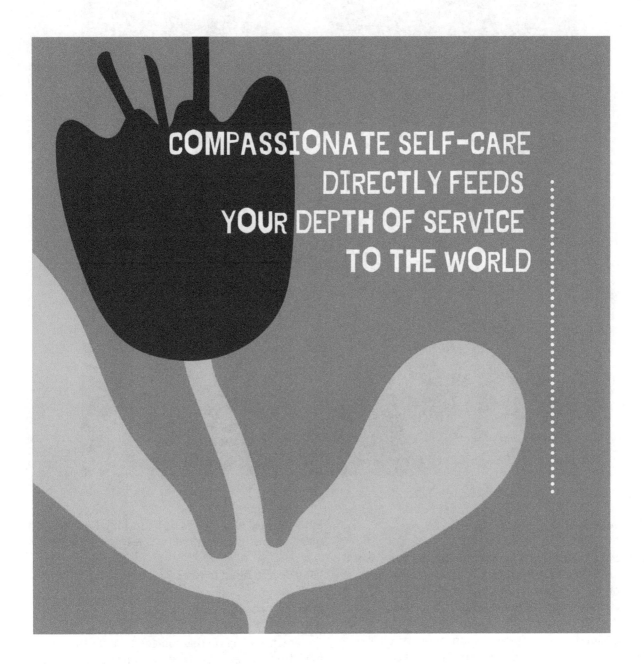

COMPASSIONATE SELF-CARE
DIRECTLY FEEDS
YOUR DEPTH OF SERVICE
TO THE WORLD

Have you discovered what you need to feel cared for?

Are you able to give it to yourself?

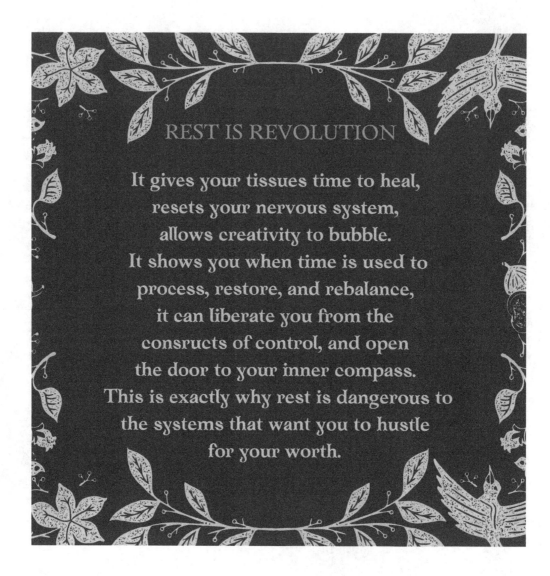

REST IS REVOLUTION

It gives your tissues time to heal,
resets your nervous system,
allows creativity to bubble.
It shows you when time is used to
process, restore, and rebalance,
it can liberate you from the
consructs of control, and open
the door to your inner compass.
This is exactly why rest is dangerous to
the systems that want you to hustle
for your worth.

You Need Rest.

Living in a culture hyperfocused on productivity, work, and busy-ness, mixed with hyper-individualism, is so hard on the nervous system. (Alarm clocks literally alarm the nervous system in order to wake up.)

When I am over-scheduled, rushed, or overtired, I feel like a cranky toddler that needs a nap. I cannot function at my best, make effective decisions, or access as much compassion for myself or others as I'd like. My creativity dips and ironically, I'm less able to ask for the support I need, exactly when I must need it.

Rest has powerful effects on the nervous system, your ability to integrate information, your mood, your communication skills, thus affecting all your relationships.

Finding small ways to rest is important. Resting in the midst of pushy, work-driven society is revolutionary.

Why do you need to rest?

Find your why.

For great reading on this subject, look for the nap ministry founder Tricia Hersey's new book, Rest is Resistance. She dives into the history of toxic work culture, slavery, and white supremacy. Learn where it all started.

Inspired by Tricia Hersey, author of "Rest is Resistance."

Go rest!

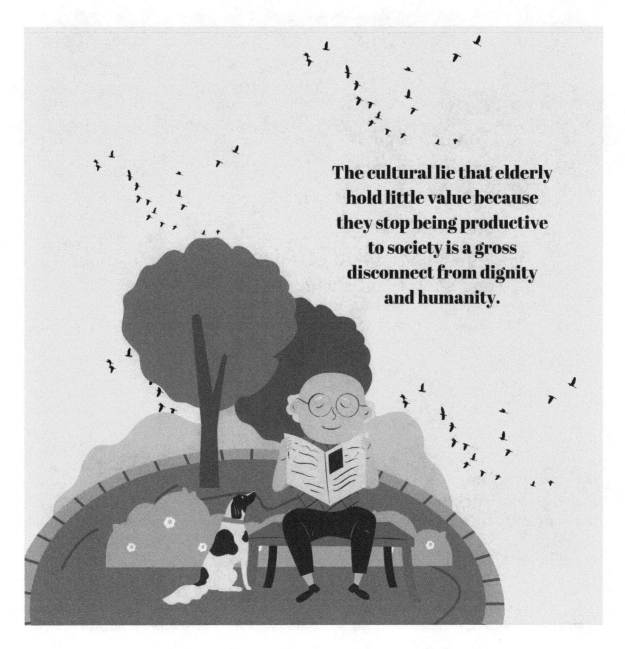

The cultural lie that elderly hold little value because they stop being productive to society is a gross disconnect from dignity and humanity.

This is one of the most heartbreaking parts of my work. To witness the lack of dignity and purpose for those placed in care homes that are understaffed, where residents are not engaged mentally and meaningfully.

I have sat with seniors who literally feel their life draining from them because of canceled programs, outings, engagement, personalization, caused by greed and politics.

After years of contribution to society, which is NOT the measurement of human value (that's toxic capitalism), they often feel ignored, dis-integrated, and worthless.

This requires a societal shift of massive proportions. In days gone by, these were the elders that were revered, honored, respected, and valued as the wise people who could teach and tell story until the moment of their death.

Of course, there are still some cultures who revere their elders, to which racism and supremacy has tried their best to obliterate. There is so much to learn. We need to start listening again to those with experience, honouring their needs, their bodies and minds and spirits, and re-integrate their visibility in our everyday society.

The epidemic
of chronic stress
has a profound impact
on the health of
individuals, their families,
and society as a whole.

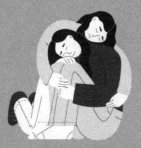

Acute stress is necessary for the nervous system to react to immediate danger.

The Yale Medicine definition of chronic stress is:

"A consistent sense of feeling pressured and overwhelmed over a long period of time.

- Symptoms include aches and pains, insomnia or weakness, less socialization, unfocused thinking.

- Treatment includes LIFESTYLE CHANGES, medications, setting realistic goals.

- Involves psychiatry, psychology.

Chronic stress slowly drains a person's psychological resources and damages their brains and bodies."

Chronic stress is unnecessary and harmful to our minds and bodies. It is utterly ridiculous that we need to treat stress with medications and psychiatry, without holding accountable the systems that create this kind of dis-ease.

Along with lifestyle changes that allow us to rest, we need the support of societal systems that make it possible to thrive in a life without the inhumane pressure that causes overwhelm.

The first step is realizing you don't need to fit into or uphold the systems that keep your body, mind, and joy suppressed.

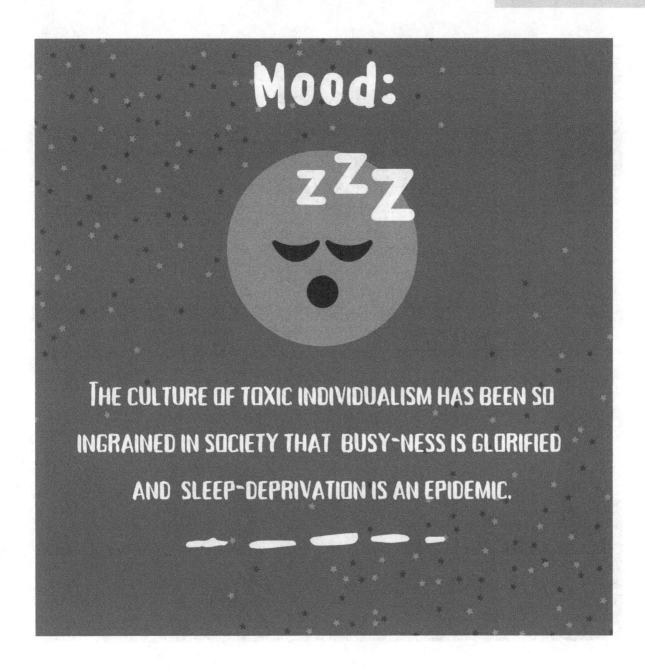

Mood:

zZZ

THE CULTURE OF TOXIC INDIVIDUALISM HAS BEEN SO INGRAINED IN SOCIETY THAT BUSY-NESS IS GLORIFIED AND SLEEP-DEPRIVATION IS AN EPIDEMIC.

Sleep deprivation can lead to exhaustion, chronic stress, chronic inflammation, brain fog, irritability, confusion, burnout, and diminished ability to handle daily tasks, which can also lead to anxiety, depression, overloaded immune systems, and illness.

It is a dangerous part of the cultural narrative. "I'll sleep when I'm dead" type of mindset is common, not only in the culture but deep within our programming.

Have you ever felt guilty for calling in sick, for canceling plans, for not keeping up with chores or children or for sleeping in or taking a nap or taking a break?

A symptom of this need to push through is often the feeling of being unworthy of rest, of respite, of deep care. I see it everyday in my treatment room. It will take collective push back to change this paradigm.

Please join me in taking the time to know what actual rest feels like and reconnect to why you need it. Much love and respite to you.

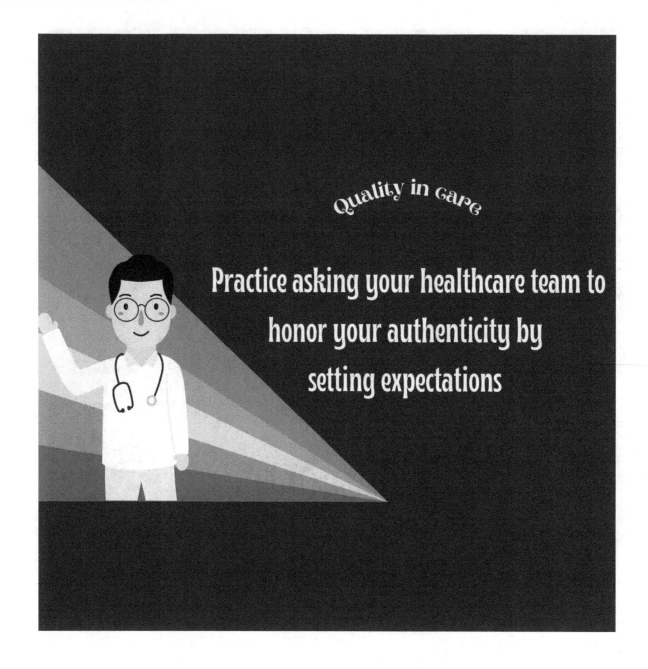

Quality in Care

Practice asking your healthcare team to honor your authenticity by setting expectations

British Columbia announced an upcoming change in the pay structure for family physicians to encourage and improve the quality of primary healthcare.

There are currently one million people in B.C. without a family doctor, and another million waiting for specialist appointments.

This change is supposed to facilitate longer appointment length with patients to address actual needs rather than in and out as fast as possible. Doctors switching from pay per visit to the new structure could be in a clinic mindset for quite a while and may need us to remind them to slow down and remember to begin creating relationships with us again.

This also could be what many doctors have been aching to do. If we put our truth forward and show them how to care for us right from the beginning of this change, hopefully it will bring about the inclusion and deep listening that we've been missing for so long, and the treatment we all deserve in order to be healthy and whole.

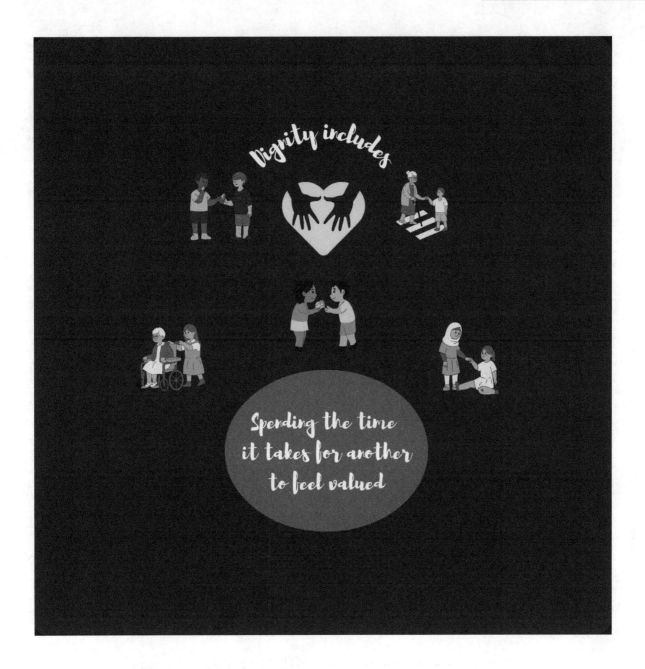

Dignity includes

Spending the time it takes for another to feel valued

You and your loved ones deserve dignity in healthcare, in housing, in community.

We all need safe spaces, safe nurturing touch, to feel heard, and to hold importance in society.

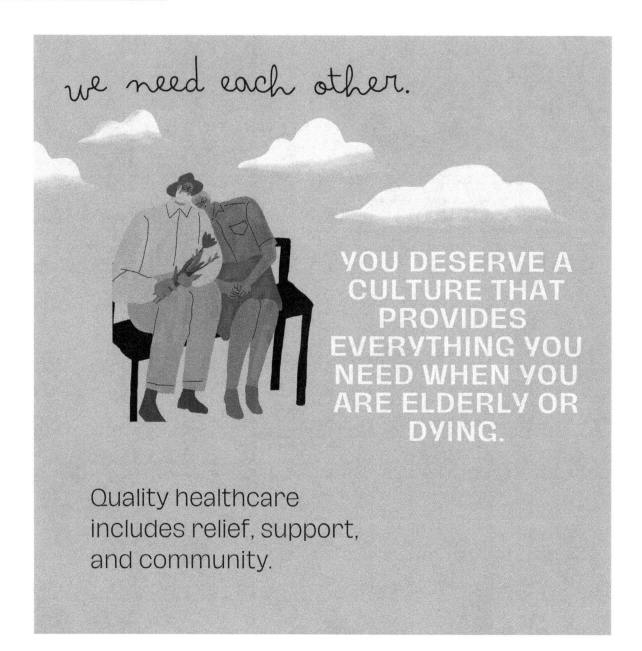

we need each other.

YOU DESERVE A CULTURE THAT PROVIDES EVERYTHING YOU NEED WHEN YOU ARE ELDERLY OR DYING.

Quality healthcare includes relief, support, and community.

The quality of care you receive should NOT be based on how much money you have saved for retirement. Since we have to pay for everything in this capitalist society, many people suffer greatly with housing, transportation, medical visits, lack of community, visibility, ageism, mobility, and accessibility, among other challenges.

And because people need to work to survive and support families, children of olders struggle with taking time off to spend time with and care for their loved ones. It's a ruthless conundrum.

A culture shift to extreme care in advanced years and for those with terminal diagnoses, includes a loving community of support, the funds to pay for necessities and caregivers, as well as frequent companionship to offer compassionate presence and nurturing touch.

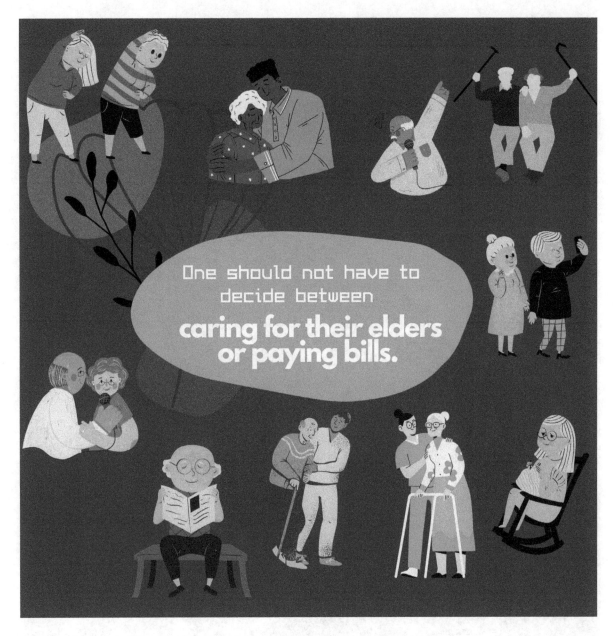

This is a very frustrating part of society's economic system. There are no built-in structures to help us pay for basic needs if we need to take time away from working to live in order to care for our loved ones.

I would really love to be able to spend more time caring for my mum who is going through a life changing/ life threatening illness right now. But if I take too much time off work, I could literally lose my ability to pay for housing.

It breaks my heart that I and billions of others don't have a compassionate support system to help us sustain our housing and monthly bills while we provide the deeply needed and important nurturing of our family.

We need healthy, loving community to care for us when we are not well or require extra help, instead of one stressed out child of a parent struggling to make ends meet while trying to get their elders to every appointment and spend quality time.

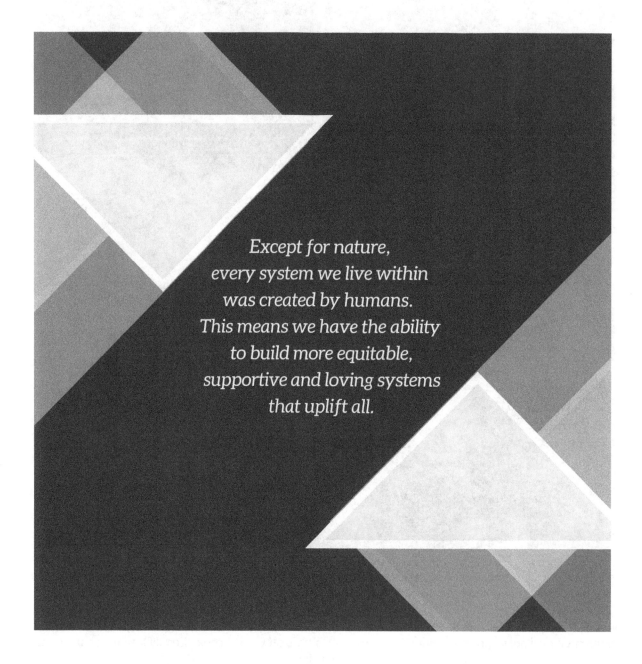

Except for nature,
every system we live within
was created by humans.
This means we have the ability
to build more equitable,
supportive and loving systems
that uplift all.

Shedding oppressive systems is possible, simply because
they were once made up by some humans at one point. It's
time to create anew.

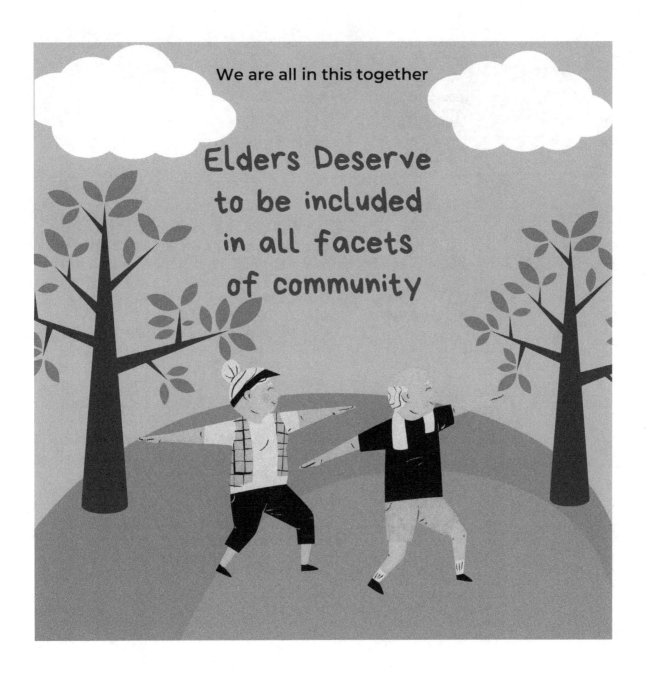

COME BACK TO ME, SHE BECKONS

COME BACK TO ME MY CHILDREN.
I HAVE GIVEN ALL THAT I HAVE TO YOU.
YOU HAVE FORGOTTEN YOUR ORIGINAL
LANGUAGE, YOU HAVE FORGOTTEN
HOW TO COOPERATE WITH ONE ANOTHER
AND LOVE EACH OTHER AS I HAVE LOVED YOU.
BE STILL FOR A MOMENT AND LISTEN.
LISTEN TO THE VOICE OF THE WINDS.
LISTEN FOR THE MAJESTIC
SOUND OF THE SUN RISING AND
YOUR COUSINS SINGING SWEETLY IN THE TREES.
LISTEN TO WHAT THE TREES WHISPER AND
THE WISDOM OF THE BUBBLING CREEK.
ALL CREATURES THAT PLAY AMONGST
MY BREAST ARE SACRED, INCLUDING YOU.
BUT YOU HAVE FORGOTTEN.
REMEMBER TO DANCE AND LAUGH,
AND LIVE WITH KINDNESS IN YOUR HEART
AND YOUR FOREMOST THOUGHTS.
LOVE, AND LIVE FOR THE BETTERMENT OF OTHERS
AND FOR ME WHO GIVES EVERYTHING TO YOU.

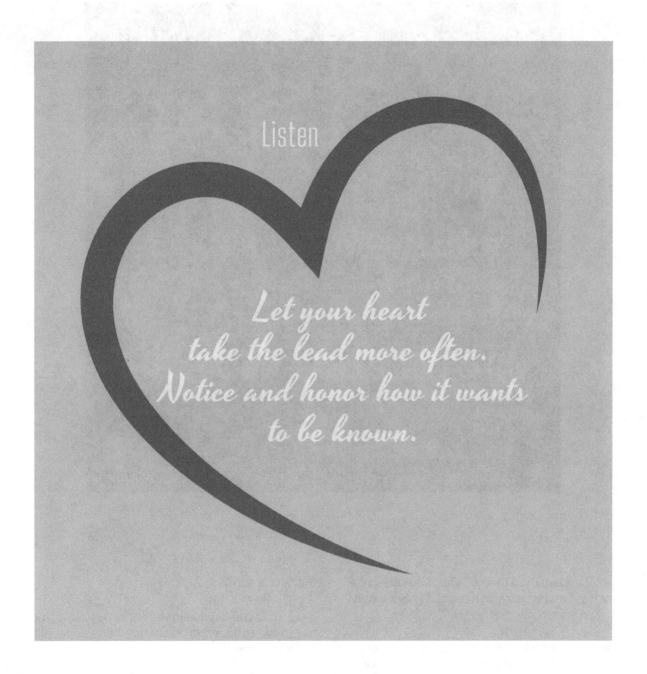

Listen

Let your heart
take the lead more often.
Notice and honor how it wants
to be known.

For a moment, or for an hour,

Still your mind as much as possible.

Listen deeply to your heart.

What do you hear?

LOVE FLOWS
FROM YOUR HEART
INTO OTHERS
WHEN YOU
HOLD COMPASSION
THERE

Wayne Dyer used to say, "when you squeeze an orange, orange juice comes out. What happens when someone squeezes you?"

What we hold inside is often what comes out. I would take it a bit further and say, what we hold inside unconsciously is what comes out unconsciously.

We have a greater ability to choose what comes out when we have awareness of what lives inside us, our automatic reactions, and how we're able to align with our own integrity. Closing the gap between habitual responses and who we prefer to be more often takes time and attention, and the courage to look within.

If you hold compassion in your heart, it is able to rise to the surface and colour how you see people and situations.

I'm not saying it's always possible to choose compassion, but it is possible to increase your capacity to act from it, to practice it, and to recognize when you see it in others.

This is a great article on compassion, how it differs from empathy, and how to increase it so that it becomes more of an automatic response.

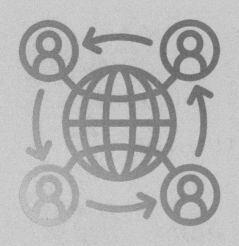

We're all in this together

When we are part of a community of support,

we are able to access a wealth of ideas and a greater capacity to meet the needs of more people.

When we are supported, we become more expansive, inside, and out.

KINDNESS IS NOT ENOUGH.

NOW IS THE TIME FOR

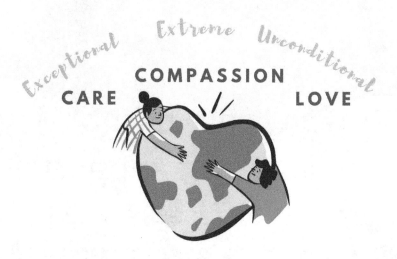

Exceptional *Extreme* *Unconditional*

CARE   COMPASSION   LOVE

There is an emptiness in suffering alone, whether alone means physically, mentally, emotionally, or spiritually.

Being held and compassionately witnessed in suffering makes all the difference. It may not solve the problem, but it resolves the ache, refills the hole, surrounds the sufferer with love and care that changes the pain.

Billions of people and animals suffer everyday. The systems of business and government do not consider this enough within the constructs we have made up. They do not consider the humanity in their decisions enough. It is too uncomfortable and unprofitable to take a look deeply at the suffering caused by systemic imbalance.

It is time to rebuild the communities that we feel in our bones, the intuitive knowing of that part of us we feel is missing. The nature within us wants to love others through their suffering. The structures outside of us do not support how we must do that. I believe there are ways to find balance between the internal and external realities and reconnect the gap that has so many holding on by a thread, one weak moment away from giving up.

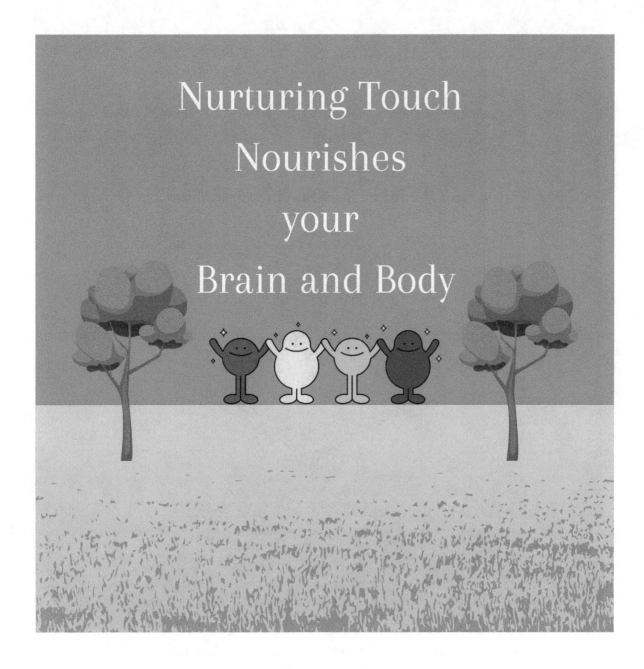

Nurturing Touch Nourishes your Brain and Body

I am privileged to work with, and experience touch all day long. Patients come to me hoping for some kind of relief, and whether that is physical or emotional, nurturing touch has an effect on both.

Touch has the ability to calm the nervous system, decrease pain, stimulate healing, and increase compassion. It activates the vagus nerve and releases oxytocin, the cuddle and comfort hormone.

You've heard that 4 hugs a day is beneficial for humans. Adding intention to nurturing touch can have profound effects. Many studies discuss the impact of positive touch.

One such study states, "Hanning described findings that four hugs per day was an antidote for depression, eight hugs per day would achieve mental stability and twelve hugs per day would achieve real psychological growth. If this is the case, touch has a greater significance than most of us would realise."

STAY IN BED FOR A MOMENT

BREATHE

STRETCH

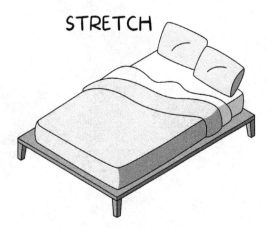

Before you get out of bed after sleeping, re-orient yourself
to the waking world.

Let your dreams slowly fall away and notice you are awake.

Take a few full breaths to energize your body with oxygen.

Gently stretch a few muscles to get blood flowing.

And if you want, hold an intention for your day.

All of this helps to reintegrate your body, heart, and mind,
and can allow for a smoother transition into your day.

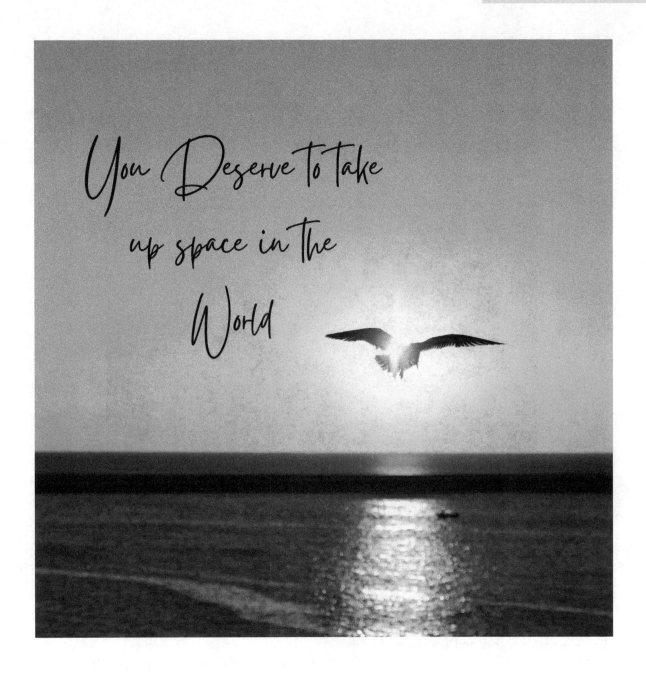

You Deserve To Take up space in The World

You Deserve to be here.

You Deserve to be authentic.

You Deserve to be supported and loved for who you are
without fear of persecution, hate or injustice based on who
you love.

You are a miracle.

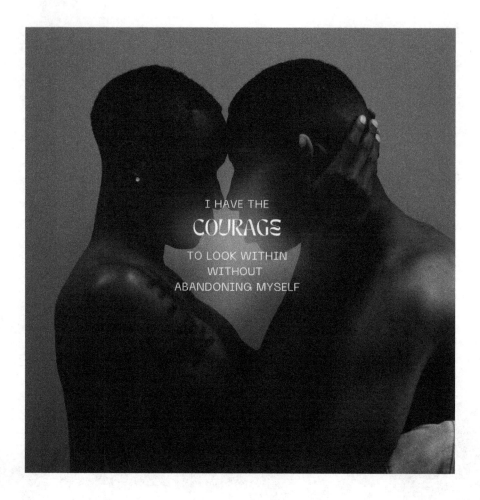

I HAVE THE
COURAGE
TO LOOK WITHIN
WITHOUT
ABANDONING MYSELF

When I was 20, I had the great fortune to be involved in an immersive personal development program. For months, we were able to dive deep into ourselves, discover who we were in the context of the world, uncover our internal operating systems, practice communication skills, accountability, and interdependent relationship, and learn to live in community.

This was an incredible experience that gave me a solid foundation to move through life, an abundance of self-knowledge, and a love for self-discovery and continuous learning.

It did NOT however, guarantee a direct path toward happiness and a struggle free existence. It was an awareness I had in my pocket that I could take out and look at whenever I remembered it was there.

Accepting this human journey, I know I will never stop evolving into new versions of me. There were times when I thought I had it all figured out, and then

I moved through different relationships, became a mama, and faced many challenges. All these involved webs of decisions and understandings waiting to be tugged on, and each time a new insight came, the entire web quivered and changed the path ever so slightly.

I see my life as a spiral of learning. Each time I come to face a similar situation, I do so with a different perspective, a greater depth of understanding. Every time I think I've done the work, something that I've never considered before pops up and surprises me, and I exclaim HA! Literally. At this point, I just accept that awareness and insight will come regardless of if I want it to.

I deeply appreciate this part of my inner world. I am grateful to be able to hold space for myself, and as a result, for others. There is fire, energy, and fierce love created when you can look inside and not run away from what you see. It's brutal, and beautiful. As Glennon Doyle says, it's "Brutiful".

I believe I am a

Good Person Inside

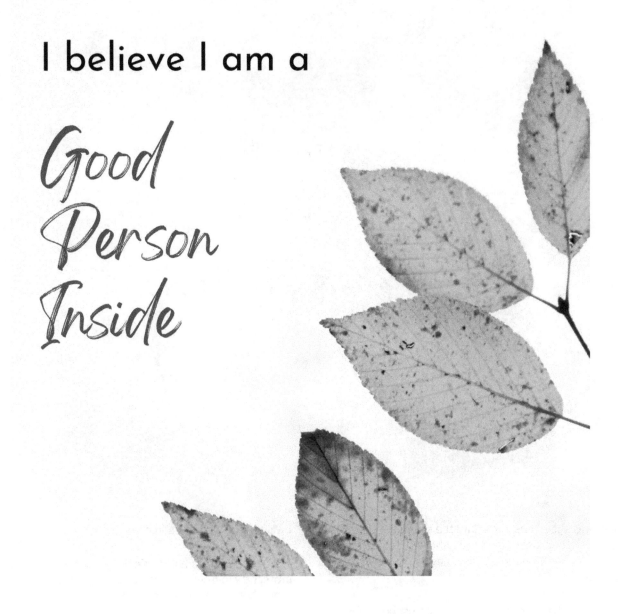

This is a revolutionary statement.

I didn't realize the power of believing this to be true. When I finally believed it and said it out loud to myself, I burst into tears.

It was emotional because I had to break through societal conditioning that told me that I didn't deserve to feel good about myself. It took the time to begin dismantling internalized patriarchy and misogyny and toxic capitalism. It took the awareness that I know better than television and other media marketing.

It took acceptance.

It also took work to realize that I am not my father, I am not my mother, and I don't need to consciously adopt the trauma that happened to them, though it was in my subconscious for a long time.

There is so much packed into our belief systems. It is SO valuable to explore and question them. Some beliefs take longer than others to shift. I am so happy to finally introduce myself to you in the belief that I am a good person. Nice to meet you.

What do you believe?

Who are you today?

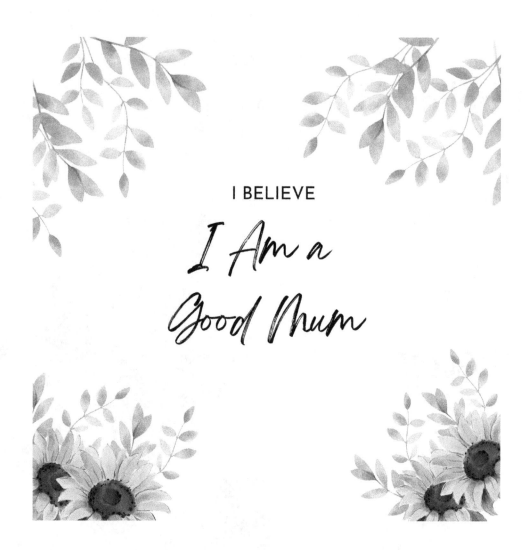

I BELIEVE

I Am a
Good Mum

This. This was a hard one. One tiny little statement that was so hard to believe because of gulit over what was 'expected' of me. I believed for a long time that I could have done better, been a better parent.

The societal lie that tells mamas that they must be perfect, that they must spend all their time being selfless, have a great career while raising children, but not work too much, plan all the events, make homemade birthday cakes, keep the house clean, take them to all the activities, talk to all the teachers, advocate for their education, read them stories, feed them healthy meals, go to yoga or the gym for "self-care", and actually sleep and look refreshed to be presentable, IS IMPOSSIBLE.

Being a parent is messy and unforgiving without the cultural pressures.

I f#@!'d up more than I can count.

I unconsciously brought my learned trauma responses and patterns into my relationships with my children.

I wish I could go back and change a few things.

Yes, I wanted to be able to do more, to give them more, to protect them from hurting more. But I could not possibly love them more than I have, and I do.

I believe that being a mama is a practice in letting go. It has been beyond beautiful, and heartbreaking, joyous, challenging, and growth inspiring. Learning about myself in the context of parenting contains my lowest moments, darkest struggles, and most amazing connections in this life.

I don't have any glamorous advice to give anyone to help make it easier. You must go through the muck; you will get dirty. Whatever parenting looks like for you, it is deeply personal, relational, and communal. There are too many of us to feel alone; ask for help. Get rest. Love them dearly. Be present...to yourself and for your children.

F#@! the clean house.

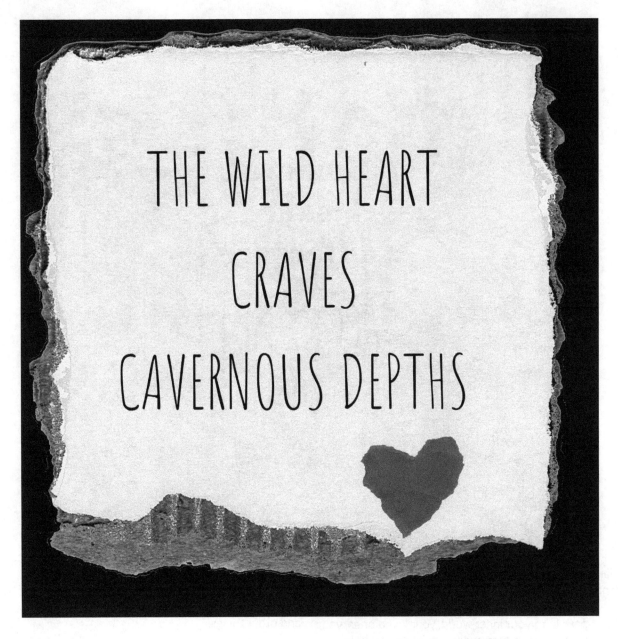

THE WILD HEART CRAVES CAVERNOUS DEPTHS

You want more.

More love, more connection, more deep rest, more clarity, more time, more peace, more justice, more wisdom.

You want to fill the void with meaning.

Allowing yourself to see these needs, to acknowledge the ache of wanting, is one step toward exploring the caverns of depth.

To peer in at the shadows under the surface, one could find loneliness, desire, fears, hope, stagnant action, ideas, creativity, lack, trauma, wonder, hurt, love, anger, confusion, loss, patterns, self- talk, awareness.

The contents of these caverns ache to be seen and held. With help, with community, with awareness, they can be held with more. The 'more' that you seek can be what arises within you when you seek to comfort what lives in that void. Your wild heart can be a guide to untangling the jumbled threads you thought you were not prepared to begin unraveling.

Your wild heart can open to your more.

Your wild heart can be your more.

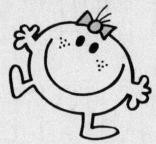

I believe
I make
a difference

Making a difference can vary greatly depending on your capacity in each day.

It can pertain to your inner world, your loved ones, your work, your art, your community, society as a whole.

Physically, it can look like caring for your body, showering/bathing, drinking water, eating, moving, breathing... or even just one of these if having a low energy day.

Inwardly, it can mean clearing mental clutter, closing loops - like deleting emails, finishing a conversation, completing a project, setting a boundary, cleaning a closet, getting closure on something, accepting something you cannot change, moving on from something that no longer serves you, forgiving yourself or another.

It can look like taking time to meditate and get centered in your energy before beginning your day. To care for yourself first, before caring for other people and other things.

I have found that when I care for and take time for my own peace, I have a much greater capacity for learning, for listening, for creative solutions, for compassion, for planning and collaboration. I receive the most beautiful feedback from my patients at these moments when I feel most open, safe, and grounded. It is then that I feel my energy affects others in positive ways. How beautiful it is to feel when others benefit from my intention. And because of this, we are both made more.

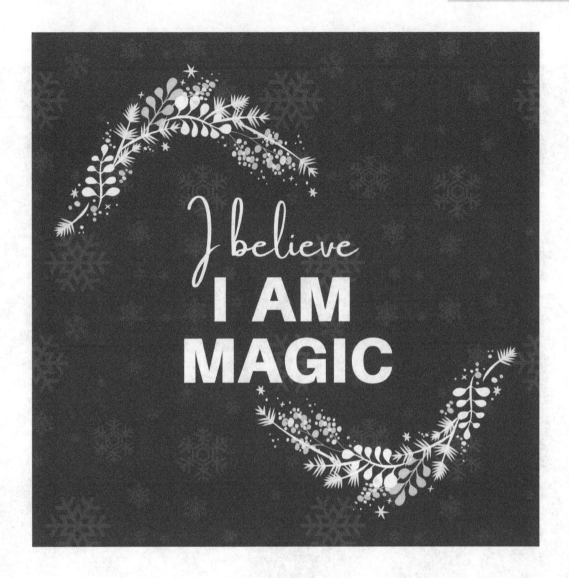

What is magic?

To me, it is creation, it is presence, it is observation, it is love, it is ceremony.

We are made of the same molecules as stars and nature and the forces that create worlds and suns.

We have the ability to create a spark so strong that alights a brand new being within our bodies and support its growth and life.

We can create nourishment for new beings from our own bodies, and stretch our tissues to bursting, and then witness the uterus contract back to nearly its original size.

Presence is transformational. When we give it to those we love, those we engage with, ourselves, it has a profound effect on the nervous system in a way that nothing else does. Being seen changes us.

Observation creates awareness and modifies the outcomes of activity. When molecules are observed, it changes their behavior. When they know they are being watched, different patterns emerge. I find this miraculous.

When we observe the world around us, and ache for justice and compassion, it can be a catalyst for change.

Love is the greatest force in the universe, able to move mountains, break down walls, and fill emptiness with richness and wholeness.

When we hold ceremony in love, in observation, in presence, we create sacredness, alchemy, transformation, and magic. We can all be magic.

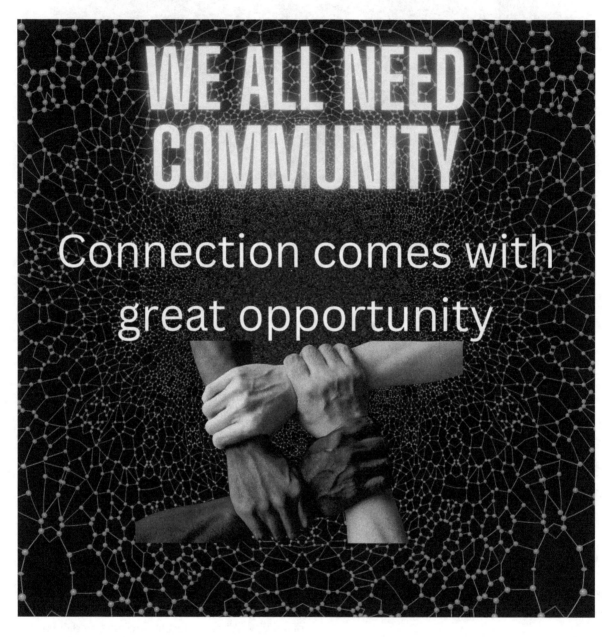

WE ALL NEED COMMUNITY

Connection comes with great opportunity

Community is necessary, it's the only way we can thrive. We are not meant to do any of this alone. Our bodies and brains are wired for touch, support, connection, nurturing, and helping others.

When we belong, when we feel loved and free to be ourselves, when we feel safe, our intrinsic creativity is engaged, and our subconscious self looks for patterns and solutions and presents imaginative ideas to our conscious mind.

This freedom makes new systems possible.

This safety encourages compassionate approaches to living with others.

These connections support a greater depth and capacity for authentic exploration and communication.

Building community is a lovely pathway to thriving together. Continually building bridges between minds and hearts has been so very positive in my experience. I have been blessed to know folks who are extremely adept at creating such connections.

What else could be possible if we had extreme support in all areas of life?

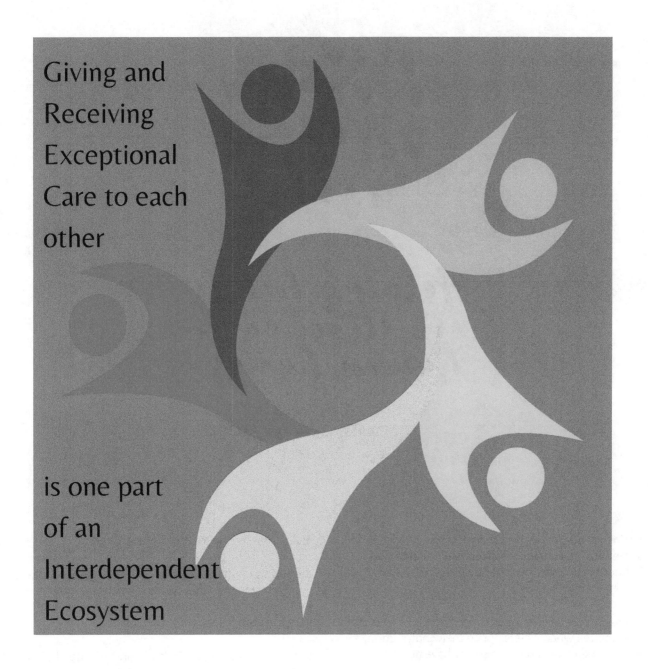

Giving and
Receiving
Exceptional
Care to each
other

is one part
of an
Interdependent
Ecosystem

If we create a circular care economy based on supporting
each other, imagine how far we can go.

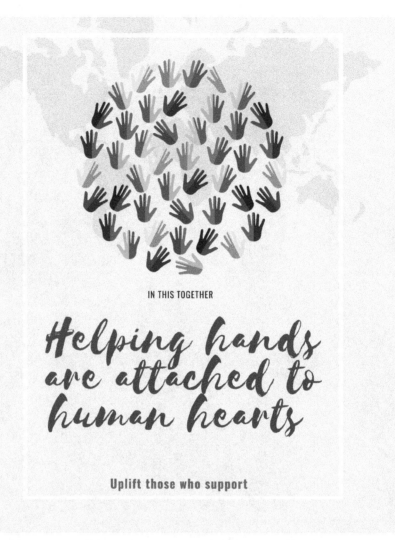

IN THIS TOGETHER

Helping hands
are attached to
human hearts

Uplift those who support

Caring for others can be a thankless job. Service is something that caregivers often feel called to do. Without acknowledgement however, burnout and bitterness may set in.

Humans have an enormous capacity for love, and often feel uplifted when others notice their contribution, and elated when thanked for how they have helped.

From the person who brings you coffee, to someone who cares for your mama in the hospital; they are all important and worthy of gratitude, verbal gratitude.

Society has room for improvement in this area. Many people walk around on autopilot and lose precious opportunity to connect. Being present when out in the world can feel vulnerable, I get it.

The feeling that comes from being seen is priceless and

giving that feeling to others is such a gift.

It not only uplifts another to acknowledge them but it connects your nervous systems when you look them in the eye and raises the frequency of their energy and increases the feelings of interconnectivity.

Kind of like the visual of the pictures of a dog before and after you tell them they're a good dog. The whole energy changes because of that interaction.

Expressing gratitude decreases YOUR stress and releases toxic emotions.

Try saying why you're grateful to someone everyday. It may seem awkward at first, but I promise you'll get used to it real fast.

And the world will be a kinder place.

LOVE YOUR PEEPS

every moment you can

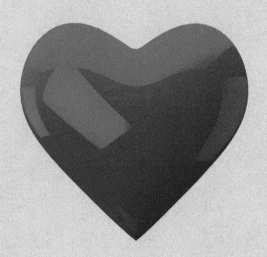

Love is forever • Life is not

Love is everything.

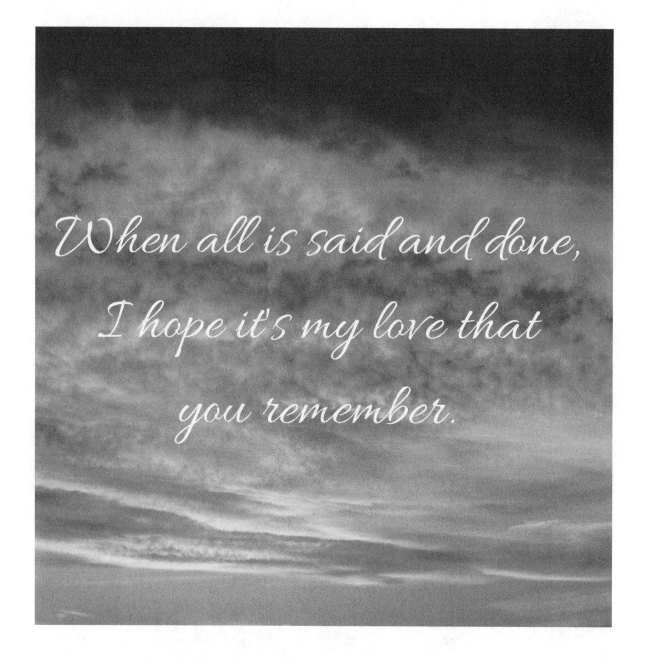

When all is said and done,
I hope it's my love that
you remember.

My mama doesn't have much longer on this earthly plane.
Please hold her in your heart and send love for an easy
transition.

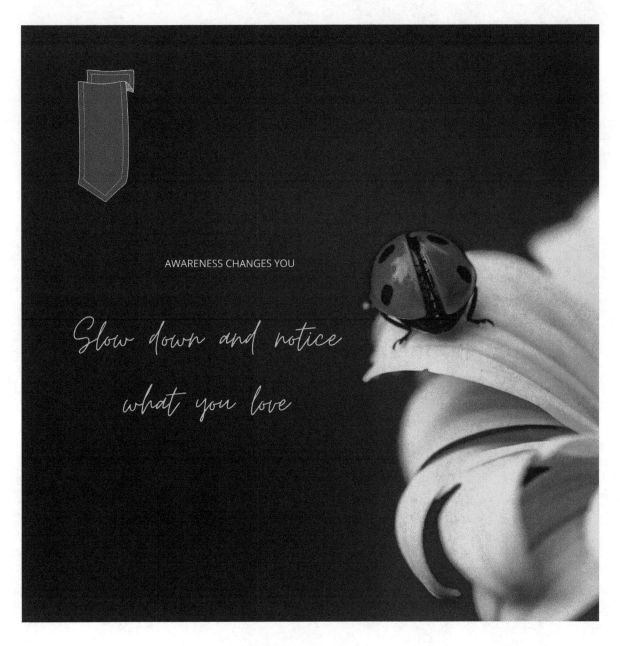

AWARENESS CHANGES YOU

Slow down and notice what you love

Awareness slows down time.

Being present and conscious in the moments you wish would last forever, helps us savor the treasures in front of us.

Awareness is to contemplate where you are, where your attention is, your thoughts and feelings about the moment, who you are in context to the moment and your relationship to it.

Time is so fleeting. Use awareness and consciousness as tools to recognize the gift of each moment and give energy to what and who you love. Love is ubiquitous, and it is a blessing to realize our own unique way of loving.

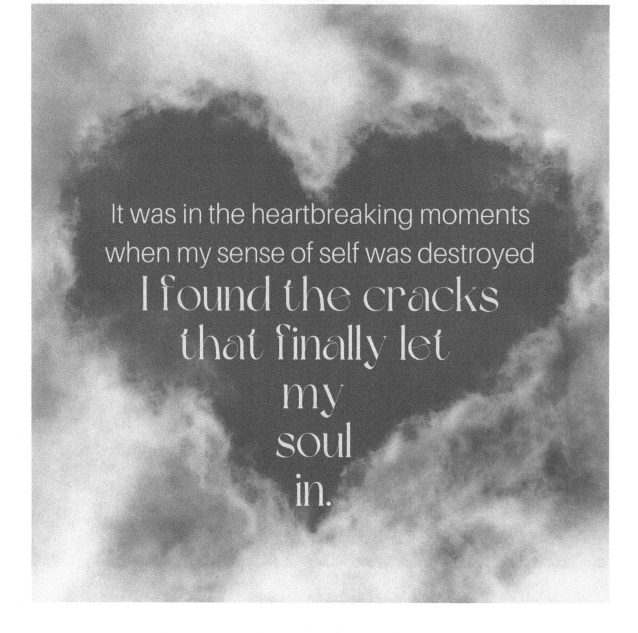

It was in the heartbreaking moments
when my sense of self was destroyed
I found the cracks
that finally let
my
soul
in.

Opening to the soul can often feel like you are breaking.
When the ego cracks, it can push hard against what feels
threatening. We can comfort this part of ourselves, while
keeping it from taking the lead.

Listen for the voice of your soul in moments of uncertainty
and fear, it knows how to hold you.

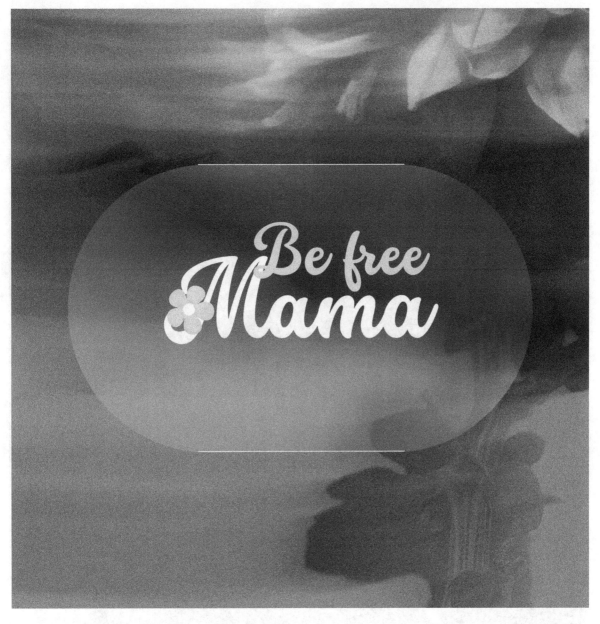

Be free Mama

Hello friends, I am sad to tell you that our Mum, Nana, friend, and beautiful soul, Joyce passed this afternoon surrounded by love.

We are also relieved that she is not in pain and know that she is with our Dad.

I want to acknowledge all of you who gave her so much love and send heartfelt gratitude to all of you who contributed to our family. Your help enabled us to be by Mum's side through her final days and weeks.

Keep the legacy of love always flowing.

If you knew her, share a story or a blessing.

Peace be with you all.

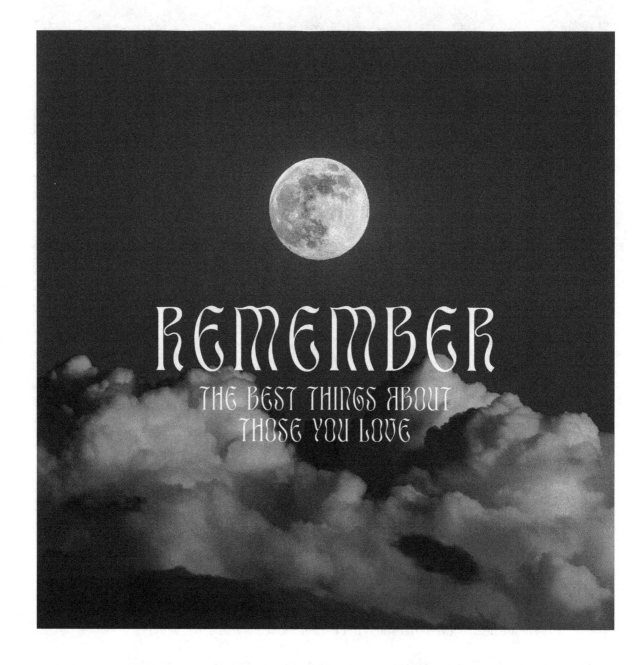

REMEMBER
THE BEST THINGS ABOUT
THOSE YOU LOVE

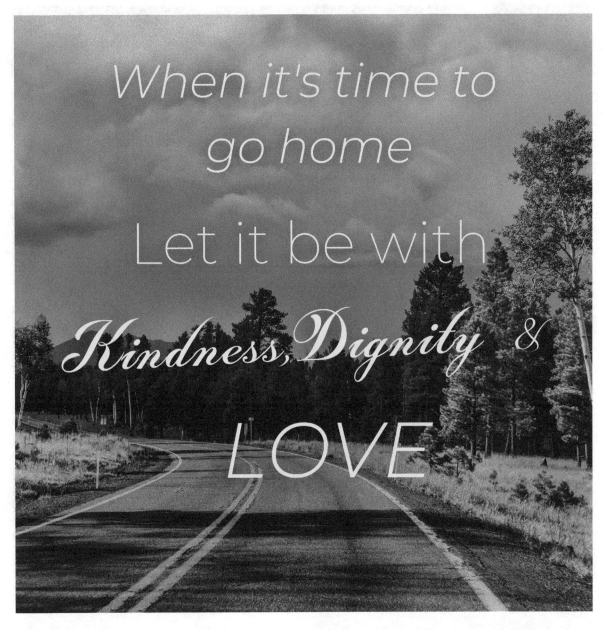

When it's time to go home

Let it be with

Kindness, Dignity &

LOVE

Providing care doesn't always equate to being caring. Many of our medical systems have become transactional for many different reasons. Caregiving provides dignity, respect, and autonomy best when it is relational.

It seems obvious and one may not think research is necessary to tell us this. However, patient safety can be compromised when caregivers lack the complex understanding, the time, or the desire to care holistically and with kind relationship.

It makes sense to me to evolve caregiving in medical systems by providing doulas, advocates, those who offer compassionate presence and nurturing touch, to patients in all stages and of all ages and abilities. Especially if nurses and doctors and care aids lack the time.

This is my aim through the one caring human initiative.

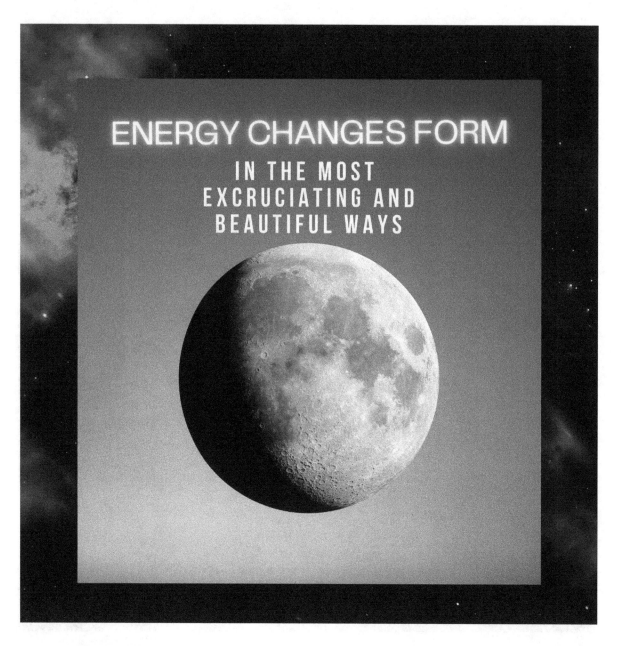

ENERGY CHANGES FORM

IN THE MOST EXCRUCIATING AND BEAUTIFUL WAYS

We are all on an energetic journey.

It feels mysterious and precious, complex, and simple all at the same time.

The cycle of life is an energy. Its nature is to endlessly flow from one state into another, from birthing a cherry blossom to the fruit to its decay.

Humans cannot avoid this nature. From birth to death, we are always changing, feeling emotion, growing physically, learning, and moving. From the tiniest particle in perpetual motion to whole societies, nothing can stay the same forever.

The journey I have great appreciation for is how love moves us and fills us and changes us. How love has impacted me from my most vulnerable infancy to holding me through millions of simultaneous feelings, to learning my value, to trusting others, through the grief of losing loved ones, has given such profound growth and capacity to hold space for myself and others.

This is a journey I would not trade for anything. I am beyond grateful for being able to experience all the beauty and heartbreak. It has been worth the grief to love and be loved so deeply.

ALLOW YOURSELF
TO BE CHANGED
BY LOVE

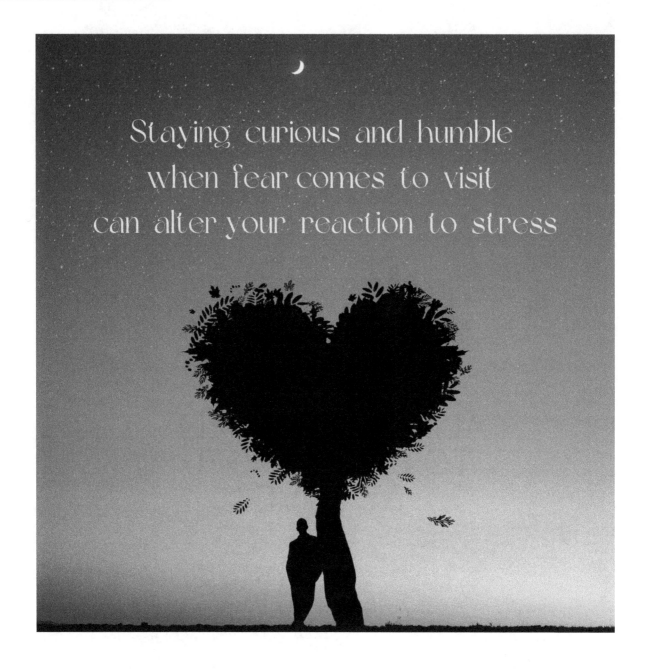

Staying curious and humble
when fear comes to visit
can alter your reaction to stress

Curiosity and humility have probably saved my life and nervous system more than a few times. I used to be easily triggered into panic and fear, maybe because of childhood trauma, maybe because I wasn't shown how to regulate, maybe because my neural pathways had laid down tracks in my brain that caused me to be reactive. Likely a combination of all these and more.

Teachers and mentors in all different capacity helped me gain awareness of my patterns and processes. The more I learned about myself, the deeper my understanding grew of emotional recognition and regulation, the greater empathy I felt for others, and I became more resilient.

Situations that would previously rattle my bones became less fearful, and I found myself gaining insight each time I faced similar feeling circumstances. Curiosity helped me build capacity for holding difficult moments. Humility helped me have compassion and strength.

I am on a journey of continuous learning. I hope to never stop. I'll never be perfect. I will still be triggered sometimes. I will be emotional and messy and often late and will love with my whole heart. And for this I have gratitude.

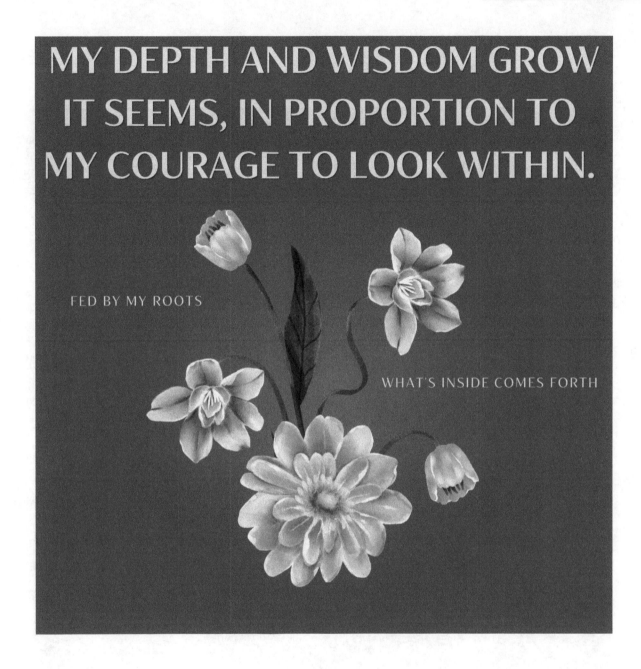

MY DEPTH AND WISDOM GROW
IT SEEMS, IN PROPORTION TO
MY COURAGE TO LOOK WITHIN.

FED BY MY ROOTS

WHAT'S INSIDE COMES FORTH

We are indeed layered like onions.

I also compare courage to the cooking of onions. The more I contemplate the beauty and complexity in each juicy layer, the greater my tears of discovery, of understanding, of shedding what no longer serves me, letting the pungent richness fill my senses.

As I apply heat and sear and simmer, these layers become translucent, releasing the sharpness of scent, allowing the focused energy to bring out the depth of flavor.

Every time you explore another piece of yourself, you are able to recognize your depth and become wiser. This can possibly spare yourself from the excessive tears of the first deep cut.

You can also then begin to recognize others that have been cooked in their own juices, the ones who hold knowing in their eyes. Once you see it, the depth, you cannot unsee it.

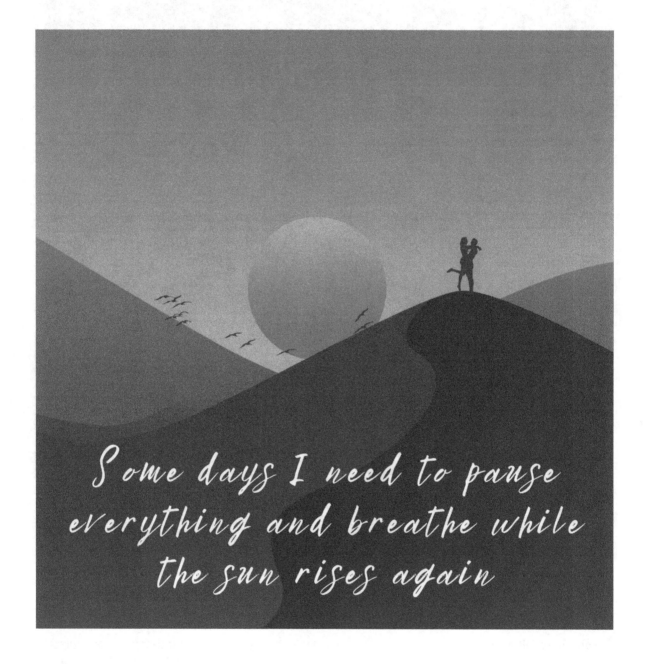

Some days I need to pause everything and breathe while the sun rises again

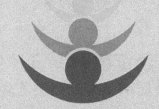

GENTLY RAISE
EACH OTHER UP
UNTIL WE ARE
WHOLE

A community is where nobody gets left behind or
falls through the cracks in the system. We all deserve
unconditional love and exceptional care. When we lift each
other, we all rise, valued, and heard.

REMEMBER THAT
TRANSFORMATION TAKES TIME
AND MAY LIQUIFY
YOUR WHOLE WORLD
INTO A PILE OF GOO
BEFORE YOUR NEW FORM IS SHAPED.

"We delight in the beauty of the butterfly but rarely admit the changes it has gone through to achieve that beauty." - Maya Angelou

The process of transformation is rarely smooth. We don't have magical tools of instant transfiguration, such as in some worlds of wizardry and witchcraft.

The human experience and journey through the murky waters of awareness, learning, growth, and change can be dark, scary, exhausting, and painful because of the uncertainty laid out before us.

Quite literally, as the above quote indicates; butterflies, and moths have one of the most destructive paths of transformation as any creature on the planet.

The butterfly is in this adult stage for only weeks in order to mate and lay eggs, though some could hibernate and therefore live for several months.

The life of a butterfly begins as an egg laid on a leaf, which hatches a caterpillar that will eat for several weeks. Once it is grown, it will enter the chrysalis, or the pupal stage, (which to me seems aptly named if compared to a human child in school being called a pupil) which can last several weeks to several months, some as long as two years.

The process of complete destruction, growth, and creation of an entirely new body and physiology obviously takes some time. The percentage of this insect's time in the pupa in relation to its entire lifespan seems to appropriately align with how much of our human lives are occupied by turmoil, challenges, learning, growth, consideration, noticing unhelpful habits and patterns and implementing change, if desired. There is wisdom in the goo.

In other words, the caterpillar endures its gooey existence and uncertain future, to eventually transform into one of the world's most beautifully regarded creatures, that does its part to further its species while giving back to the greater ecosystem and serving the circle of life.

SPRING
WILL COME AGAIN

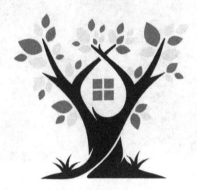

SNUGGLE IN TO THE DEEP
STILLNESS OF THE MOMENT.

LET THE LIGHT OF LOVE
WITHIN BRING FORTH THE
GRATITUDE, WISDOM, AND
PATIENCE TO SUSTAIN YOU.

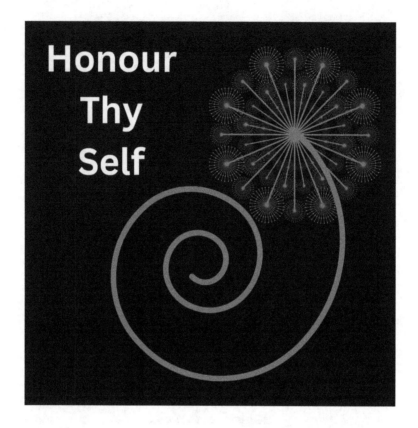

Honour
Thy
Self

It is time to practice what I preach.

Winter is a time of slowing down, of hibernation, of looking within and deeply listening to the call of the soul whispering incantations to nourish the body, mind, and heart. It draws on the dark to encourage deep rest. Then, it brings remedies and renewal, underground growth, and flow of inspiration toward new beginnings.

My family and I have had this time of beckoning deep rest turned upside down with the illness our mother suffered, the worst from October until she passed December 9th. Our energy sapped from worry, grief, and so much time spent in the hospital. The ability to rest thwarted as calls to loved ones, paperwork, preparing final arrangements, and gathering up and re-organizing mum's house took priority.

Bypassing the need for extreme downtime to grieve has compromised my immune system and left me with a chest infection, bronchitis, brain fog, and no energy going on 7 days during the holidays, has been a poignant reminder that I am human and the need to honour my body and soul is required for optimal health.

I have been disappointed to cancel appointments with my patients and disappointed with society's economic system and insurance corporations that allow the sick and grieving, self- employed folks to fall through the cracks of financial sustainability.

I also am disappointed that I did not follow my gut regardless of economic consequences.

So, this week, I am honouring the need for deep rest. Though it needed to be sooner, I will nurture my body's desire to begin healing.

I keep receiving these lessons to practice honouring the self. I humbly admit to not being perfect, not listening when I know what to do, and awkwardly navigating the cold waters of grief, the winds of change, and the belief that comfort and warmth will once again inhabit my body, mind, and heart.

Sending love to all those wandering humbly toward wholeness, may you soon find peace.

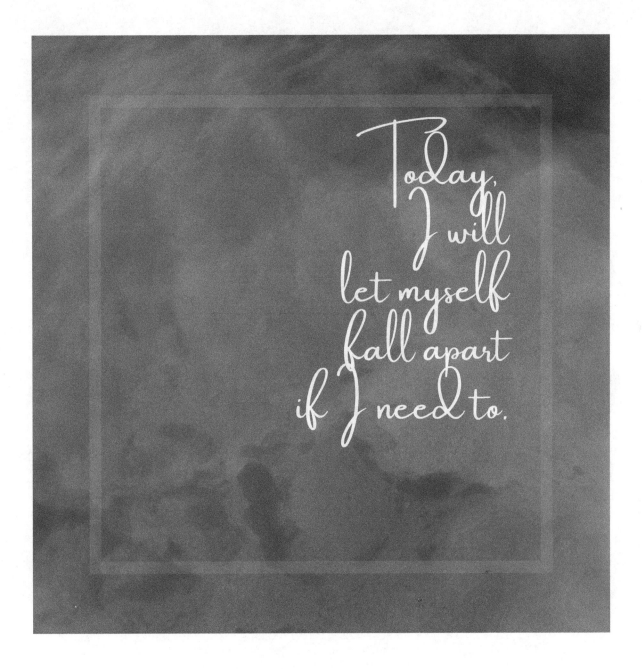

It is ok to fall apart, to be grief stricken, to not know what to do, or how to move forward.

I don't fall apart so that I can put all my pieces back together. I let myself crumble because to not would mean ignoring my vulnerable humanity. Raw emotion is freeing. It drops the falsehood of keeping it all together, of needing to prove your worthiness.

You are worthy because you are here. You are worthy because you feel everything. Your truth is beautiful. It is meaningful.

Acknowledge your beauty and worthiness.

Let go of the rest.

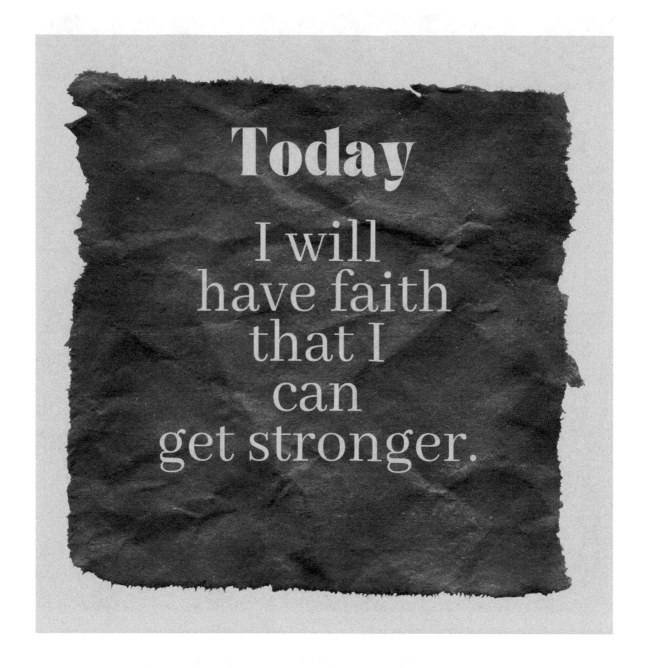

Today
I will have faith that I can get stronger.

Today, I am resting from the utter exhaustion of the last few months, my body had to shut down for a while. I understand, it's been rough on my body and my spirit.

I have felt glimpses of energy beginning to return to my blood and my breath.

Today, I feel like I will be okay. Soon.

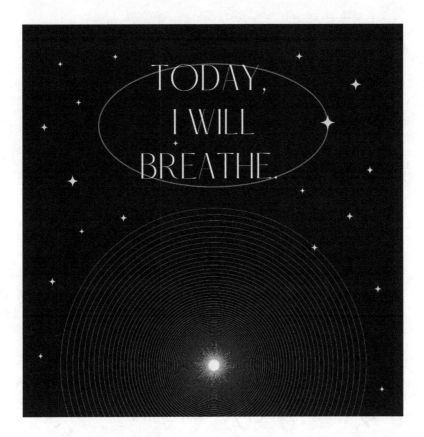

Moving into a busy week, it's so important for me to ease in slowly. If I rush in without awareness, I know from experience that my body and mind systems become shocked and out of sorts. That then makes me grumpy and not at my best. This is unhelpful when I spend most of my days offering help to others.

To feel my best, I love to start my day slowly and mindfully. I wake earlier than I would need to if I were to jump right in.

I lay in bed, appreciating the softness and warmth. I take slow, intentional breaths to wake up my mind, my circulation, my digestive system.

When I'm ready (which is sometimes a long time), I will rise and go to the kitchen and put on the kettle. I measure out aromatic coffee for my French press as the water begins to boil. I like to add powdered nutritional mushrooms and ground cinnamon to the coffee grinds for immune health.

I intentionally breathe in the soothing scent and imagine it moving through my body, imagine it nourishing my cells. Setting this intention prepares my system to receive the benefits of the delicious concoction.

Noticing how my body feels when I inhale the aroma allows me to intuit whether it feels good for my system, or if it doesn't smell right to me today. If it doesn't bring my body ease and joy, I will make something else. I love tea as well. Smelling and paying attention to the reaction is a valuable reminder that our bodies are incredibly wise. We're built for intuition for recognizing when something is off before ingesting it. For survival.

This is a deeply ingrained system. People have forgotten about this ancient, built-in wisdom. This is what our senses do. They help us discern what will be health-giving, and what could be dangerous. Intuition and breathing are linked. We all breathe, but we don't all acknowledge the intuitive sense.

With my coffee, I also love to ingest a few pages of a book that holds great depth and insight to wake up my mind and imagination. This helps me connect to the deepest parts of me, my wild nature. This brings my creative and critical thinking systems in line with my breath and my flow. After I serve myself in these sacred ways, I am ready to serve others.

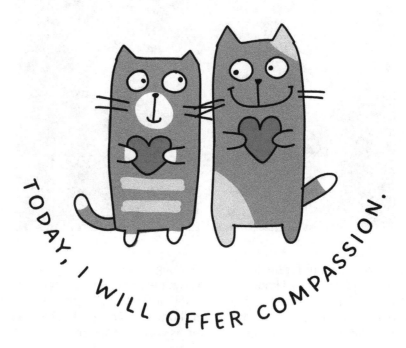

TODAY, I WILL OFFER COMPASSION.

When I give compassion to myself, I receive acceptance.

When I give compassion to another, I receive connection.

When I give compassion to a child, I receive love.

When I give compassion to community, I receive belonging.

When I give compassion to an animal, I receive loyalty.

When I give compassion to nature, I receive life.

When I give compassion to the earth, I receive a home.

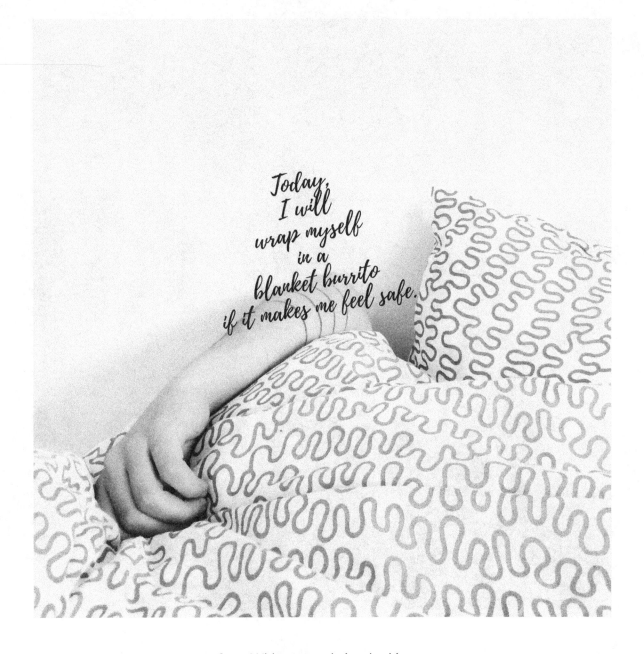

Today,
I will
wrap myself
in a
blanket burrito
if it makes me feel safe.

Cozy. With a cat curled up beside me.

I might read. This is my win today.

I hope you find coziness today.

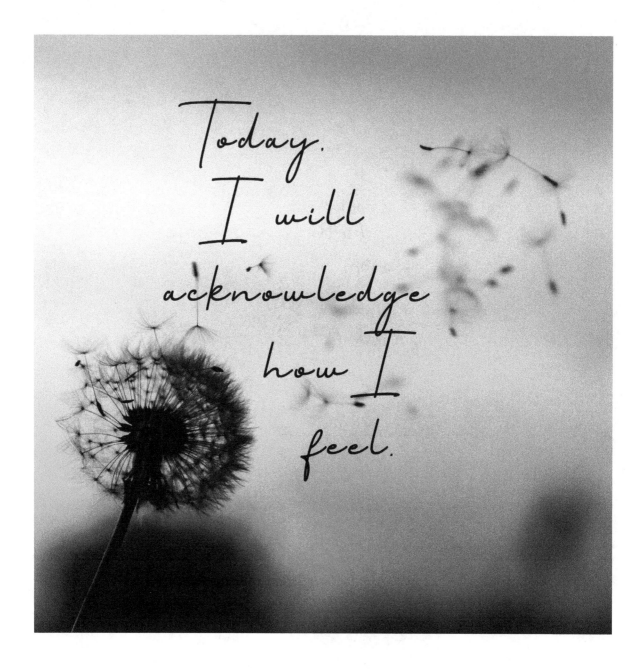

Today,
I will
acknowledge
how I
feel.

One dandelion plant can grow up to 5,000 seeds in one growing season: one wind carrying waves of possible new life.

Similarly, our hearts and bodies can hold hundreds of emotions in the span of a day, that can turn into seeds of awareness, discovery, and connection when we pay attention to them.

Acknowledging how I feel provides the opportunity for reflection, understanding, and growth. However, I believe simply recognizing what's bubbling inside is a beautiful process of feeling our capacity and depth. We are incredibly powerful beings. Emotion can be a superpower.

Waves of emotion can spread our truth, allowing vulnerability to create connection, and belonging. This honours the universe born between people when we trust our humanness and emotional processes. The possibility of new life.

Brené Brown shares much insight on emotions in her book, Atlas of the Heart. I highly recommend.

TODAY, I WILL SAY I LOVE YOU A MILLION TIMES.

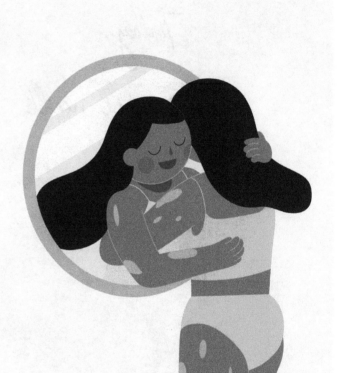

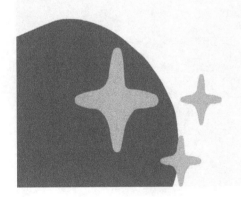

I am a paradox. A messy puddle of hot and cold, at the same damn time. A mushy mix of hormones, menopause, tiredness, joy, love, clarity, compassion, healing, awe, and gratitude.

I am finally starting to feel my body righting after bronchitis, breathing deeper, brain fog lifting. It is miraculous to move from despair and fear and lethargy into peace, calm, and joy of being alive again. It's like metamorphosis.

Today, I'm so thankful for a body that knows how to heal, and a soul that holds the wisdom of divine timing, the deepest grace, and the voice to show me what I need to thrive.

You are a miracle. You have a wise body. You have a heart capable of great love and endless depth. I love that about you, and I love that about me. I choose to love this whole messy package. I will look at my reflection and feel love. I will say I love you to more people, animals, and nature more frequently, and also to myself. I love you, and your messiness too.

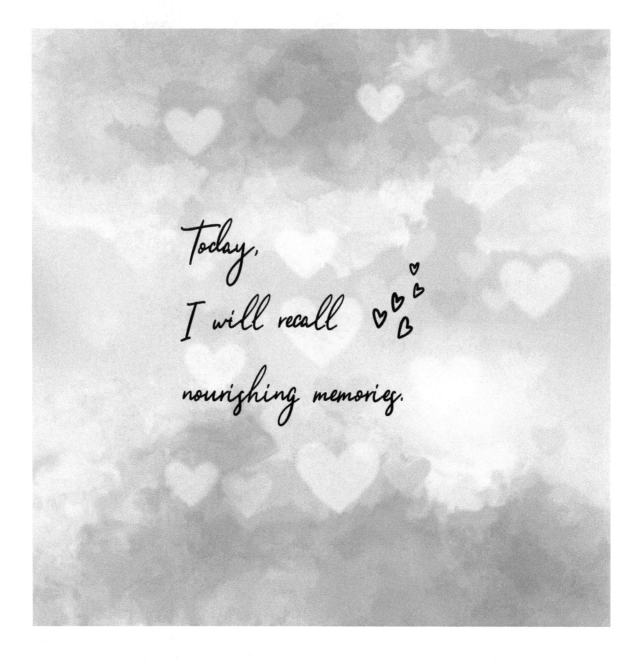

Today,
I will recall
nourishing memories.

We can create sensory experiences that re-engage
the positive emotions we felt in a previous moment by
intentionally thinking about memories that meant a great
deal to us.

It is enjoyable to occasionally be lost in a beautiful memory
and can nourish our bodies and neural networks as well.

Savouring these memories, over time, can improve mental
health and decrease the amount of time we focus on self-
deprecating thoughts and behaviors.

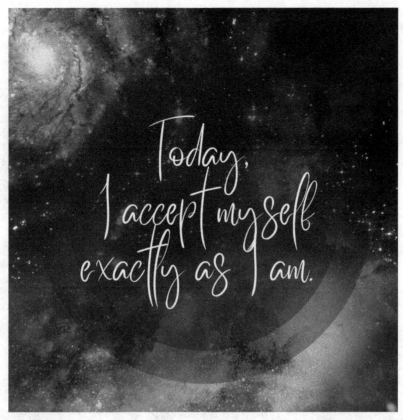

This is a hard one.

We have been taught by our systems, by culture, by our traumas, by our own brains often, to look for what's wrong. What's different. Our programming says if we don't fit in, we risk our survival.

This is why it's so easy to think there is something wrong with us, instead of recognizing and trusting what FEELS wrong around us and in how we're being treated. Trusting ourselves is challenging against these odds.

Sometimes, it seems I'm missing something. Like there is more I should understand, more I should be doing, like I should know exactly what this hole is that I need to fill.

For many, this void is a longing to know oneself deeply, to connect with the soul, the wild nature that we fear so. For many, it's a desire to return home to a place we can feel but cannot see. We look around every corner, hoping for a glimpse of what feels real, what gives meaning to wholeness. And for others, it's the drive to get as far away from themselves as possible.

Navigating this void can be a perilous journey. There are endless obstacles to become stuck on. It can be helpful to grasp perspective each day before traveling these waters.

What helps me most from getting lost when looking deeper are these things:

(And I'm definitely not successful every time)

1. Awareness - noticing where my mind is going and how my body is feeling at the same time.

2. Intention - consciously choosing if I have the time and space to explore at the moment. If I do, I will journey. If not, I intend to place it on the back burner and plan to come back to it when I'm able.

3. Compassion - allowing myself the grace to fumble through imperfect thoughts, feelings, and actions until I reach one island of perspective. And then choose to rest there or continue on if I have the energy.

4. Pause - consciously choosing a point to put down this work until another day. To gather what insight came this day and to ponder that lightly for the next little while, on and off. Stopping to rest is very important to integrate every time I learn something new.

I hope this is helpful.

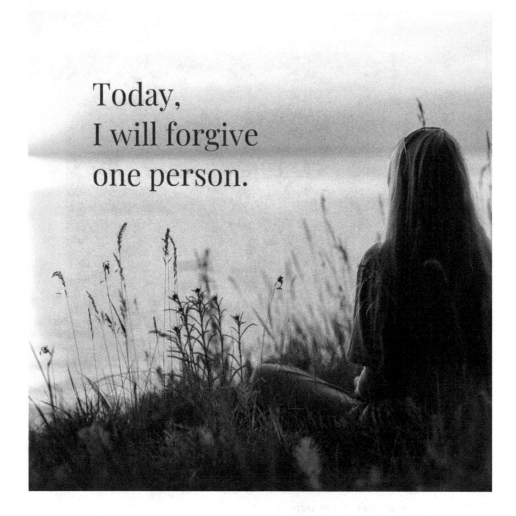

Today,
I will forgive
one person.

There are different kinds of forgiveness.

One kind means to close the books on something, such as forgiveness of a debt, closure of an account, to end a story.

This is useful in order to declutter the office, the accounts, or the mind.

Another kind can feel like an obligatory high road. One that feels forced, expected of one who has been hurt or wronged. This is the one that can feel like gaslighting if there has been no attempt to listen and understand what would feel like reparations to those who have been harmed. If this is you, please know that you NEVER need to forgive from a place of obligation. (Unless it is to appease for the sake of survival in the moment, in life-threatening situations. In which case, it is not true forgiveness, but a safety concern.)

Our society has been known to be sadly deficient in holding abusers accountable for their harm-doing so as to not upset the status quo or change power dynamics. (There are several social justice organizations available to help folks in a plethora of circumstances. If you need help finding one, please reach out to me.)

Sometimes, we need forgiveness for closure in our own minds and hearts. This kind has nothing to do with the one who does harm and everything to do with the one who desires relief. Relief from carrying the burden of victimhood, of feeling unworthy of safe, thoughtful treatment, respite from it consuming our daily thoughts and energy. To create the space, we need to move on and live life unburdened by the weight of something that sapped us for probably far too long.

This kind of forgiveness is just for you. For your healing. For your peace of mind.

And often, we need to forgive ourselves for suffering, for not knowing how to navigate unknown territory, for reacting out of fear or trauma. This can be the hardest step for some. We may judge ourselves more harshly than anyone else.

Please give yourself grace.

You can always learn more about what helps you feel most aligned, alive, and safe.

"How are you?" "Fine. Good. Ok. Alright."

Why are these our default greetings? In passing, when there is scarcely time to respond, let alone hear the answer.

It seems silly to ask a question that we have no intention to follow through to its conclusion. How are you has become superfluous, rhetorical. It's no surprise, however, in this time crunched society that we offer a polite salutation without thoughtful attention.

We've been taught to rush and that all we have time for is an empty greeting with no real connection. Our time doesn't feel like our own. Personally, I have an extreme dislike for rushing. I used to think time was not my friend, but I realized that the pace of life is what turns me off.

Moments are my friends. Eons are my friends. Wallowing in the forest is my friend. Luxuriating in a fantastic book or contemplating poetry are my friends. Unproductive indulgence is also my friend.

When I'm hoping for an undistracted response, I like to change my questions. Instead of how are you, I'll ask, "What's good today?", "what's on your mind/ heart today?", "What are you looking forward to?" I looove to make connections this way. People don't expect to hear questions like, where is your compass pointed today?

Robert Fulghum once asked his readers to replace their wristwatch with a compass for a week to see how their default thoughts might change if their focus was different. This is brilliant. It takes us out of the autopilot, which risks us missing our lives.

It's a good practice to consider our default questions and answers to others and for the way we talk to ourselves as well. Notice, and then shake them up if they feel worn out and ineffective. What is your purpose and intention with your greetings, your conversations, your work meetings, your philosophical explorations, and your heart to hearts?

Connection is what we all need and crave. If this feels absent or inadequate, use these moments we often miss because of our conditioning. Use awareness and intention as a default for a week and see what changes in your life.

Today, I will ask a question and listen deeply for the answer.

Connection is magic.

Whether I'm asking for support or offering it, my nervous system still lights up in a good way. I notice that my heart engages, my senses sharpen, my body becomes present, my brain readies.

It may feel vulnerable or awkward or perfectly natural. Whatever the emotion, the fear of opening subsides once the first step is taken.

We need connection as much as we need air to breathe. Our nervous systems are highly linked, and through connection, even brief positive interaction, we can exercise the large and extremely impactful vagus nerve.

The vagus nerve regulates the heart, lungs, and gut. This tells me that connection can have a healthy effect on the immune system, digestion, breathing, and blood pressure.

Interacting with another in a meaningful way drives a sense of belonging in both parties, regardless of the reason.

Sending love to you.

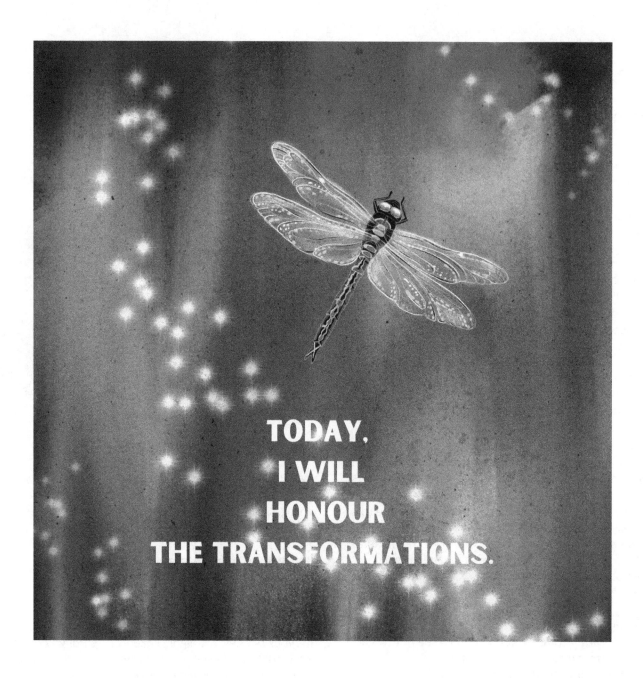

**TODAY,
I WILL
HONOUR
THE TRANSFORMATIONS.**

Every day, there are thousands of transitions. 86,400 seconds in a day that die and are reborn. Life and death are our nature, our humanness, part of our culture.

Though current society fears aging and death and tries to hide it away, so we don't have to look it in the face, it is what brings joy to the moments we remember to feel alive!

There are many big moments to celebrate, to carry, to nurture, to get through. There are also 86,400 small moments every day that we get to honor the life/death/ life nature in ourselves. Every second transforms into the next.

One second can mean the difference between living and dying, between falling and flying, between fire and ash. The dragonfly grows its wings by moving the Lifeblood of its previous moments outward to create the structure that sustains its transition to an expanded life.

When I honour my ordinary moments, and the nature of my transformations, I live an expanded life. I am changed. Love is the magic that carries me through every second. May you feel love, expansion, magic, and change every day. I see you.

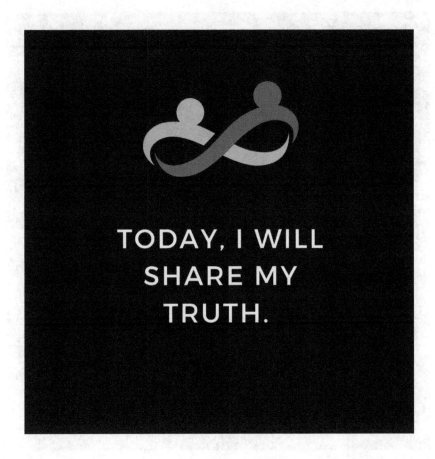

TODAY, I WILL SHARE MY TRUTH.

The truth will sometimes set you free.

It might be painful, it might be a relief, or both. It may challenge or offend others. How others see the truth you present is not up to you, and you can't change how someone else reacts. It's possible too, that you may not fully understand the great impact your authenticity could have on others. Your honesty may save a life, even if it's raw and unpolished. Maybe especially so.

I listen to several podcasts and have heard others speaking their truth. I have been inspired and emotionally turned upside down by some of the stories. I always seem to learn something about myself through the eyes of someone else. From brave souls who just talked about their journey. They can't know the impact their words have had on me, and I'm so grateful that they shared it anyway.

I'm going to be a guest on a podcast next week, talking about some of the childhood traumas that shaped my life. I imagine it might feel raw and scary, but also brave. I'm looking forward to the insight I gain from the experience. My hope is that it touches the heart of someone who listens to my words, makes them feel less alone, and encourages them to discover and speak their truth as well.

Some of the things I may be discussing will be abduction, abandonment, and how financial issues and moving frequently in childhood created an unusual, unquenchable homesickness in me that made me physically sick whenever I had plans to travel or go away for even just a weekend.

It was a long, tumultuous journey back home to me. The good news is, I finally recognized that some of my fear reactions came from these deeply embedded belief systems. And once you understand something like this, you don't unlearn it. It always seems to take me in a healing direction. And the journey is ever unfinished, and this I am grateful for.

The point is, that is ok to be where you are at this moment. It's ok to not know, it's ok to have seconds or minutes of recognition and clarity and be confused the rest of the day. It's ok to need a sounding board, a therapist, a friend who listens deeply. It's ok to be needy, it's how we're built. We are human and we all have needs. We're meant to be picked up by our community when we need uplifting. And if we don't have the right communities, we need to create them. We are meant to see ourselves in context with our environment and through those we love. I didn't learn all these things by myself. You don't have too either.

Love to you.

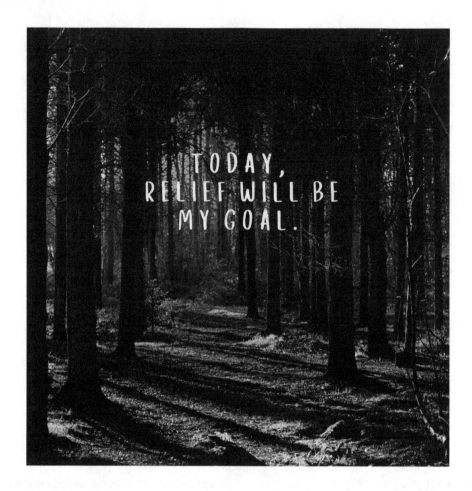

TODAY,
RELIEF WILL BE
MY GOAL.

When there is relief, there is less resistance. Relief transforms us like alchemy. Finding relief when there is fear feels like peace. When there is pain, relief causes unclenching, a physical relaxation from holding your breath, an exhale.

When I treat patients on my massage table, it's easy to detect when relief sets in. There is a moment when breath flows out easily, and the body spontaneously sinks into the table, muscles become less rigid and more mushy. It's easier to work with muscles when they are not contracted and rigid. In the same way, a mind is able to hold creativity and openness not when gripped by fear but when it can have a bit of softness to it.

When I'm anxious or worried or stuck in a fear-based reaction, I look for a little crack in my mind where I can feel a tiny bit of relief. A glimpse is all I need to remind me that relief is possible, that I'm capable of feeling peace and healing again.

Epiphanies happen occasionally, but most often, relief comes in tiny steps or micromovements. It's very difficult to move emotionally from anxiety to calm, sickness to wellness, or devastation to joy all in one step. It takes time and self-compassion.

This doesn't mean that challenging emotions are bad. All emotion has validity and value. Emotions have power. Feeling everything (and sometimes feeling nothing) is a result of paying attention to the world around you and the world within. You don't have to experience emotion the way you think other people do. What you feel is your truth.

Nature is magic. The sunrise every morning is magic. Buds emerging on branches as the ground and air become warmer is magic. You, in your nature, are magic too. Relief, when it comes, can feel miraculous, unbinding, and sometimes unsettling.

Moving through one emotion leaves a hole or space for another to settle in. If we can choose the next thought or feeling intentionally, it feels a bit like directing the flow, laying a path of stones that cradle the movement of your lifeforce for a second. It's not something to perfect. It's a dance to experience.

Love to you.

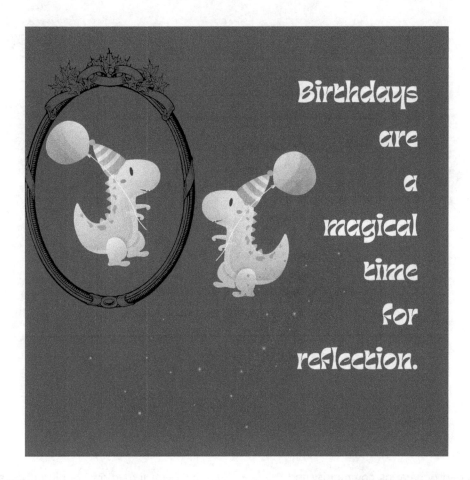

Birthdays are a magical time for reflection.

It's very common to look back at past years and iterations of our lives when we arrive at another full circle.

I briefly wondered this morning if the earth celebrated her full rotations and cycles around the sun, and immediately thought, of course she does!

Each morning, evening, and season, we are witness to her beautiful celebrations of ebb and flow, strength, and surrender in her unabashed wholeness.

Dancing with the sun, moon, and stars, sharing her dazzling light shows and rainbows.

Holding tender plants underground while they hibernate and giving them encouragement to let loose their buds from her incubator in the spring.

She is a brilliant mother, praising and loving all her babies, animals, and plants alike, demonstrating how to nurture and shine, offering unconditional bounty to all who take shelter in her home.

I've learned a lot from her throughout my life, this year even more, it seems.

From saying goodbye to dear ones in physical form to feeling cradled in my grief and joined in joyous dance, she graciously holds me in all my seasons.

That presence is so very powerful.

I aim to give and receive and love and celebrate as Mother Earth does.

I strive to hold others through their seasons, unassuming and gloriously gratitudinous.

I truly appreciate each of you for being here on this planet, traveling with me along our paths, seeking to celebrate moments and seasons in yourselves and for one another.

You are here to witness the magic of your budding.

Be present for it, celebrate it, give it your breath, dance in rapture.

We have so few breaths left in these bodies.

Life on this planet is a miracle, be here for it all.

Love to you in all your miracleness.

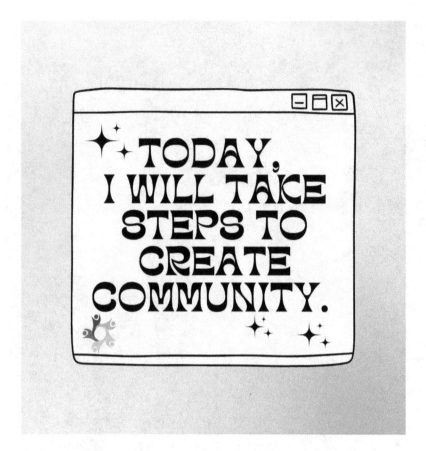

Your body is a crucial part of creating community and finding your peeps.

You can find your intuition in your gut and in the signals your body gives you.

Every choice you make is an opportunity to practice listening to your inner wisdom.

Asking questions and listening to what your body says can support you in making the right choices for yourself.

For example, think about deciding between two items on a menu. Imagine the smell and taste of one item and then the other while paying attention to the reaction your body has. There may be a subtle feeling shift between the two. One could feel more mouth watering than the other. Sometimes, I can actually feel faint heartburn when I do this, signaling to me to stay away.

With some choices, you might feel your body tighten, physically back away, or feel dread. In other choices, you may feel excitement and a full body yes when an opportunity presents itself.

An important step in creating anything is imagining what it could look like and how you WANT to feel when immersed in it.

First, it's helpful to know your intention so you understand what you'd like to align with when making a decision. (It also helps to know your non-negotiable values for this process)

Second, listen to your body signals regarding each step toward connecting with new people and opportunities.

Recently, I had a full body yes... actually three of them. All of them, opportunities to connect with others in community.

One, a musical revue with a community I deeply love and respect and gives me space to fuel a passion of mine.

Two, the opportunity to take a course with my son that will allow me to spend precious time with my child and is focused on health and education, combining a whole bunch of value-driven awesomeness.

Three, an invitation to speak my truth to a larger community, on a podcast, allowing me to connect with others in a way I've never done, and a chance to trust myself and listen to my intuition.

There are countless ways to connect with your own values, then reach out to others through that lens. It may be the gritty part of you that needs love or the caring human wanting to nurture others. Feel it first, then act.

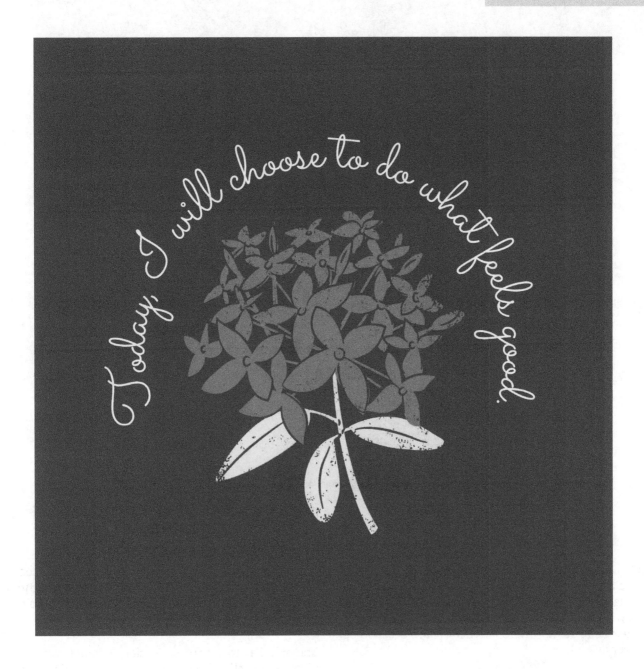

Today, I will choose to do what feels good.

What feels good?

In the words of Sonya Renee Taylor, "An acorn doesn't say to itself, I need to find some water. It just allows water to flow in because that's what is inherently good for its growth."

Humans can be extremely adept at blocking what inherently helps us grow. Societal conditioning contributes to internalized voices of patriarchy and not-good-enough-ness.

What I'm aware of this morning is that when I recognize and let go of the other voices telling me what I should be in order to be acceptable, I can more easily hear my soul.

Living from a space of whole self consideration, acceptance, and love; my inherent nature, good things are drawn to me.

Giving myself a moment to breathe before getting out of bed, a slow cup of coffee before the day starts. Infusing my mind, heart, and body with magic and presence and health and peace. Allowing in that which bolsters my sense of integrity and connection to myself before interacting with others and within a society that wants me to be different.

Remembering to let goodness find me, let miracles find me, to hear my innate self isn't easy. It's a practice in letting go of the external that has insidiously and subconsciously become our internal measuring sticks.

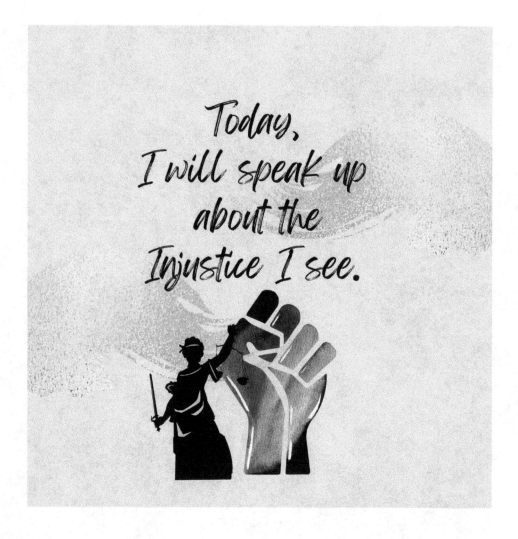

*Today,
I will speak up
about the
Injustice I see.*

When I'm connected to my integrity and values, I more easily see and feel the connectedness of everything. I see the imbalance of power in systems that view the white cis hetero thin rich functional male body as the ideal for everyone else to strive toward in order to have acceptance and power over others.

I see racism, ageism, ableism, and patriarchy as symptoms of this imbalance. Human dignity is one of my top values, and when I witness the violation of it, my heart breaks.

Paying attention to these feelings can be difficult and can also light the fire of righteous anger. Ruminating in anger itself is unhelpful of it stagnates. But anger that sparks the desire to serve others, to help others, that calls to action, can be exactly where change begins.

One of my purposes is to bring compassionate presence and safe, nurturing touch to folks in care homes, hospice, and palliative hospitals. The elderly and the dying are populations who often feel ignored, forgotten afterthoughts, hidden from the hustle of our societies.

Viewed as unproductive and undesirable, not because this is true, but because our culture has become so frightened of their own mortality that they can't bear to look at aging and dying in the face.

The only way to a more just society is to notice and speak up about injustice. By having open conversation within us, in our homes, our communities, in our systems and workplaces.

Sonya Renee Taylor says, "You're living in someone's imagination right now. You may as well make it your own." This means that everything in our cultures and societies were created by someone. And we dream dreams with parameters given to us by our upbringing and what we were told we could strive for. But because all of this was once just an idea in someone's mind, everything can be changed.

Notice what's around you with love. Speak up if something doesn't feel right. Gather your peeps.

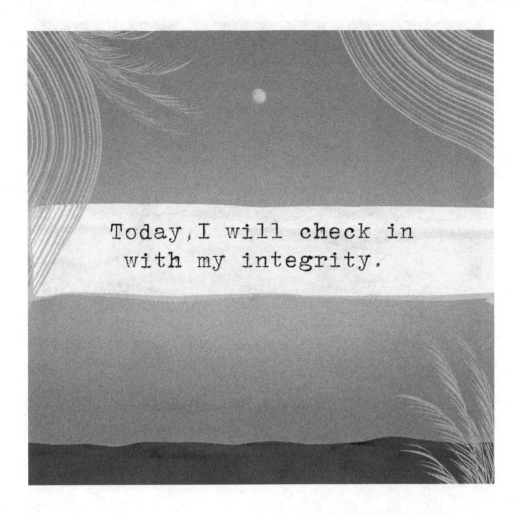

Today, I will check in
with my integrity.

There are many times I have abandoned myself. Sometimes, it was because I felt my physical or emotional safety was in danger. Other times because I didn't have or didn't know my boundaries. I kept quiet for financial security at different jobs. Most often, however, it was to try to avoid others from abandoning me.

I found situations where I compromised myself more devastating and frequent the more I ignored the signs my body and mind sent. This spiraled into shame as I hid parts of my life from family and friends so I wouldn't be judged for my choices.

Staying with an (ex) husband that was an addict and emotionally abusive. Financial failures and stress. Not being able to support my children for a few scary months where I had to ask for social assistance. All of it horrendous and shame-inducing, perpetuating the desire to hide the truth from others.

I've worked for companies that compromised my integrity every day just being there. Until it became too much for me to hold, I suffered silently until I broke.

Brené Brown says, "Shame can't live where there is

compassion." This means talking about it with a trusted other can help dissipate shame and give tremendous relief once shared.

There are countless small ways we don't validate our own truth. Saying I'm fine when we're not, putting up with racist, misogynist, or ignorant language or behavior without calling it out, not asking for what we desire, or ignoring our boundaries.

It takes a lot of awareness, personal check-ins, and deep work often. Practicing listening to myself and getting to the heart of my truth has been difficult at times, easier at other times. Having the courage to follow through when we finally hear what matters most to us can be even more challenging. But if we listen to the pokes we can't ignore, it becomes easier to recognize the subtle nudges.

Holding myself with respect helps me remain intentional about checking in with myself. And it's interesting that when I check in with myself daily, it contributes to holding myself in respect and love, too. It goes both ways. I hope you can always align with your integrity, listen to your intuition, and trust your soul.

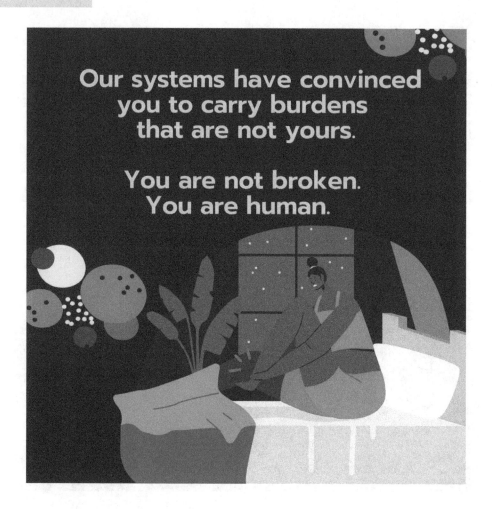

Our systems have convinced
you to carry burdens
that are not yours.

You are not broken.
You are human.

Your heart, gut, and nervous system are built to notice the blatant and subtle things going on around you and react internally. This may happen at a subconscious level. Your conscious mind may not recognize as acutely how you are being affected by what your body observes.

Your body notices everything, even if you can't put some of it into words. Many have been taught to ignore emotions that arise, especially if they don't match what can be externally perceived in the moment. We absorb much more information than we physically see.

Many of our systems, medical, educational, political, etc... create the dysfunction and disparity that we adopt as our own and as our fault. When our basic human needs are not met, it can lead to fracturing of self-worth. You deserve and need to be valued, cared for, safe, and in community of some kind to bolster your sense of self.

I'm very close to many people who often feel anxiety and depression. Feelings have been divided by our society into "good" and "bad", "desirable" and "undesirable", "acceptable" and "crazy". We've been socialized to pile extra feelings of

shame and guilt, just for holding human emotions in our bodies. We are blamed for not keeping in all together when it's our support systems that are lacking, in favour of toxic individuality and power over others. No wonder or bodies feel such discrepancy. It's effing confusing.

I resonate with Glennon Doyle in her book, Untamed, when she talks about trying to feel grateful when we thought life would be more beautiful than this and feel guilty for not being happy in life with "good enough". We feel deeply when we pay attention.

Life is hard, and we sometimes feel a thousand things at once, and sometimes we dissociate and feel nothing. This is a super valid reaction to what your body and mind are perceiving! Emotions are not meant to be categorized & pathologized. They are meant to be felt. Sometimes, it feels ok to just observe them, and sometimes, they spark action. Only you can know what's right for you.

It's hard to always trust the wisdom of our bodies. Getting help, going within, and learning to listen are all ways to hear our deepest truths. Take your time.

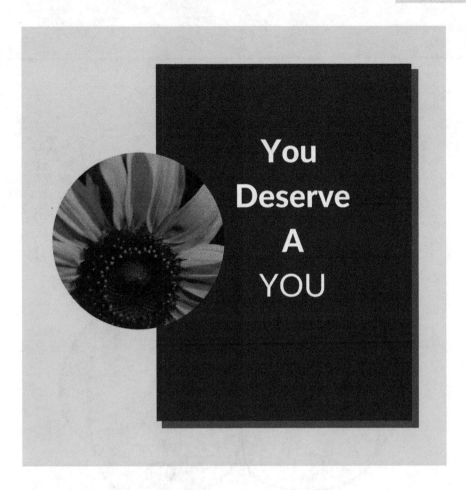

One of my patients said to me recently, "You Deserve a YOU". What she meant was I deserve be cared for and have a massage treatment from someone like me. She consistently feels relief and calm after our appointments together.

After she left, I thought about how profound a statement that was. In many ways, I would love to experience another me to feel what others feel when I care for them. To have deep discussions with, or to explore my mysterious soul with.

I can also understand this statement from a different perspective, one that contradicts our societal conditioning as women to be selfless. I deserve a self. I deserve a deep, loving, chaotic, emotional, sad, joyous, desire- filled, always evolving, compassionate, subversive, questioning, wondrous, authentic, magical self.

I deserve to recognize my vulnerability and my most infected wounds, to feel my innate wisdom and to know sacred communion with the world. To feel individuality and creativity, and also universal interconnectedness.

Our selves are a part of the whole, the flow of nature, made of stars and organized dust and consciousness. Looking

at a Sunflower, one might not guess that it is a beautifully organized system of hundreds of parts living in harmony with each other. It looks flawlessly like one organism. Each lovely ray floret looks like a petal sprouting off the edges and the tiny disc florets fill the inside portion. All individual flowers themselves with different purposes, for a common goal.

The ray florets don't reproduce but are bright and long to attract bees to the disc florets, each of which grow a seed. Each of us have hundreds of parts working in harmony to live. We have different layers that can somehow manage to birth ideas and humans. We can feel a multitude of sensations and emotions. We experience cycles of birth, life, and death, not only in the length of a lifetime, but everyday and in every breath.

From death comes new life, as each flower dies, so a seed is born. Can we fathom to view each human life as we perceive a Sunflower? With awe and reverence for its beauty and simplicity, audacity and colour, life, death, and rebirth? We are all held, together, as part of a perfectly flawless universal organism. Connected by our unique and individual experiences and perspectives. You deserve to know this YOU.

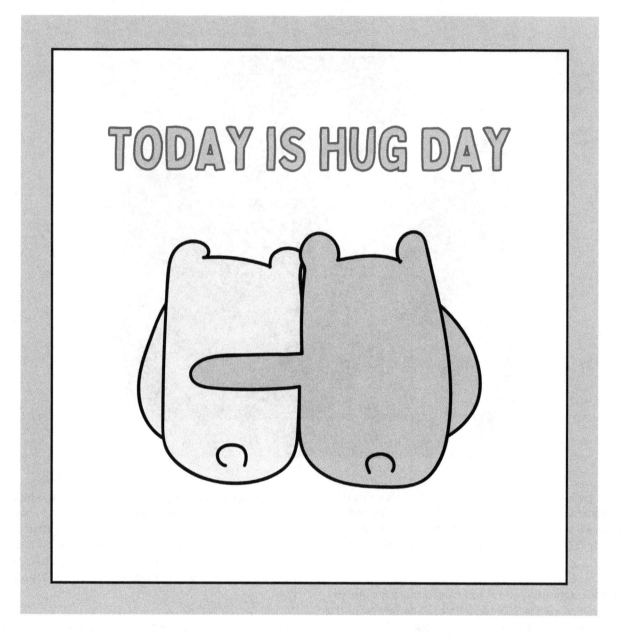

TODAY IS HUG DAY

Hugs are the healers of the world.

Safe, nurturing human touch is essential for life. Babies die without it. Our bodies and nervous systems were built for it.

Hugs are magical and mutually beneficial. You can't give one without receiving one.

They are a portal from the body to the soul. It is said that a hug that lasts more than 20 seconds releases oxytocin, a hormone that increases well-being, happiness, love, connection, bonding, and decreases stress. A true body-mind-heart connection.

One year, I wore a shirt at the Vancouver Pride Parade that said "Free Mom Hugs," and I'll tell you what a blessed day that was! I could not even count how many gorgeous connections I made over just a few hours. The trust, the emotion, the love that flowed from so many human hearts filled my cup and my soul that day.

Asking for a hug can feel vulnerable. Your need for touch is your body craving connection, trusting that takes courage sometimes.

Find some folks to offer hugs today. And remember that consent is always necessary first for the other to feel safe.

Love to you.

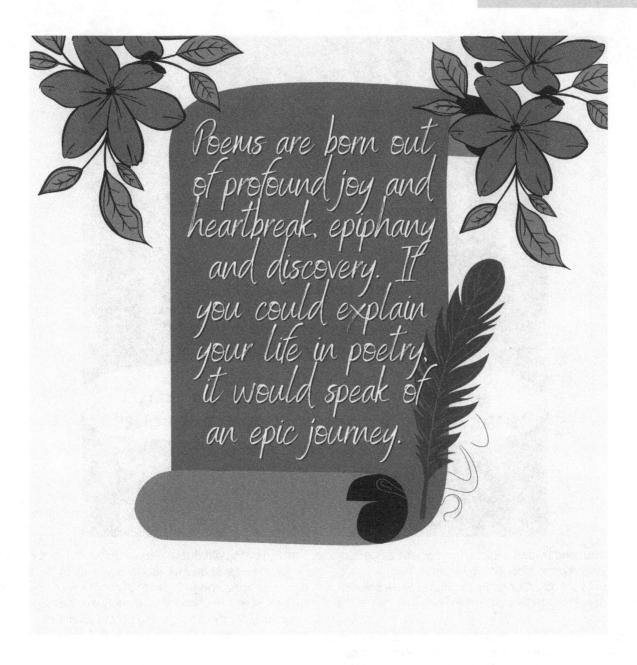

Poems are born out of profound joy and heartbreak, epiphany and discovery. If you could explain your life in poetry, it would speak of an epic journey.

As a writing exercise once, I decided to write about a very difficult time in my life in another voice. I imagined myself as a young girl in a Medieval Era, using language that reflected the day, and spoke of my experience in terms of an adventure.

This was powerful to me in re-framing the context in which I saw myself and the way that I suffered, was supported, or not supported, and provided an alternate lens to look through. It also added a dimension of connection to an alternate me and of understanding of her deepest desires and fears. This led to empathy for myself and for what others have gone through, making them who they are today.

Seeing yourself from a different perspective can be helpful to your self-awareness and compassion. I highly recommend trying to write yourself into poetry. It can be fun and remind you of your creativity and other parts you may have forgotten about.

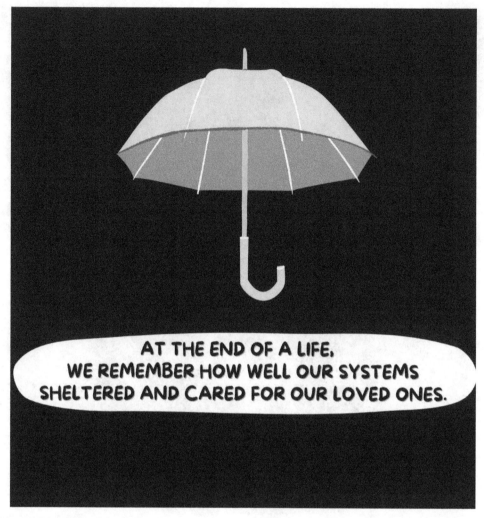

AT THE END OF A LIFE, WE REMEMBER HOW WELL OUR SYSTEMS SHELTERED AND CARED FOR OUR LOVED ONES.

We are surrounded by and immersed in societal systems. We rely on interconnection, communication, and cooperation every day. Our social structures were created and operational long before we arrived here.

Our predecessors did what they thought appropriate at the time when implementing systems such as healthcare and education. Though they thought these structures worked for the benefit of all, they were built through a colonial and biased lens. And because we teach and perpetuate what and how we are taught, it takes courage, strength, and creativity to step out of oppressive bias and see through hearts of compassion, trust, and humanity.

For many years, I have witnessed (and likely you have too) injustice in our systems. I have seen children treated poorly or worse because they don't learn or see the world in a "convenient" way for the school system. I have seen patients in the healthcare system mistreated for asking questions, for being confused or frustrated, for needing help, for not having enough money, for not having the "right" colour skin or heritage, or for being an older.

Sadly, growing old doesn't equal respectful care in many circumstances. Economic inequity can mean the difference between aging and dying with dignity or with apathy. Are these systems overloaded or inadequately funded? Are they structured for the people who access them or for business efficiency in mind?

When our loved ones are facing the end of life, our hope is to provide ultimate compassion and dignity in their last years, months, and days. This is difficult for many due to financial and systemic barriers to access and care.

The experiences that our loved ones, and eventually we, will face, will only be as good as our systems allow. We often think of their last moments, whether we are present or not. We hope they didn't suffer too much. We wonder if we could have done something better. Many folks die in peaceful surroundings with loved ones gathered. Many do not.

I want to offer myself as a building block to more equitable and compassionate systems of caring for humans. My heart won't stand for anything else.

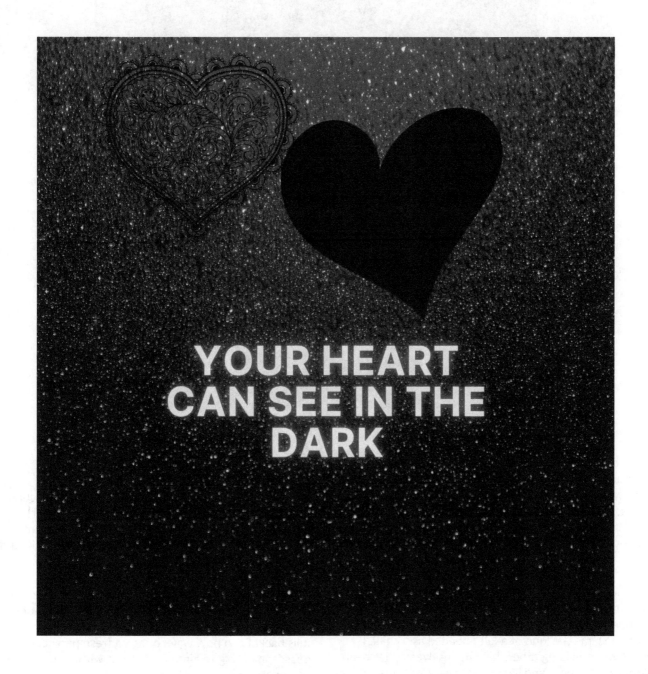

YOUR HEART
CAN SEE IN THE
DARK

Even when you think you're lost, broken, or alone, your
heart of wisdom knows exactly where you are.

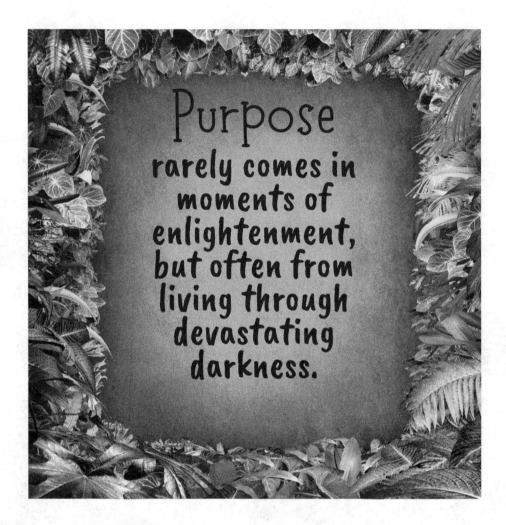

Purpose rarely comes in moments of enlightenment, but often from living through devastating darkness.

Purpose can grow from within us like a sunrise, brightness overcoming the shadows, slowly using a canvas as big as the sky. Sometimes, it appears as quickly as a flash of lightning, giving small bursts of clarity and then darkness again. Circumstances can be difficult and sad from traumatic experiences, even when you have no conscious memory of them.

For example, if you've heard of the archetype of wounded healer, that fits me perfectly. I gained a fear of abandonment from situations in my early years, and because of this, I believe I became the kind of adult I needed as a child. I have a love for helping others heal themselves. It has been a journey of darkness and light, tears, fears, and great relief. And it continues. Our wounds can often become our gifts to help others.

Sometimes inspiration comes from a mentor, teacher, or something you're drawn to and decide to try. Even when it comes this way, I believe there is a longing for the flow of our soul river that beckons us to jump in. When we listen,

life presents us with opportunities for expansion.

It may not feel like passion or destiny, but simple curiosity. It may be creative or grounding, uncertain, or heart-wrenching. It could be speaking to a crowd or silently holding someone in their darkness. It may feel awkward or could feel like home.

Purpose might be constant for some, but in my experience, it has an ebb and flow. Like a cave on a beach that fills to bursting when a wave comes in, then empties as the tide pulls back. Each new wave bringing fresh perspectives and ideas; something to learn from, to sit with, to challenge, or to accept.

However, it's not always the growth that gives us a reason to go on. I find the emptying just as important as the filling up. These moments provide rest, reflection, and integration. I cannot fit one more drop of knowledge in me when I'm at capacity, so it is, sometimes the emptying that allows purpose to show itself.

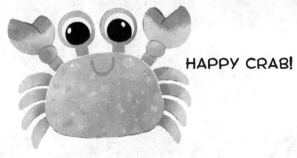

I DON'T WANT TO BE PRODUCTIVE FOR A CULTURE THAT JUDGES MY WORTH BASED ON MY OUTPUT.

I WANT TO FEEL INNATELY WORTHY AND TRUST THE INTEGRITY OF MY OWN TIMING.

FEELIN' CRABBY

HAPPY CRAB!

Toxic capitalism that reduces people to numbers and productivity is abrasive to my soul. It repels me with great force when I am treated this way. In fact, I am much less productive in a system like this because I am so miserable that my soul won't let me forget it. It pokes and prods and tugs at me until it consumes my conscious awareness, and my body wants to escape as hastily as it can.

I can't imagine that I'm the only one who feels this way. Actually, I know I'm not because of the conversations I've had with past colleagues of toxic work environments we were subjected to together. One place was so overtly about profit mongering that I'm surprised I made it so long, though it was likely because it was wrapped in a somewhat humanitarian guise.

Another job was fun for a while until I came to know that many there had become corporate zombies, counting the days to retirement, and living for their drinks on weekends. I could not risk being put under this spell.

There are several others I could recount, but you probably get the picture. I'm happiest in my daily life when I have space to breathe and connect with myself, with nature, and with others on a deep level.

I understand that there is so much to be done every day to make this world run. But the nagging question in my mind is always, "for who"? Who do these systems benefit? There is no doubt that I have gained much from capitalism. I wonder, though, what more has been lost because of it.

Financial wins have been great for billionaires, but at what cost to their hearts and spirits and deep connections? I'll never know. What I perceive, however, is that corruption is present when you let those who contributed to your wealth suffer the consequences of this imbalance of power and money.

Integrity is when there is alignment of mind, body, heart, and soul. Imbalances for long periods of time can upset the whole system. This applies to humanity, culture, structures (physical and social), and our own human bodies.

In order to thrive, we need to take our time connecting to what is truly important and essential to our souls. A fraction of a self is not my idea of a fulfilling life. Wholeness is.

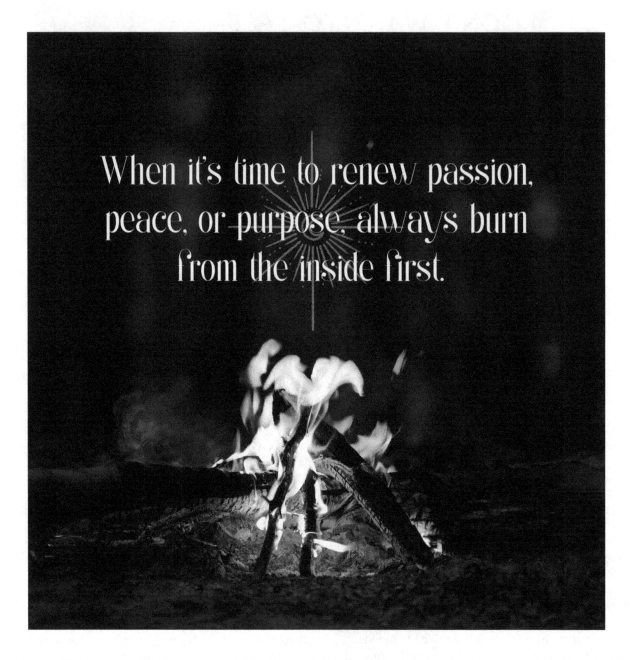

When it's time to renew passion, peace, or purpose, always burn from the inside first.

Renewal serves us in many ways.

To renew is often defined as refreshing, rejuvenating, or restoring something faded or disintegrating.

It can mean examining beliefs, behaviors, or boundaries we thought to be the truest form of who we are and deciding to evolve to a truer space in mind and heart.

The most effective way to feel integrity is allowing it to come from deep within. Alignment comes from frequent and honest listening to how we feel. It is what resonates with your soul, the darkest incubator of your wildest and wisest self, your core, the most consistent and unending part of you.

We feel emotional pain when we are not aligned with this part of ourselves.

This is also where passion and purpose come from, where peace comes from, and where courage, curiosity, love, and joy are born.

Before integrating what outside pressures demand from you, go within and burn away the debris that is taking up vital space and sucking energy away from what truly means the most to you.

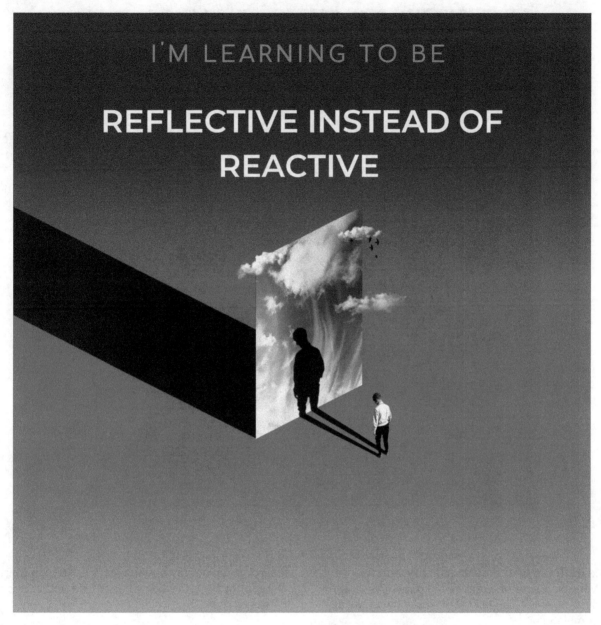

I'M LEARNING TO BE

REFLECTIVE INSTEAD OF REACTIVE

Though I've done a lot of work to become aware of my internal reactions over the years, there is always room for growth. It is an ongoing journey to be intentional about how I prefer to feel and to cultivate a life that allows me to inhabit these feelings often.

I remember Wayne Dyer saying, "When you squeeze an orange, orange juice comes out." It has been said by many others as well that what we have inside of us comes out when we are squeezed. When we are stressed, tired, hungry, unaware, surprised, or depleted, we tend to react in a way that shows our insides, what we're made of, or what has been building over time.

If there is bitterness that hasn't been resolved, that can emerge. If there is fear, it can shape our interactions. Though, if we have awareness of what is going on for us internally, we can better understand if it is applicable to the situation in front of us.

Shadow aspects of ourselves that we haven't fully accepted have a way of showing up when life presses down on us. Being able to hold awareness of the stirrings within is a step toward understanding what drives our ship when we're taken out of familiar waters.

Wholeness is a never-ending and worthy journey.

Self-reflection is a powerful tool in your growth and evolution.

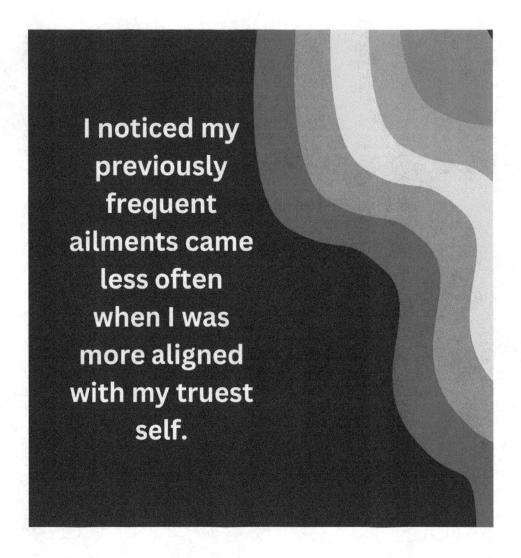

I noticed my previously frequent ailments came less often when I was more aligned with my truest self.

Telling the truth can boost your immune system. Alternatively, being out of integrity can put stress on the immune system, which can lead to sickness over time as the stress accumulates.

I used to get sick A LOT. I used to get bronchitis at least the times a year, plus colds and flu. Not that I was lying, but I was not living my truth or saying what I meant or honouring my heart or my body. It takes courage to live in integrity in a society that can be so judgemental of truth-tellers. Our systems don't support honesty at many levels of interaction, so much so that we don't even realize it often.

From saying you're ok when you're actually feeling horrible or sad to staying at a job you hate or feel undermined at, we all experience misalignment at some point.

I've been vulnerable to folks who took advantage of my openness and desire to help others, and it certainly took me many lessons to figure out what feels good and what

doesn't, and what my boundaries are. Though these things may continually change, my core truths and values remain the same.

Each experience has helped me grow into a person who recognizes my intuition. I trust my body more, to tell me what it needs. I listen to my heart far more than I ever used to. I can honestly say I haven't been very sick for many years now. Except for a couple weeks after my mum died, I've been pretty healthy for a few years. Even when I had covid, symptoms didn't last very long. When Mum was in palliative care, I didn't feel I could honour my need for rest, sleep, or proper nutrition, which is why my body got so run down.

I believe we can build up our systems of support so that we are healthier individually and collectively. We could feel better emotionally, physically, and psychologically if we were encouraged to live in integrity and speak our truths.

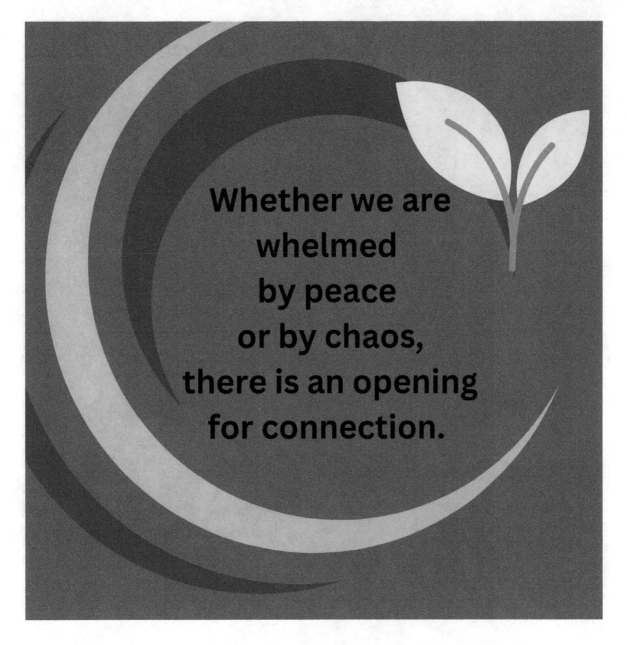

Whether we are
whelmed
by peace
or by chaos,
there is an opening
for connection.

When your inner nature gives you a gift that whelms your senses, your intuition, your emotions, you are engulfed in the moment, fully alive in the experience.

A moment that is juicy and human obliterates the blocks of apathy and fear and "proper" behavior. The moment your authenticity bursts out of you, it makes you more whole in an instant. It allows threads of connection to be tugged and followed. It creates the space for the bigger life you've been wanting; it moves the creaky, old door guarding the void that needs filling.

Connection doesn't have to be elusive. We have the opportunity every day to pay attention, to say what we mean, to point out what we feel, see, hear, or touch.

Our senses experience hundreds of things every moment. Speak what you notice out loud to yourself, to another, to an animal, to the universe. Find significance and meaning and miracles in it all.

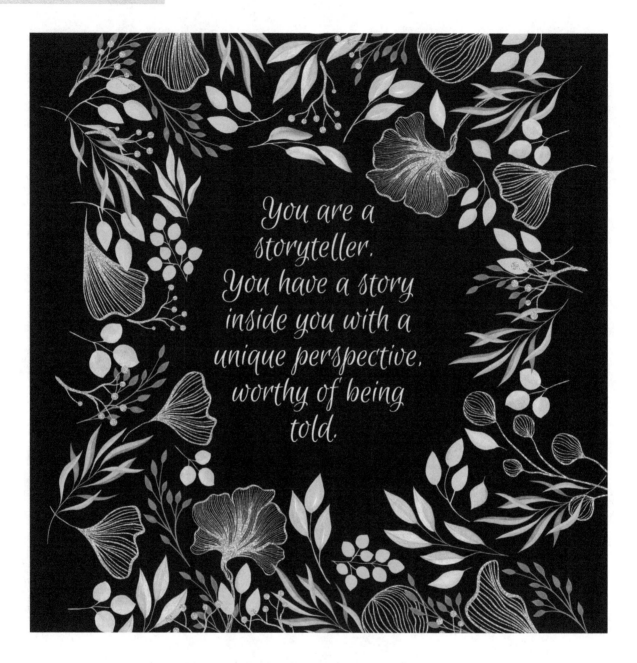

You are a storyteller. You have a story inside you with a unique perspective, worthy of being told.

Most everyone on the planet who has expressed what is inside them in language has been human. Many people discount what they have to say, share, discuss, or express because they don't feel worthy in some way. They may believe that their story isn't interesting or feel they don't have adequate skill or training to write or speak about what feels important.

This was me for a very long time. I felt nobody would care or listen to my words, thoughts, and ideas because I don't have a writing degree or a masters in a subject that I have life experience in. Imposter syndrome kept my words and thoughts hidden for a long time. I used to be terrified of being judged, of being called a fraud just for sharing perspective on my own life.

Though fear still sits under the surface, I try to comfort it each day and write anyway. Books and stories are made of words from the unique perspective of someone's life experiences. And everyone knows something a little different than everyone else, whether that is your outward life or inner imaginings.

You are qualified to tell your story because you are human. You have no idea who needs to hear your words or how it will impact others. It is only necessary to share what is true for you to leave something beautiful in this world.

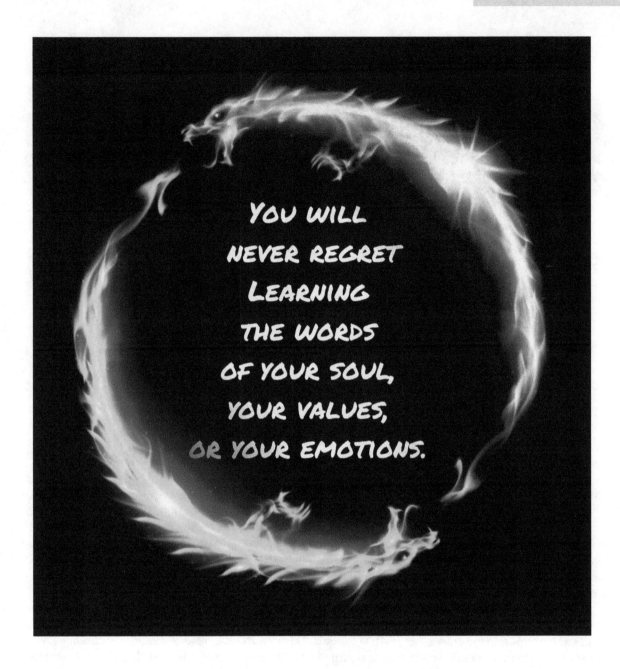

YOU WILL
NEVER REGRET
LEARNING
THE WORDS
OF YOUR SOUL,
YOUR VALUES,
OR YOUR EMOTIONS.

In past relationships, I didn't have the language to articulate the feelings that were SO big inside me, they would come out in repetitive words that ran around in circles and tripped over each other. This would feel so frustrating that I would end up just crying and not being able to explain myself. This would leave me feeling flaky, embarrassed, misunderstood, and unworthy of love in the moment.

It took many years, countless books, hundreds of difficult conversations, dozens of jobs, a few mentors, several personal development courses, meditation, and deep listening to my soul to learn what I value most, and the words that resonate with my hardest emotions.

In other words, it can be very challenging to describe exactly what we mean. However, there is not one day that I regret the time spent and the learning I experienced to be able to express more succinctly who I am and how I feel. It's an ongoing journey that has given me much confidence, consistency, peace, ease, and relief.

Authentic words of the heart can be very limited unless we begin with curiosity for a language that lands precisely in the shape of our feelings. It's a beautiful thing when that happens. It feels like word alchemy that transforms ambiguity into clarity.

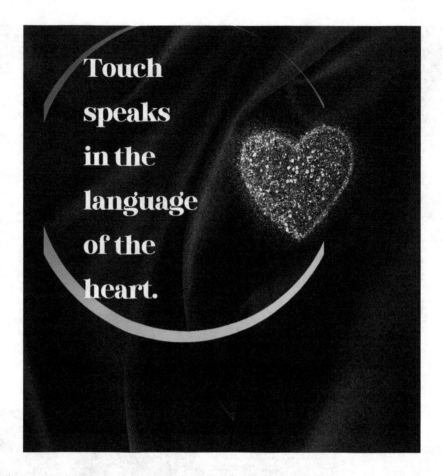

Touch speaks in the language of the heart.

Verbal language is usually outward facing when communicating with another.

Touch is an inner experience. You cannot give touch without also receiving it. In its basic form, touch is intuitive. Human nervous systems are wired for it, therefore crucial to our health and well-being.

Touch can feel comforting or invasive. It can bring up memories and stir emotions. In my work as an RMT, informed consent is extremely important and necessary for safety, nervous system regulation, and for intention to be known. Consent before touch builds trust in a therapeutic relationship, bodily autonomy is respected, and allows a starting point for healing in any capacity to begin.

There is an exact map of your entire body in your brain. The neural pathways that have been well worn use a larger space in the brain. This can help increase skill level, create habits, both healthy and destructive, and deepen thought patterns.

Emotions may be realized through the touch of any part of the body. Feelings may arise consciously or subconsciously in relation to certain areas. For example, I had one patient become tense and feel uncomfortable when I treated over a specific spot on her right shoulder. She was uncertain at first why this feeling came up, but after some time, she remembered it was an area that a condescending family member would put a hand when talking down to her, leaving her feeling judged and hurt.

Becoming aware of these feelings helped her start a new story about this spot, one related to care and ease of tension. This can lead to eventually carving a new neural pathway from that area and shrinking the area used in her brain for the triggered reaction.

Safe, nurturing touch is such a gift, it goes beyond verbality into a felt language that can be difficult to describe. Touch holds layered nuance that makes sense in the heart and soul, if not the rational mind. We have an ancient longing for touch built into our every cell.

One caring touch can change someone's whole world, wake up a heart, create a connection, bolster a sense of belonging, and make sense of emotions.

Everyone deserves a loving touch and to realize their full capacity for speaking from the heart.

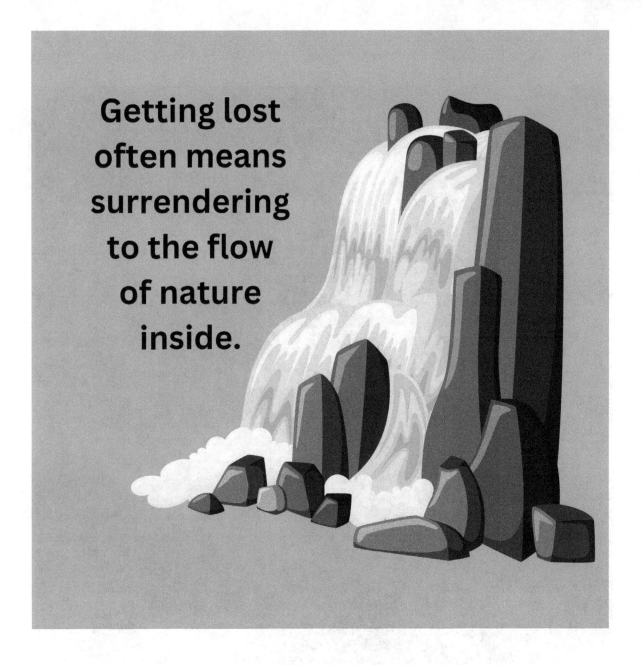

Getting lost often means surrendering to the flow of nature inside.

Performing in an energetic and fun show this week with amazing peeps has been a great way to get lost in the music and the flow of nature inside me. The moment is alive and becomes wondrous when I'm sitting right in it.

It's a beautiful way to let my soul flow through me and share it with others.

Being in nature, immersing myself in the sounds and smells of forest, dirt, and flowing water creates peace within me and connects me to the same feeling of wonder, groundedness, and presence.

Surrendering can feel scary, often when we are vulnerable to forces outside of us, however, when we surrender to what's inside soul-fully, surrendering feels like connection.

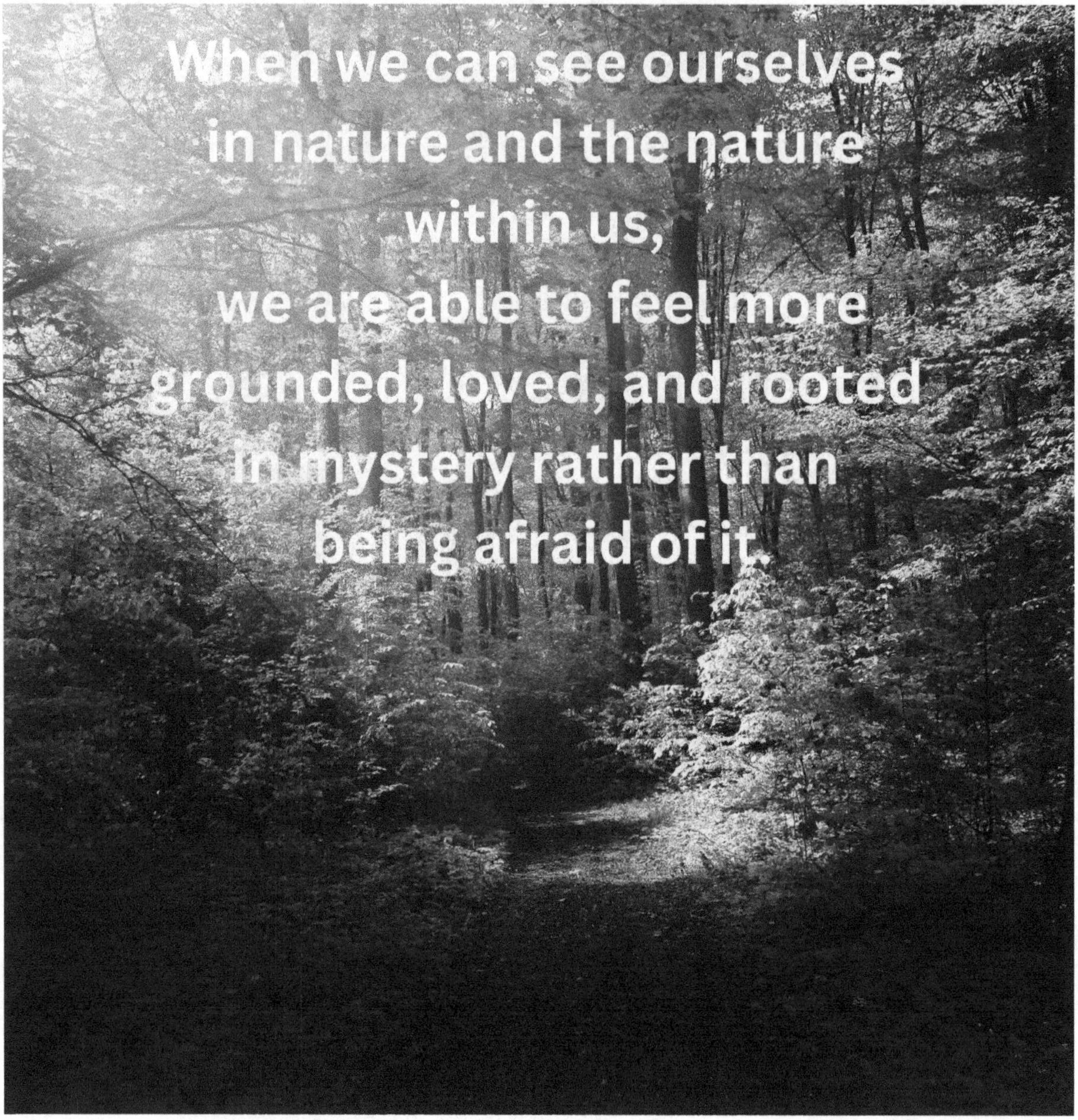

When we can see ourselves
in nature and the nature
within us,
we are able to feel more
grounded, loved, and rooted
in mystery rather than
being afraid of it.

Nature reminds us where we came from, reminds us of home.

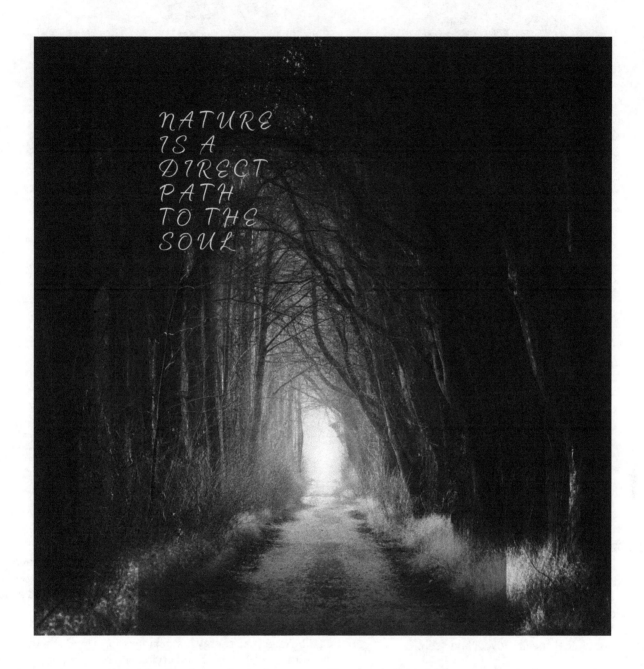

NATURE
IS A
DIRECT
PATH
TO THE
SOUL

We are drawn to pure authenticity. You know the feeling when someone is being truly themselves. They are magnetic. It makes you want to be near them and bask in the awe of their glow. It gives us a glimpse of who we want to be.

Trees, forests, bodies of water, waterfalls, mountains, and deserts all have powerful sturdiness, unwavering authenticity. We are made of the same bones and lifeblood. We have an innate trust in their connection to themselves and thus are drawn by their magnetism.

They remind us of who we are and who we can become, and urge us, dare us to be authentic. They speak to the nonphysical part of us that honors and loves our undiluted truth.

They are kin. Listen.

Other direct lines can be found when getting lost in creativity, connecting deeply with another human, or communing with animals. Getting lost often means surrendering to the flow of nature inside.

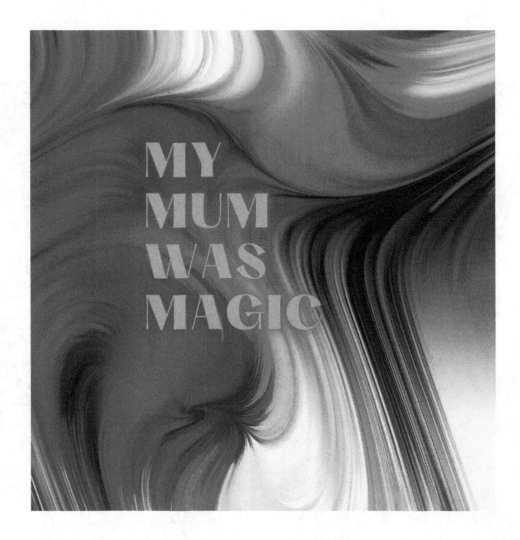

Today, we celebrate the life of my mama.

1941-2022

Mum had a beautiful way of looking straight into the hearts of others. She loved connecting quickly and deeply. Connection and quality time with loved ones were her dearest values and her love language. She wanted to make those she knew feel special, loved, and seen.

She was master of the long goodbye and had the warmest hugs. She was known for adopting new family members anytime she could. Her heart wouldn't stand for anyone being alone on holidays or special occasions. The only requirement to joining our family was a hug and a smile, and maybe the occasional afternoon of learning how to jive in the living room.

She had great empathy and could see when I was struggling with emotionally raw feelings, and like magic, was able to draw out the depth, meaning, and beauty of sitting with

my feelings and allowing me to explore in a safe space, and discover what my next step could be. It was a powerful gift that she shared with hundreds of people in her healing room. Helping those who worked with her to discover their truth, their power, and their ability to heal in the most tender ways was her passion, her mission, and was a wonder to witness.

I believe that energy just changes form, and she is still here with us all, laughing and crying and holding our hearts. She left a little magic along her path in life. Magic that touched so many. She has friends all over the world who were changed by her presence.

My gratitude and love go out to all who loved her and hold her in their hearts.

"Keep love in your hearts and share it exuberantly with everyone you meet, everyday. " - Joyce Graham

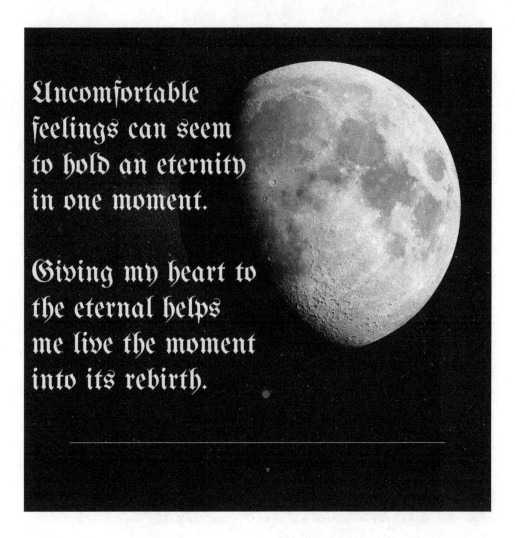

Uncomfortable feelings can seem to hold an eternity in one moment.

Giving my heart to the eternal helps me live the moment into its rebirth.

Just as the dark side of the moon lives in shadows, our difficult emotions often do as well. It can be excruciating to live in darkness. That's why the darkest nights always feel the longest. The hard emotions, when every sense is heightened or dampened, wanting to scream, feeling suffocated by feelings pressing down on the breath, unsure how to stop the suffering. When talking to others does not offer relief, feeling through the discomfort of each moment, trying to remember self-compassion, is the only way I have found to dissolve, surrender, and live into another moment of precious emotion.

I have been pressed by intense emotion and sensitivity for the last while. Struggling my way through feelings that seem 100 times stronger than I'm used to. Not different emotions, just much more powerful. So painful sometimes that it feels like I'm birthing myself into a new being. I have often thought of emotion as my superpower, though recently it can feel like an explosion of death and rebirth. One moment feeling like eternity, or weeks feeling like seconds.

How do we have the capacity to experience this cavernous depth, this indescribable awareness, this paradox of lightness and heaviness, of flow and stagnancy, power, and weakness, all in such a fleeting ray of sunshine or in the breath of wind upon your face or in the whisper of a dragonfly moving behind your ear.

I don't know if this intensity will remain with me for the rest of my days or if it will fade. They say everything shall pass. We'll see. Trusting the movement is difficult right now. And that's where I'll be, I guess, for now.

If you feel called to share your depth, awareness, or uncertainties, please do. I'd love to feel not alone in the wonders of seeking emotional understanding.

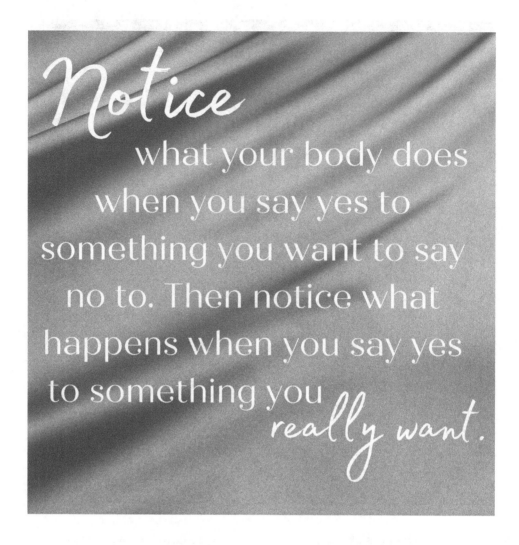

Notice what your body does when you say yes to something you want to say no to. Then notice what happens when you say yes to something you *really want.*

I recently needed to make a significant decision that, at least for a few years, would shift the trajectory of my life. I feel like I've become fairly practiced at tuning in to my body to discover the sensations of yes and no. I trust my intuition, and the body is a great barometer for decision-making.

This time, however, it was so subtle that it was difficult to discern which way I was leaning. So, I discussed, imagined, made pros and cons lists, and still was uncertain. I think it was unsettling because I could visualize going in either direction and making it work. In fact, I would love a life in which both were sustainable for me.

Ultimately, I had to choose. The moment I made a decision, my body instantly relaxed, and that was the first indication that I made the right choice for me. It was then that I realized I was following my joy instead of a deeply ingrained belief that I'm only good enough if I have certain things.

Tuning into the body isn't easy for everyone. Practicing

this is a fantastic tool and often another layer of wisdom. Sometimes, it's very evident what the right decision is. Other times, it's difficult to hear. Moving backward in the scenario can be helpful, and sometimes, we have to jump in before gaining insight from our choices.

I love what Glennon Doyle said on a recent podcast, "I don't want to love my body, I want to love WITH my body."

This is to say our body, mind, and spirit can't be separated. Living and loving with our whole selves lets us feel less alone instead of judging each part of us as a separate thing and connects us more with those we love. The "i" that notices my aliveness includes my body, mind, thoughts, sensations, longing, beliefs, emotions, and soul. Making decisions from my wholeness, conscious consensus from every part of me, feels right.

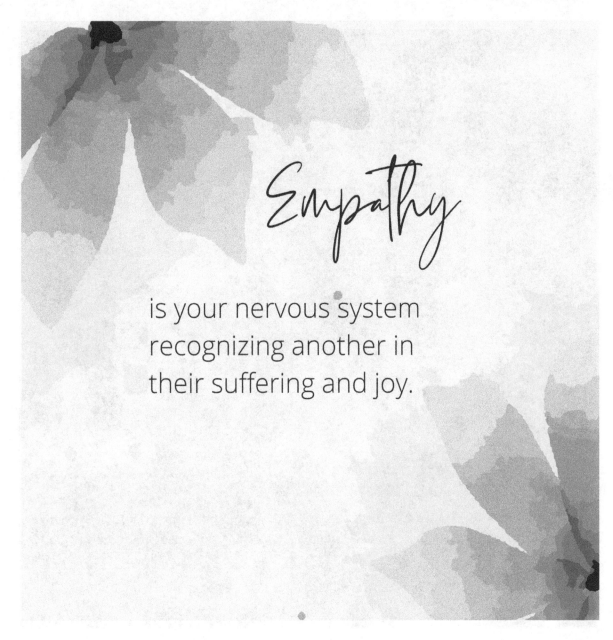

Empathy

is your nervous system
recognizing another in
their suffering and joy.

If you could see into people 's hearts and not be scared by what you recognize in yourself, would you look away so quickly?

If you knew that holding the awareness of their suffering or joy to reflect understanding back to them might change their experience of the moment, would you linger with them?

We rush away so often from situations that feel uncomfortable. What's is more uncomfortable than the feelings that arise when watching someone suffer?

Many people have the capacity for empathy, but do not know how to carry it.

Holding space for another is being able to sit with our own discomfort for short periods of time. We are able to expand our capacity for holding another's truth through practice, awareness, and curiosity.

Expansion can often start with self-empathy. We are taught to bypass and mistrust our own feelings for the sake of propriety, conformity, and productivity.

Emotions are not an easy fix and take time to muddle through. Having empathy and holding space for yourself and others can be an act of revolution and evolution. What is a more powerful gift than sharing dignity and understanding with another?

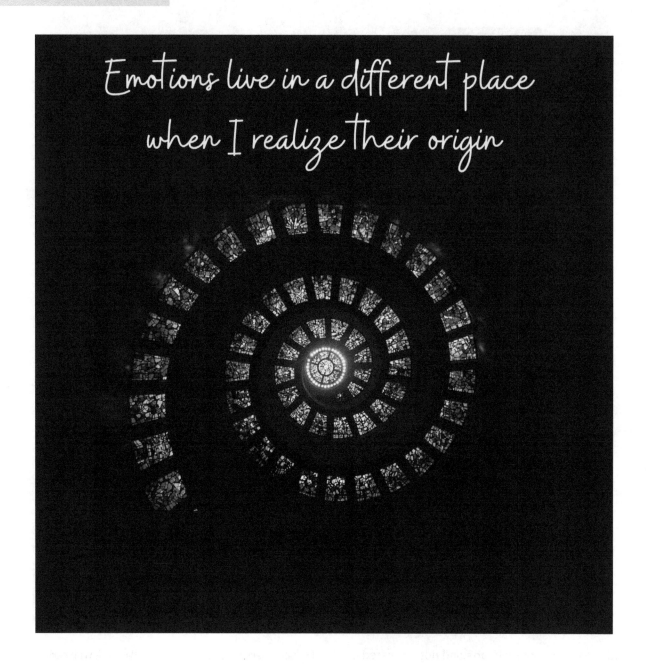

Emotions live in a different place
when I realize their origin

Every emotion I experience is rooted in some other moment. At my age, it's rare to have a feeling arise that I haven't felt before. So, when a familiar feeling comes, I recognize it like an old friend.

Sometimes, I will fully react in body and mind to the emotion, and sometimes, I can watch it as it arises. Other times, I have to muddle through it for a while before I realize I'm wallowing.

It is a powerful process to sit with an uncomfortable feeling and contemplate when I first felt it in my life (something I

learned from Dr. Gabor Maté). This helps me realize that what I'm reacting to could be more intense because it triggered the memory of a feeling in my body.

So, it's not only the present moment I'm being influenced by, but my entire history of feeling that feeling. Through this process, I'm learning how to be reflective instead of reactive. It helps me live in emotions differently. It adds a little grace to challenging moments, each time I am presented with the same feeling situations in the spiral of life.

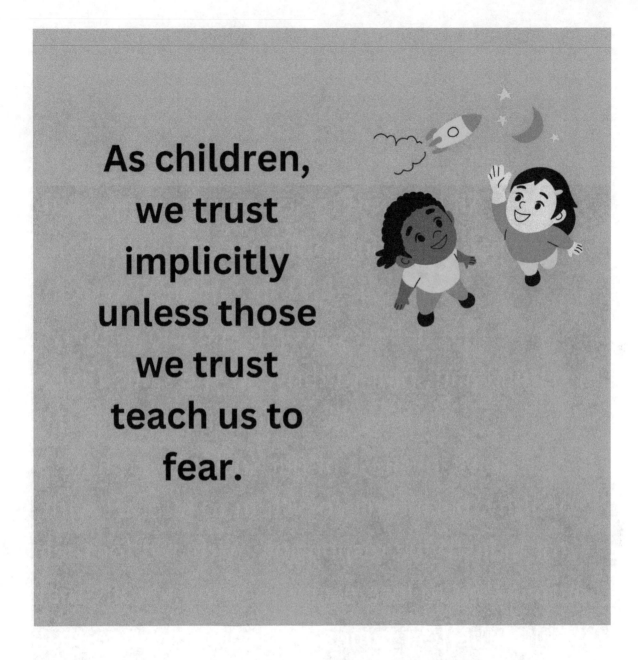

As children, we trust implicitly unless those we trust teach us to fear.

Compassion is the antidote to fear.

We are raised within systems that teach us to assimilate or fear being outcast. We are raised by people who are often indoctrinated in these systems much longer, and to find any who have not been touched by fear is rare.

I'm not talking about clean fear, such as reacting to an imminent threat, but fear that keeps us worried or regretful. The olders in our lives do their best, hopefully, to see through the guise of this pain and fear, but it isn't easy. Each generation may be able to move a little further into the consciousness that we create our own fear based on what we were taught to think and believe.

This is why connecting to our own deepest truths is so important. It can lead us to relief and understanding. Talking about this with others has revealed for me, that most of us have been living in the same dream of lack and unworthiness. Having compassion for ourselves and others as we slowly rise out of fear and into connection is a great gift. Lead the way.

All I want is to see parents supported properly in order to support their children, to be cared for in a medical system that believes people and allows body, mind and spirit to thrive at the same time, to have free education to raise the consciousness of our societies, to have a healthy, balanced ecosystem to interact with, for industry be responsible with and for their output, and to love each other so radically that it shifts the fear mindset to one of love so that we can nurture ourselves, our communities, and the diversity all over the planet. Too much?

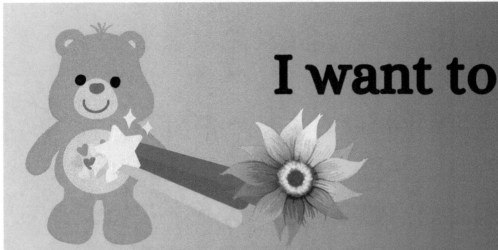

I want to

fix the world's problems with the fierce beams of love that come shooting out of my heart. Like a care bear, but in real life.

Throughout my work with others, I've been called a Soul Doula, Señorita Amor, Human Ativan, and some other fun things.

It took me a long time to realize the value in my softness, my compassion, and my unwillingness to back down from advocating. Love is a physical force and an emotional fierceness. Love literally changes dynamics and opens hearts, ears, and minds.

Like flowing water can shape rocks and contour the world around it, love has the same capacity. Ever transforming with gentle strength and softness.

Love is the s#@t.

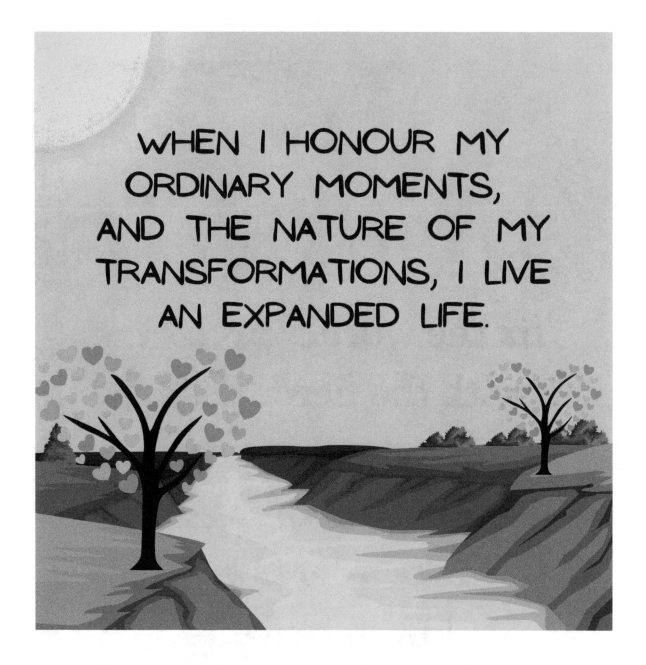

WHEN I HONOUR MY ORDINARY MOMENTS, AND THE NATURE OF MY TRANSFORMATIONS, I LIVE AN EXPANDED LIFE.

When I notice my actions, my thoughts, my feelings, I live into each new moment with the ability to reflect on the extraordinary of the ordinary. Awareness, for me, holds the magic that allows me to see the incremental changes within me that lead to transformation.

I can be changed in an instant by a hug or a smile, a sunrise, or a snowflake. When I reflect on the growth and connection of the last 2 months, I notice the small, ordinary moments that shifted my perspective.

One word, one shared look of recognition, one hand squeeze, one high five, one giggle, one lyric, one song, one bowl of soup, one by one, they add up to trust, to joy, to love, to opening the heart, to understanding myself more. I live into expansion moment by moment by simply noticing.

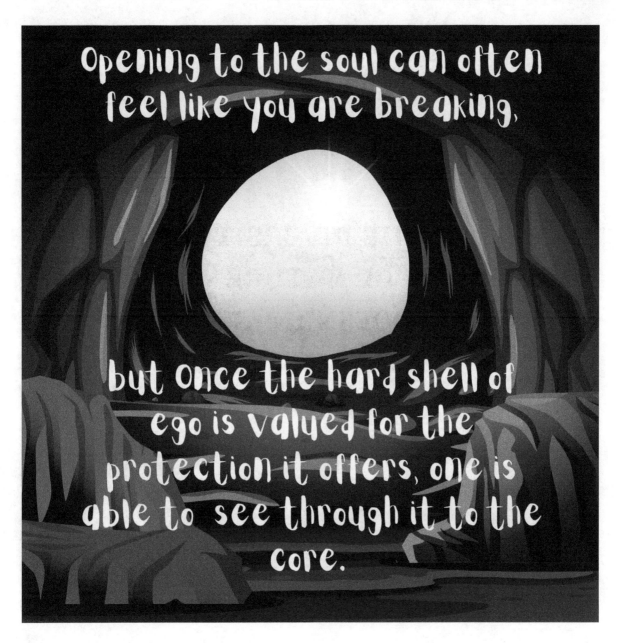

Opening to the soul can often feel like you are breaking, but once the hard shell of ego is valued for the protection it offers, one is able to see through it to the core.

Vulnerability arises in innumerable ways every day. It's a magical interaction between yourself and your deep inner world and between yourself and the outer world you are a part of and connect with moment by moment.

There is a spectrum of vulnerability, I find. What is high on the spectrum for me may be no big deal for someone else. Some days, getting out of bed or interacting with others can feel like too much. Performing on stage for some is an exciting kind of openness that combines a character with your own personality.

We all have capacity for different levels of vulnerability. Recognizing when to safely breach a comfort level varies by the moment and could possibly result in growth or understanding. It can be tricky to navigate the balance, or it can feel just fine to operate from one layer most of the time.

Our egos have an important job in trying to keep us safe from harm. I find it impossible to have zero ego as we grow and develop in an interdependent community, and it is a necessary protector. Acknowledging and accepting all our layers, I believe, gives us access to our unique synergy that creates the energy and flow from which we move in the world. I am grateful for my ego and for my vulnerable, loving heart. I live an expanded life when I love all parts of me.

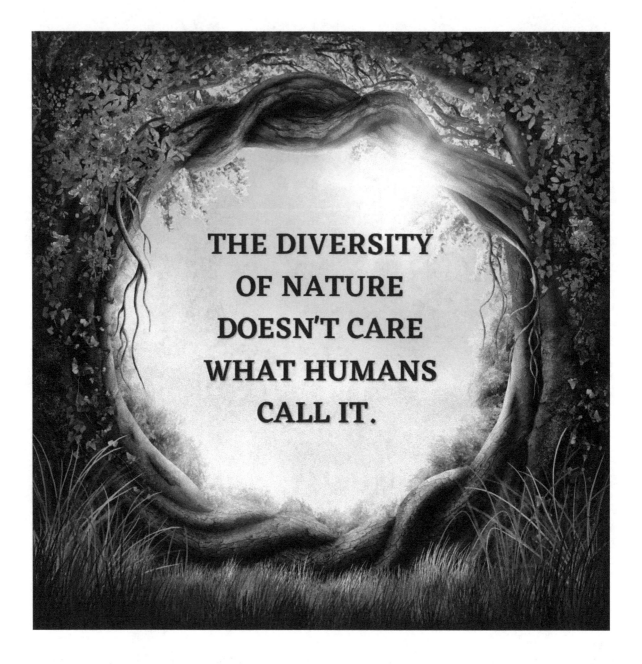

THE DIVERSITY OF NATURE DOESN'T CARE WHAT HUMANS CALL IT.

The human brain craves patterns in its environment in order to feel safe. This is one reason for naming and labeling everything. We see recognizable shapes in clouds, we have scientific names for every single thing on the planet, and we read people's faces everywhere we go.

In nature, the labels don't matter. A flowing river or a forest of trees would not have an opinion about or feel hurt if we called them by a different name or judged them in any way. They would go on being themselves, living in their nature, sharing their miraculous divinity with us.

Humans possess this ability as well. Our inner nature is the part of us that always feels connection and flow, doesn't care how others perceive us, and has no need for labels. It's where we experience awe and meaning. This part of us is called the soul (haha...see the irony in labeling that part of us?). It is what it is. We are in this together.

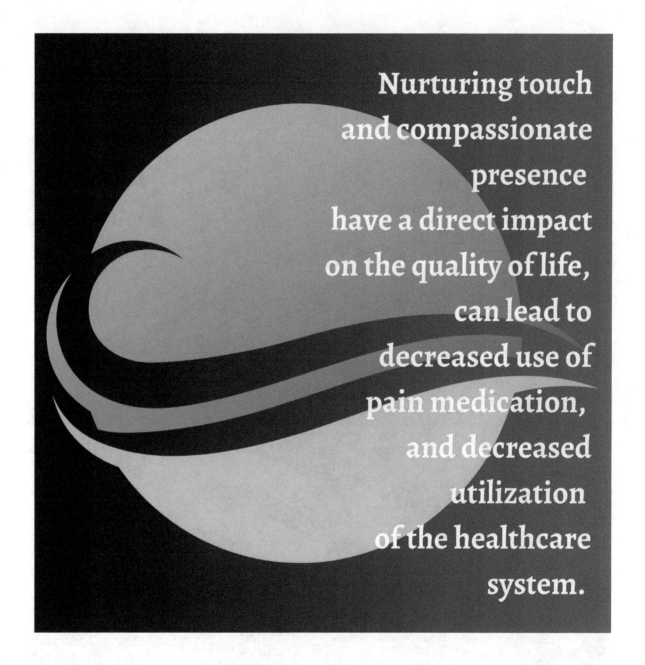

Nurturing touch and compassionate presence have a direct impact on the quality of life, can lead to decreased use of pain medication, and decreased utilization of the healthcare system.

Having just one person to connect with during a stressful time is calming and can regulate the nervous system. Adding compassionate touch can increase these effects.

A wide-reaching,
caring community network
for vulnerable seniors
is possible,
and worth
investing in.

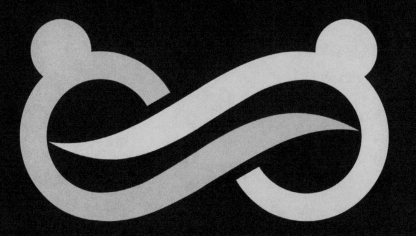

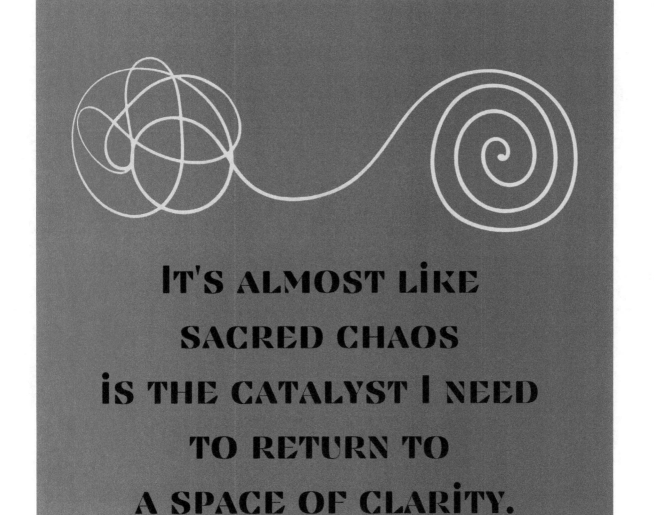

IT'S ALMOST LIKE
SACRED CHAOS
IS THE CATALYST I NEED
TO RETURN TO
A SPACE OF CLARITY.

Chaos lovingly reminds me to find my center despite the
storm around me.

Like a tree, welcome all creatures who rest and shelter under your strong branches, and those who find respite in your depth and wisdom.

Be a storyteller of your truth. You cannot know the impact
your life may have on others.

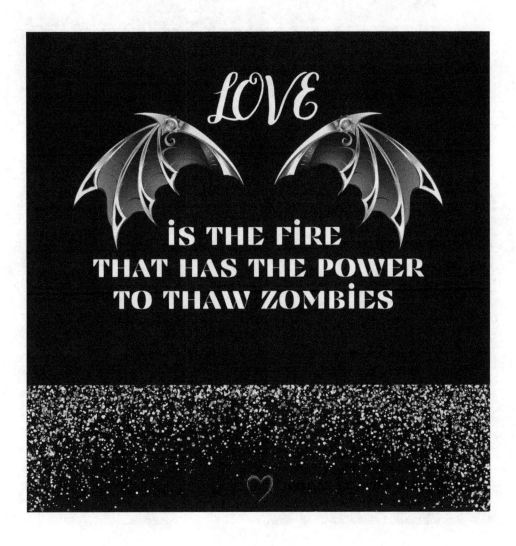

LOVE

IS THE FIRE
THAT HAS THE POWER
TO THAW ZOMBIES

Once upon a time, I was a zombie. I don't know if you've ever known one, or perhaps you were one also? I was shut down, disconnected, and was running on auto pilot. It was a combination of being deeply unsatisfied with my circumstances in life and trying not to know it.

The best thing in my life at the time was my young children, though my soul kept telling me I needed more in order to fill my cup and love my children from a place of wholeness, rather than relying on them for my happiness. I wanted to be an example of following my joy for them instead of teaching through my actions that they should remain small and settle for unhappiness.

It took an astute acquaintance, connection with a dear friend, an insightful book, and some belly dancing to help me shift my perspective and gently blow my spark back into flame. Even though I hadn't fully acknowledged it yet, the deep longing was calling me to realign with myself.

Receiving love from others helped me feel my worth. We're often told that we can't love others until we love ourselves. But we don't love in silos. We cannot do love alone. We are complex, multi-layered, interconnected, and interdependent beings that gain perspective by interaction and relationships. We live in perpetual context.

We are moved by feedback. We can do what we want with the opinion of others, but when someone gives you love wholeheartedly, it shatters the cold mirrors that hide our vulnerability, and the broken shards can finally reflect back to us what we've wanted all along. To feel alive, to feel seen, accepted, and loved. To thaw from the dead-inside feeling and realize we're allowed to be whole.

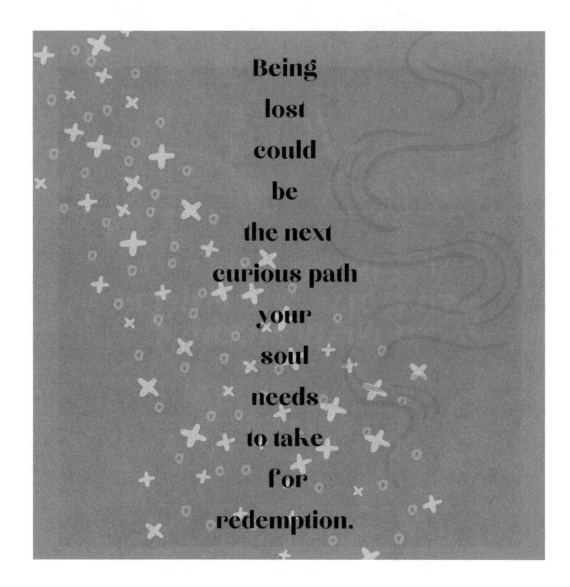

Being
lost
could
be
the next
curious path
your
soul
needs
to take
for
redemption.

Life seems to be a continuous cycle of feeling lost and then some clarity. Being scattered and then grounded. Being anxious and then calm and back to anxious. We are constantly moving and evolving, so of course, it feels like this.

Leaning into the discomfort of uncertainty has been a life struggle for me. I have often felt like I will self-combust if I can't figure something out, especially if it's important to my heart.

I'm very good at sitting with others in their pain and sorrow and confusion, suggesting they breathe into the discomfort. Being on the other side of this advice is oh so much harder. I had a friend recently revel at the chance to offer my words back to me.

The experience of being lost, however difficult, leaving bits of my heart crumbling outside of my body and leaking out of my eyes, is also delicious in a strange way. I can see my heart from different angles and notice things I hadn't before. I can choose how I want to scoop myself up and hold my pieces. It feels like a terrifying and worthwhile adventure to a new evolution of me. It can feel like redemption, but not the kind that saves you after life is over, but the kind that is accepting of all that is now. It is peace within the storm.

We are in a constant state of dying and rebirth, in every moment. It takes so much courage to remain aware through the ebb and flow. It's also ok if we don't. We possess different capacities at different times. I have so much love and respect for you who are in the space of feeling lost at this very moment. I see you.

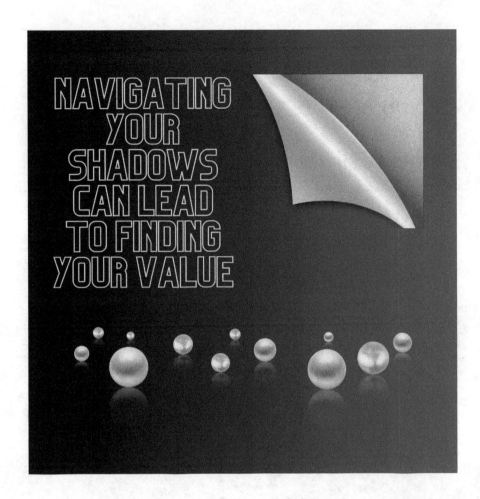

Peeling away layers that we have kept in the dark for so long can be one of the hardest things that humans do.

We hide these thoughts, beliefs, and desires for fear of judgment and fear of the pain it may cause to face them.

It was likely a protective reflex that made you subconsciously hide them away in the first place. Somehow, you got the message that these parts of yourself were not conducive to getting the love and acceptance your little you needed for belonging and safety.

But now my dear, is when your truth needs to be held in the light of the conscious mind and heart in order for you to feel belonging and safety. We can't feel fully accepted until we are fully seen.

Where do you start when navigating your shadows? Beginner baby steps.

1. You breathe...like actually breathe.

2. You look at parts of yourself that are hardest to face, just to observe. What makes it difficult to look at? Is it because you feel shame surrounding the subject? Has it been too well hidden? Is it confusing? Does it feel complicated and time-consuming? Observing your thoughts, feelings, and beliefs about this one part of you is one way to inch it toward a dim light; light that hopefully doesn't scare it too much and send it fleeing back into the depths.

3. You taste, but in tiny little bites. Too much too fast can be overwhelming. Opening your thoughts and feelings to it for a short time, WHEN you have the time. If you don't have time, and it comes up, try acknowledging its presence and promise to return soon.

4. You open your heart and mind at the same time. That is, if you're going to be thinking about it, you need to have the presence of your heart also. This helps to bring compassion to the process.

This is not to say that you mustn't just feel sometimes. Being immersed in wordless emotion can be super helpful and cathartic. (It's just hard to turn off the brain sometimes)

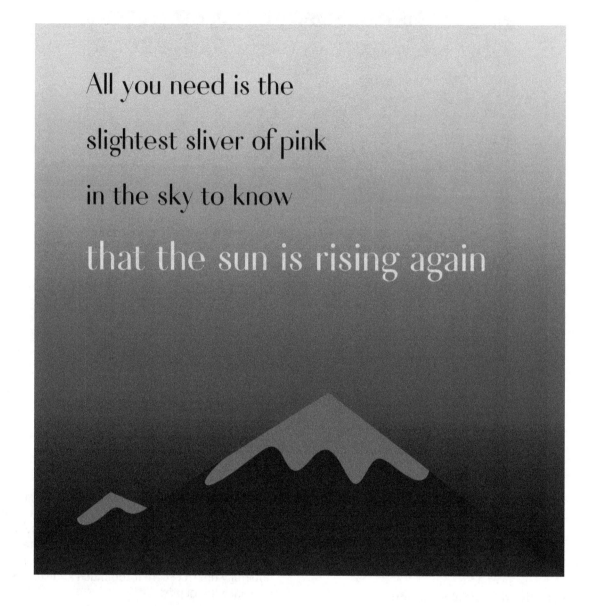

All you need is the
slightest sliver of pink
in the sky to know
that the sun is rising again

Opening to your truest self feels like a sunrise. There is just the tiniest touch of lightness in a small part of the sky at first. Then, a sliver of colour, be it pink or gold, that begins to show itself. The colour expands slowly, at its own natural pace. The sky above you begins to brighten, and more of what surrounds you becomes visible, illuminated, the light seeming to come from inside the earth.

As the light grows, it touches you, changes you, fills you with a sense of awe and wonder. Soon, spectacular colours of all shades are bursting overhead and all around you. It is wondrous and beautiful to behold. And then the brightest light in our solar system peeks over the horizon, and life changes as we know it. The light touches everything in our frame of view.

It's a miracle to me that it keeps happening, and I get to witness it so often! It's like a breath of fresh air. I feel the same awe and privilege when I witness my own or another's expansion into understanding more of what's inside. There will always be shadows in different places, based on where the light is being directed. They are there to discover or explore or just sit with whenever we are able to adjust our eyes for a while.

If you've seen that glimpse of pink in the sky once, you know what happens the next time you see it. All it takes to know your growth is that inkling of your soul, the slightest glimpse of your truth. Opening comes like a breath of fresh air when you've witnessed it just one time. The journey to yourself begins with one sliver of light from within.

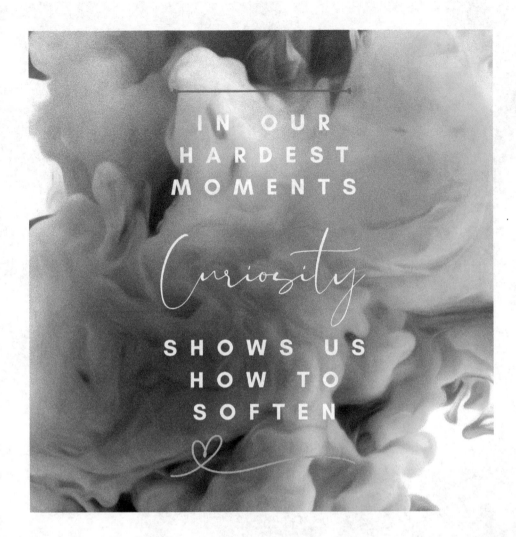

IN OUR
HARDEST
MOMENTS

Curiosity

SHOWS US
HOW TO
SOFTEN

Becoming curious helps us see past fear and to look through the eyes of compassion. This matters because when we are activated by fear, the rational brain is impaired and can be difficult to calm once it takes hold.

It can be a challenge to remember to get curious when we feel scared, so I like to make it a habit to ask myself all kinds of questions during every state of mind and heart, and in this way it's just something I do often.

In her books, Byron Katie suggests we ask ourselves when we are suffering from a particular thought, "Is this true, can I be sure that this is true?" So much of our emotional suffering, as well as excitement, comes from thoughts that we perceive as negative or positive, bad for us or good for us.

Think of one of your consistent thoughts that make you feel sad or worried or mad. Now, look around at where you are and realize that in this very moment, you are safe and reading a post on social media. You are being supported

by the surface you're sitting or standing or laying on. So right in this moment, ask yourself if how you feel reflects what is happening now, or if it's a projection based on what happened previously or what MIGHT happen in the future.

Even during dire circumstances, such as being by my mum's side in palliative care, when I got curious about my thoughts, feelings, and my mama's life, strangely, I became more present. I could hold her hand and feel the softness of her skin, feel the strength still in them, and notice the scent of her that had been present throughout my life. These were precious moments that I may not have noticed if I was crumbling in fear and worry.

It's not a perfect antidote to feeling fear, of course. Nothing ever is. Fear is a useful emotion. But constantly living in the past or future isn't helpful and can make us miss the precious moments that we live for. Letting curiosity drive some of our minutes, hours, and days can move us right out of the grips of suffering and into wonder, love, and compassion.

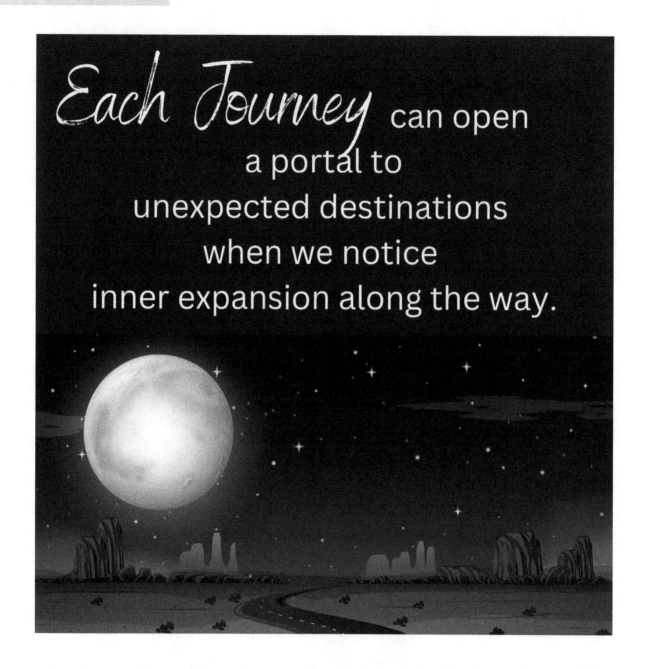

Each Journey can open
a portal to
unexpected destinations
when we notice
inner expansion along the way.

Paying attention to the expanding desires inside me constantly leads me to surprising insights and outcomes. One path forks into many and learning how to connect each path feels like pure joy and creation. One idea builds a foundation for the next.

I have experienced this state of flow in unexpected moments. In conversation with others, when energy expands, and synchronicity explodes. When singing with my cast, and we hit that perfect state of oneness within a song and feel complete bliss. When writing a succinctly beautiful sentence. When learning a new concept and having it so deeply resonate that it brings unexpected tears.

I love the feeling of expansion so much that I look for opportunities to experience it. This is also supported by my love of continuous learning. Trusting the language of my soul is the best way to find the fun, lean into learning, and follow the joy.

It's terrifying to imagine shrinking back into a life of stagnancy and smallness that feels cut off from the nourishment of expansion. Remaining open is vulnerable and sometimes scary, but oh, so much more life-giving, heart-filling, and soul aligning. The juiciest paths are lined with stars and made of unknown mysteries within, waiting to be discovered.

Our capacity for holding space expands through practice, awareness, and curiosity.

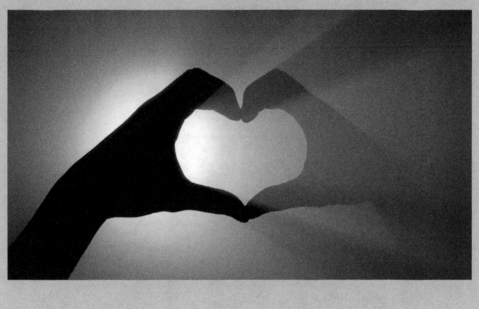

Our nervous systems love to be in familiar surroundings in order to feel safe. This doesn't mean that we can't go out and experience new things and different places. We need to attune our bodies and acclimate to what might feel experimental.

Just like slowly building muscle, we can push our comfort levels a little bit at a time, taking breaks when it feels too much, and trying again when we feel renewed.

Humans have different proclivity for being in the presence of suffering. I commend those who work every day, saving lives, being there in people's most vulnerable moments, or while they take their last breath.

Empathy often arises when spending time with those who are dying. When I started treating people in hospice, I was asked how I could handle it. Besides holding dignity in high regard, supporting those at the end of life is tempered in moments of discomfort and sadness, grace and compassion, and genuine interest in the human I have the privilege of serving.

Building capacity takes patience. Like building muscle, it doesn't happen all at once. Holding space for the truth of others is a gift that allows them to feel seen and heard and valued. This can be shared both in our personal and professional lives. It can be personally challenging, which can offer great expansion of our hearts and nervous systems by means of holding space for our own emotions and discomfort. Self-discovery, self-compassion, and consoling conversation with friends help to repair our hearts when rest is needed.

Providing nurturing touch to the elderly and the dying offers deep relief psychologically and emotionally,

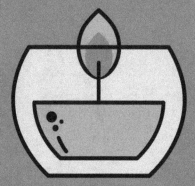

shows them they are important and reaffirms that they still belong.

As a Registered Massage Therapist, this is what I do. I've seen the profound impact of nurturing touch. You don't have to be a massage therapist to provide this, however. Anyone can hold loving intention while offering a safe touch with consent.

So many who have lost significant partners rarely feel the warmth of someone holding their hand and may not even realize how deeply they crave it until someone does exactly that.

Sometimes, it makes all the difference in helping another feel seen, valued, and calm. Our nervous systems all react to how others treat us, notice us, or ignore us. Being a source of compassion and touch is a healing thing, whether someone is dying or just wanting to live more fully.

Healing

takes place on many levels, and rises from a biopsychosocial aspect, which is a combination of biological, psychological, social, economic, educational, historical factors and belief systems, among other things.

If you've never heard of this before, it is just a fancy way to say that all of our life experiences contribute to our perspective on everything, including illness and healing. While wading through what we believe to be true, it's so helpful to examine these different layers and clear out bias, upbringing, and societal expectations. Paring down to bare bones frees us to fill our hearts with conscious beliefs, values, and actions. This is part of discovering how to align with our truest selves.

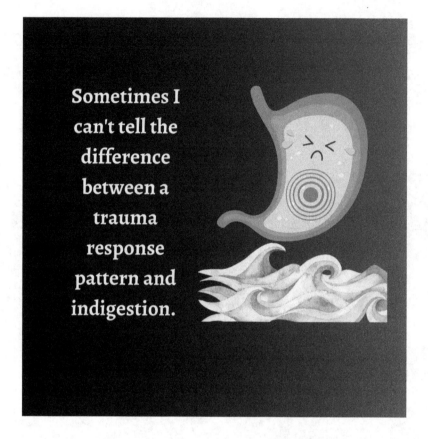

Sometimes I can't tell the difference between a trauma response pattern and indigestion.

Unusual topic today.

I'm trying to figure out my body's signals. It can be hard to discern the difference, sometimes, between feeling anxious because of past trauma patterns, and my body compass feeling I'm straying away from the integrity of my soul (such as physical symptoms sparking the slow burn of fear). And sometimes I wonder if I'm just having indigestion. All 3 options are a possibility. Yesterday, I ate a couple of handfuls of expired peanuts. A friend recently had a heart attack. And I'm going away, which has its own issues.

It's worrisome when physical symptoms begin simultaneously with anxiety. I'll be traveling soon, and my history has been to manifest some illness to stop me from leaving. This pattern came about, I believe, from a time in my childhood when belongings or people that I loved had disappeared by the time I got back home. This happened for several reasons, one being a repossessed storage unit where the lack of payment prompted the auctioning of our precious things while we were away. This is devastating to a child. We moved A LOT during my formative years, and I think this also contributed to a deeply ingrained fear of leaving a place in case what I loved was gone when I returned.

I've noticed this tendency has greatly diminished over

the years. I no longer become sick. However, I do notice flutters in my belly and occasional heart palpitations. I find it interesting that anxiety can feel like a heart attack. An aching heart can affect the entire body's nervous system, causing physical pain and suffering.

The trouble is that not listening to the directions of my soul can create the same symptoms. Fear can cause anxiety. As can a disruption in the gut.

So how to tell the difference?

I haven't found a quick solution. I don't know if there is one. I do know there are rarely instant fixes to these sorts of things (besides antacid). Time is relative, and the soul will not shrink to fit into human constructs.

Hopefully, this feeling will teach me something, or move along soon... or both.

I'm hoping to gain insight through it all.

In the meantime, I will practice breathing, listening, and trying to eat smarter.

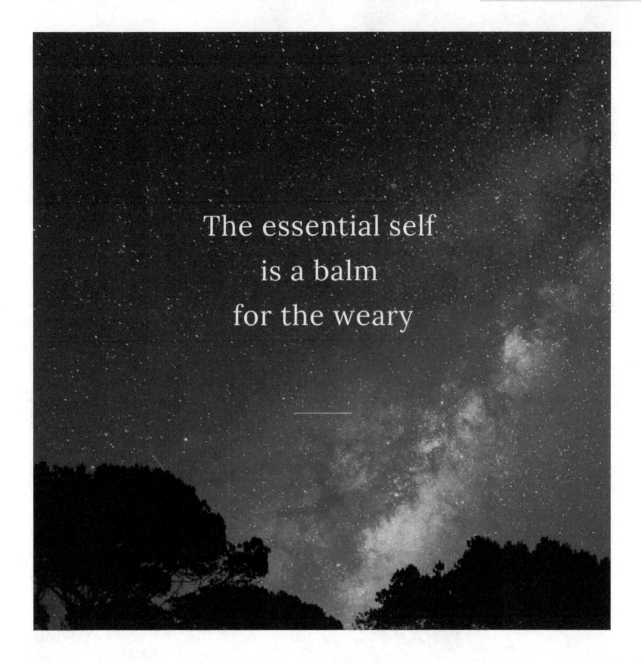

The essential self
is a balm
for the weary

Our essential being, our spirit, soul, and deepest wisdom is always turned on, flowing, like a river that permeates the world, the universe, giving its endless energy to us. For many, it can be a struggle to hear this part of ourselves, as we get wrapped up in our daily grind and hustle. If we become quiet and notice its existence inside us and all around, for a few moments throughout our day, awareness washes over us again.

It is a lively, energetic place to create from and a soothing place to rest and rejuvenate. It knows you to your core, sees your fears and excitement, it understands you in your truest form, and in your most confused moments. It loves and holds you through all the bumps, learning curves, and through your seeking for wholeness and belonging.

The connection is always available to us. Jumping into the flow is an ever-expanding option. We are infinitely whole and belong indefinitely. We have been conditioned to not believe in our own vastness or trust our deep wisdom. But once we peel away the layers of acculturation, we can't close the curtains completely to the awareness bubbling under the surface.

Feeling this connection is the only way to get through some days. When doubt and exhaustion take hold, I feel held in safety and reassurance and accept that life has big waves that overflow and recede. There is a difference between being weary from traveling down the path of hard truths and the exhaustion of inauthenticity. I much prefer the one that feels aligned with my spirit.

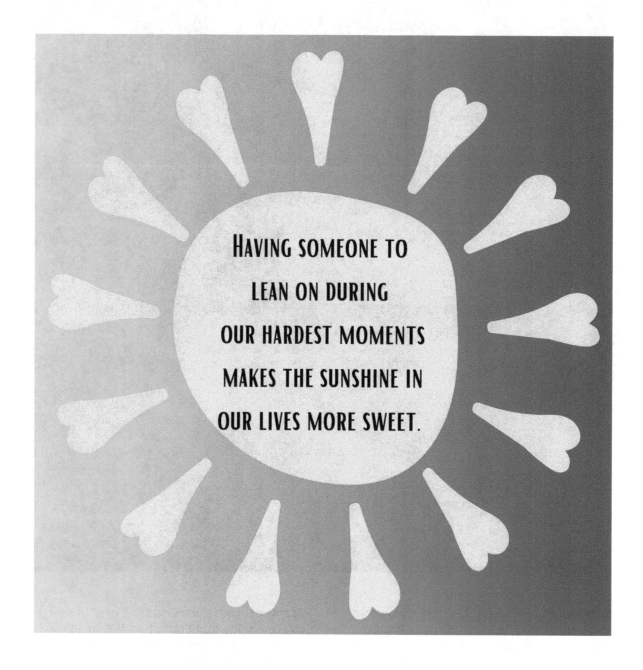

HAVING SOMEONE TO
LEAN ON DURING
OUR HARDEST MOMENTS
MAKES THE SUNSHINE IN
OUR LIVES MORE SWEET.

It's an honor to be able to offer softness in people's hard moments and be a reason for someone to smile and feel lightness in their heart.

I am thankful for countless moments and humans that provided a loving cocoon for me to accept and repair my body, heart, and spirit. Each time has helped me feel the sunshine on my face with more significance and gratitude and made me aware of the innumerable angels there are on earth.

I hope this kind of love opens hearts and spreads compassion all over the world more and more every day. I'm feeling grateful today that I'm able to share this with a dear friend right now.

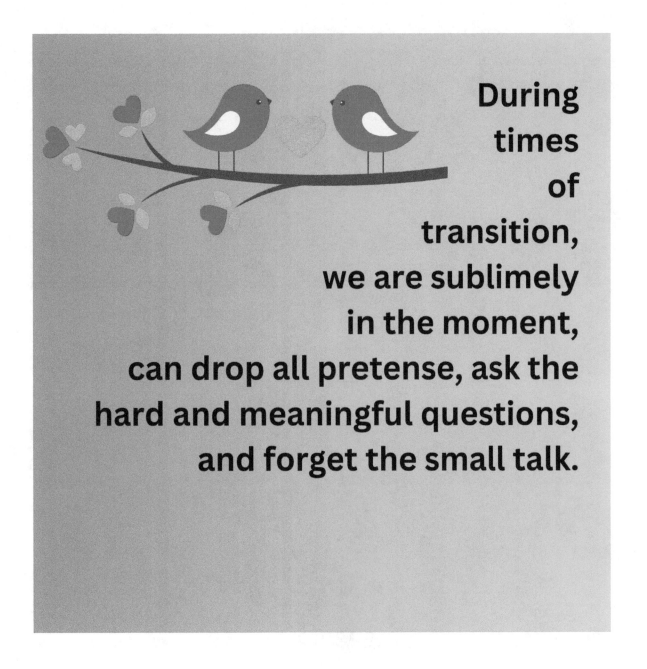

During times of transition, we are sublimely in the moment, can drop all pretense, ask the hard and meaningful questions, and forget the small talk.

During times of change, heartbreak, or newness, though they can be unsettling, we are often able to see through old patterns, and our perspective can be shifted as much as our circumstances. We drop the need to placate, let ourselves feel righteous anger, grief, relief, and in brief moments, morph into a truer version of who we are.

We can shake off the dust and debris of a former iteration and dream of who we want to be next. Somehow, when we lose our footing, it helps reinforce our soulful roots and see paths in front of us that hadn't been touched by light before. There is magic in the transition that can lead to transformation. This is alchemy of the soul.

Spaciousness

and

stillness

feel more like home as we lean into expansion

Heart-fully/ thoughtfully easing into the day allows the space for my heart and mind and body to hear each other and focus on the same stream. Expansion is a gift of that alignment, whether that means rest or action. Intention gathers consciousness, stillness deepens it.

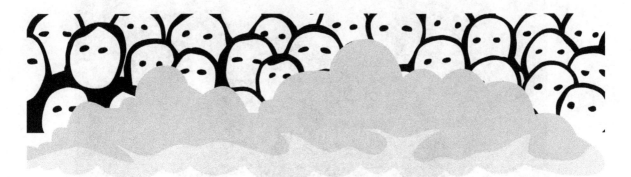

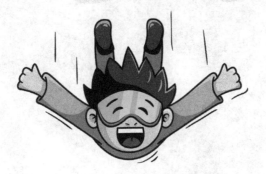

Like an elimination diet but for people

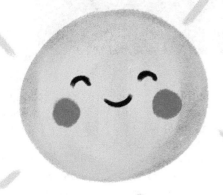

We don't always get to decide who surrounds us when we're out in the world, but we do have a choice when we're not at work or some form of it. Obviously, there are exceptions, but what I'm getting at is that we don't have to fall into false expectations and can keep our own joy in mind when tempted to move toward something that doesn't fill us.

Getting to know who you really want to spend your energy on can be like an elimination diet. During the covid shutdown, I didn't see anyone except for my partner and children. Then, slowly adding others back into the mix, I was able to feel into whether my body said yes or no to how I felt in their presence, or even just when thinking about them.

In this way I was able to add value more consistently to my life in terms of fulfilling relationships and leave out the ones that didn't feel right to me.

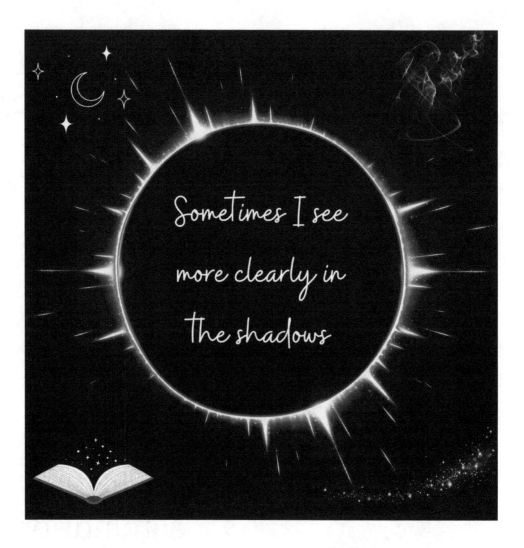

Sometimes I see more clearly in the shadows

t's interesting what happens when we let our eyes adjust to the darkness. There are beautiful things that live just out of the gaze of direct light. Moments when you still remember your dream in the space between asleep and awake, the sweet feeling when you make a decision but haven't told anyone yet, the ecstasy of longing before you confess your feelings, the knowing glance of safety with a loved one, the squeeze of a hand that nobody else can see, the agonizing love you have for your child.

Also in the shadows are our layers. The thoughts and emotions just under the surface, the deeper parts that others don't always have access to but for a trusted few, and darker spaces that we don't often open a portal for. Then, there is the deepest river of soul, connected to oneness, always flowing, always living inside, always there to align with. This river supports us even when we aren't aware of it. It shows us subtle direction to our truest self when we tune in. Although, it can also get very loud if we haven't been able to pick up the signals.

The eclipse this week has been very potent. It could be dragging past events and lessons up to the surface again. This doesn't mean you must experience them all over again. It may be enough to acknowledge them and let them float on by, like watching a movie. If dramatic things resurface, we don't have to engage, but understanding them from a higher perspective could help release them.

This week has also brought lightness and joy to many, finally being able to shake off feelings and situations that no longer serve us on our path.

Humans have the capacity for such beauty and loving power. We can shift our awareness from sunshine to shadow and from darkness back to lightness whenever we decide to. We can lead with our bodies, our minds, our hearts, our souls, or our entire wholeness. It doesn't matter which, all we need to do is adjust our eyes.

You are not at the
edge of the river,
waiting for
inspiration
in order to jump in.
You are the river,
the flow is always
inside you.
Ease into
your nature
to feel it.

While I was sitting outside yesterday, listening to a podcast, I felt in a calm state of flow, afternoon sunshine glowing on my face, content kitty laying in the grass, both of us enjoying this relaxing moment.

The cutest little fuzzy bumblebee circled my head and landed on the ground beside me. It sat there, trusting its nature, and began cleaning or preening itself. It reminded me of a cat when it repeatedly licks a paw and moves it over their head or eyes or ears. The tiny bee's knees stroking the fuzzy jet and golden plumose.

It felt like a moment of trust and connection between three souls and within each of us. Humans can learn so much by emulating creatures and allowing rest and communion to be present in our daily lives. I'm grateful for this moment. It reminds me to trust. Clarity comes after the tumult, every blessed time.

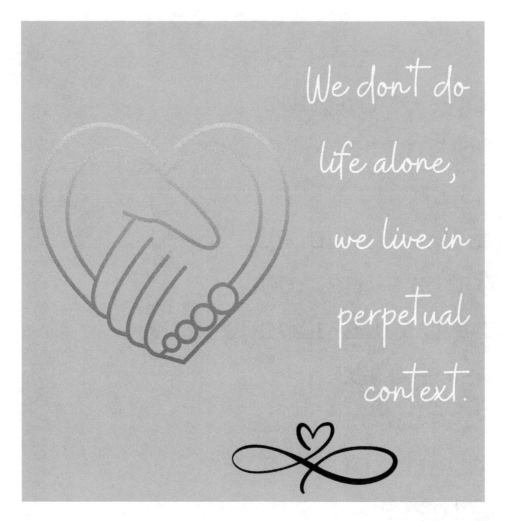

We don't do life alone, we live in perpetual context.

Humans are born from relationship and into relationship. Our species cannot survive without care both within the womb and once in the outside environment. Our bodies and nervous systems require touch and nurturing in order to survive, grow, and lay down neural pathways that promote healthy development.

As infants, we search for loving faces to know if we're safe. As we grow, we mirror and respond to others to learn about who we are. We learn how to talk to those surrounding us based on the family dynamic we were presented with. These turn into beliefs. We adopt the lens we look through very early in our lives, and unless we question it at some point, we continue to carry these perspectives with us everywhere we go.

Our belief systems can bring us joy and show us beauty. They can cause suffering and grief. And often, a bit of both. It's how we are built. We experience the world around us from the context of our relationships and seek out those we resonate with. We also have our own inner nature and deep wisdom. Sometimes, when we explore the depths, we find our upbringing in alignment with us at a soul level, and sometimes, the two are way off.

Then, we can begin a process of soul searching and discovery. The vibration of alignment feels like ease and relief to me, even if the context is a challenging situation. The tension of a small gap between where I am and where I want to be, can be juicy and full of energy, pregnant with potential. A large gap can feel excruciating. Separation from oneself is painful.

Relationship is what has always brought me back from the painful beliefs holding me away from myself. I look for the compassionate faces to mirror when I need more softness and encouraging faces when I want to feel empowered. I look away from the faces of hate and unwarranted judgment.

We can't control the context into which we were born, but we get to decide who's faces have influence in our lives now.

It is empowering to feel the safety of others holding space for us to explore our truths.

It always amazes me when an incredible group of humans come together to support one another in the most authentic and heartfelt way. It hasn't always been easy to find, though it is the kind of space I love to be in.

Since the first time I experienced this level of support and intentional exploration, I have been continuously trying to cultivate more of it in my life. These conversations may be with one person or an entire group, though they hold a thread of honesty and unconditional love that helps me feel safe and seen and challenged in the best ways. They share with me a loving mirror, an open mind,

an inquisitive, and curious heart.

I discovered again yesterday that I love to be this for others so much, in a cohort of incredible folks coming together to practice this. Of course, I'm not exactly what everyone needs, but I am focused presence, and sometimes, that makes the difference in someone's day.

I continue to learn to support others and be supported by calling in community and being authentic as I'm able. In this endeavor, in living my truth, I hope to allow others to do so as well.

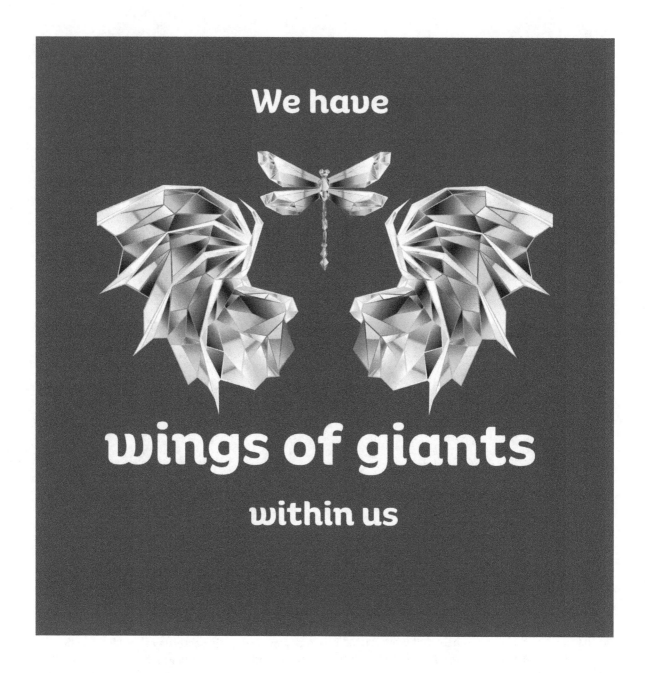

We have

wings of giants

within us

We are the seeds, the seedlings, the mighty protectors, and the fallen, standing in community together.

We are the egg, the playful infant, the adventuring adolescent, the fierce and nurturing mama dragon, and the wise old dragon all at the same time.

We are the imperfect learner, the seeker, the guide, the connected creative, the mover and shaker, the medicine elder, the precocious lover, the confused and the confident, and the death-bed wisdom sharer in one lone breath.

You are this, and so much more.

Can you feel it?

CW: talk of birth control and reproductive health.

There are some incredible healthcare providers for whom I'm incredibly grateful. Human service comes with variability of quality, which means patient treatment can depend on personal and professional bias, belief systems, and a plethora of other subjective factors. Even though doctors take an oath to do no harm to their patients, harm constitutes many different things for different people. It is subjective. The only way to know for sure if you've caused harm is to humbly ask the person in question how they feel about the specific situation.

I always find it best practice to try to find a caregiver that fits with who you are and what you need, if at all possible. A person whose presence you feel safe to be honest with. I know this seems next to impossible in some situations. There are as many different treatments as there are massage therapists, physiotherapists, or other allied healthcare professionals. This goes for physicians as well. It can be a rare find to encounter the perfect fit. That doesn't mean, however, that we have to accept poor treatment or worse.

As I move through accepting and healing of my shadows, I recalled a specific year I was unfortunate enough to have two doctors, a few months apart, who were less than compassionate. I was 19 years old and went for a full check up with the man who had been my mum's doctor for decades. He was patriarchal and opinionated, constantly sharing his views with his captive audience. He even had the audacity to show up at our house several times to try to convert my parents to his religion.

The expansive doctor's office had 3 floors, and the waiting room looked like a combination of a museum and a sanitarium, filled with black built-in oval shaped, padded, high-backed couches and tall circular magazine racks in the middle of each round of seats, and fake marble covering the walls. It seems an appropriate metaphor for the medical treatment I received there; archaic and controlling. During my appointment, I was going to ask about birth control until he decided to preach abstinence to me based on his own religious beliefs, not bothering to ask about my thoughts on the matter, regarding my own body. I was shocked into silence, didn't challenge him as I would have now, and felt disappointed in myself for not calling him out. I just never saw him again.

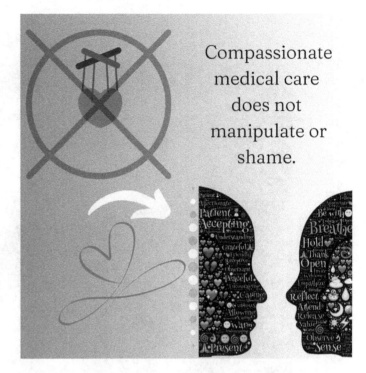

Compassionate medical care does not manipulate or shame.

A second doctor a few months later was disrespectful enough to laugh in my face when I asked for a pregnancy test, calling me stupid for not being on the pill. I remember just crying, felt attacked, unable to explain that the last doctor I saw didn't believe in birth control, and he was the very next doctor I had to subject myself to. He gave me a prescription and I never saw him again either.

I don't know why they felt compelled to mistreat their patients, but I do know they caused much more harm than any short-lived accidental physical injury. These incidents and beliefs were burned into my psyche for 30 years, whispering doubts of my intelligence, ability to make decisions, and my morality. This kind of long-lasting harm has been caused forever in the history of people, I'm sure.

Self aware and compassionate doctors and healthcare providers are what you deserve, what everyone deserves. You have agency to decide who you trust to care for your wellbeing. A shift from ignorance to compassion throughout all systems would be a dream, but it is especially needed in our healthcare and education systems.

Human-centered care creates compassionate care.

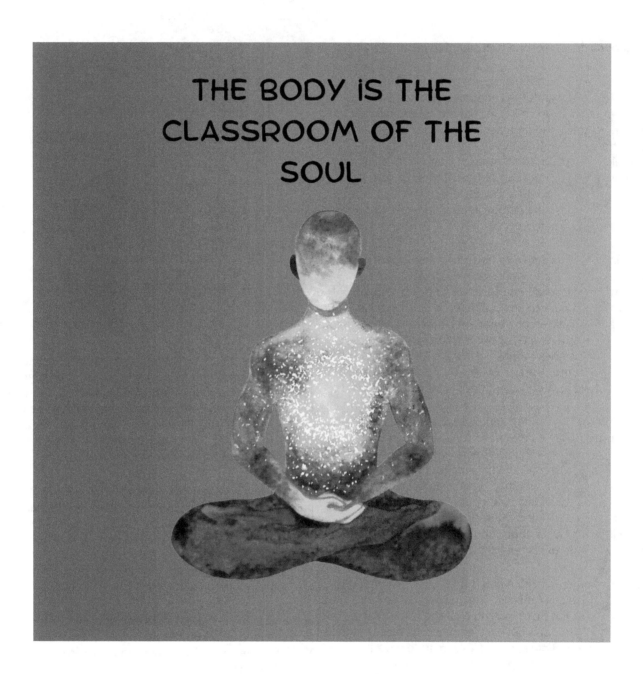

THE BODY IS THE
CLASSROOM OF THE
SOUL

It's humbling to witness the body moving through emotions
and sensations, in the process of healing, releasing,
remembering, and returning to stillness. It's a gift to hold
space for another's pain, fear, hope, and love.

Full circle moments and closing loops feel good, even if
they're also hard.

Since we will all eventually face the end of our lives, why aren't we better at providing the best quality of life to those going through it now?

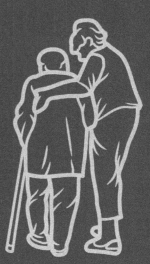

Is this the best we can do?

I believe our communities and societies have the capacity for a much greater quality of care.

How we evolve

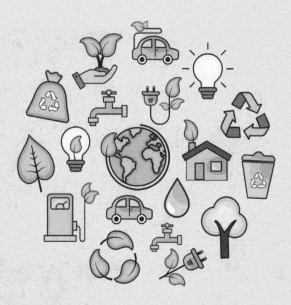

depends on our environment,
what we aim to learn,
our consciousness,
and how we choose to act.

There is so much that humans don't know about the evolution of the body, the evolution of the soul, how the brain regenerates and transforms us and maybe has its own evolution within the changing layers of time. Or how what we call mystical or magical or miracle comes upon us like epiphanies, but we can't explain why.

I don't believe we'll ever know all the secrets of the universe, or figure out the nuance of common sense, but we do know we were meant to live in community.

Physiologically, we need each other.

Emotionally, we need each other.

Spiritually, we need each other.

At least in order to survive, grow, and thrive.

Even someone who lives in the woods by themselves had to rely on others in the form of nurturers, educators, and societal support in order to get there.

We are all born to a human with a womb, whether or not we are raised by them. Community gives us the gift of life. We can observe this in many species on our planet. Love, nurturing, and support is our nature.

Let us reclaim it. Maybe we can evolve into a less fearful, more compassionate species.

I have compassion for all the parts of me affected by things too big for my conscious mind to process.

I have compassion for the parts of me that survived best when trauma was put in a separate space, under the cover of darkness for weeks, months, years, or decades, until my capacity to allow, soften, and heal these fractures, grew.

My shadows have been a deep and busy place, and have fortified pathways to and from my darkness, ossifying the knowing in my bones to create stepping stones that now allow safe passage in and back out of my depths.

I feel joy in the ache. My depths hold many rivers, my flow of source, the pull of longing, the heartache of the bittersweet, overwhelming love, laughter, sorrow, grief, and movement. I love my shadows.

They live in the back of my mind and in the fundus of my belly, in the curves of my heart, just under the surface of my skin, and in the deepest ocean of my soul.

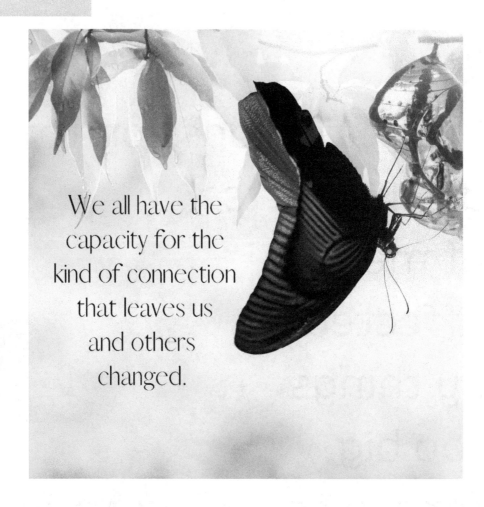

We all have the capacity for the kind of connection that leaves us and others changed.

We put up emotional walls, we avoid eye contact with people we pass, we focus on our phones instead of the world around us. I know there are some terrible things we don't want to look at, because being present with our discomfort is hard. Vulnerability is also hard. We may have been told not to talk to strangers, which is really an ambiguous suggestion. Instead, we could have been told not to get into a creepy van with a man promising you candy or a puppy.

This is to say some of our fear of connection may have come from our programming. Our hesitations stem from how we learned to survive and protect ourselves when we were younger, whether it was told to us by another or began in our nervous system in response to our surroundings. All of this is ok and served a purpose.

It takes courage and awareness of our internal reactions to look past our comfort, our invisibility, and decide to connect with someone.

Yesterday, I was at a care home that I go to weekly to help rehabilitate a patient after a fall and hip surgery. When we were done for the day, I turned to leave, and a woman in a wheelchair caught my eye and waved me over.

She spoke Italian with a few English words mixed in, so it was difficult to grasp what she was excitedly saying, even though I speak a little Spanish. She was pointing and emoting with her hands.

Because of this, her facial expressions and understanding some words here and there, I was able to chat with her for 5 minutes and hear that she was frustrated that the dining room staff wouldn't try to understand or believe her when she asked for something.

I didn't have any answers for her, but I looked her in the eye, stumbled over a few Spanish phrases that she seemed to understand, and gave her a few smiles and compassionate head nods. As she reached for my hand, she looked relieved and grateful that I had taken time to see her and listen. Then she said mostly in English, "Come back anytime."

I don't take these interactions lightly. I am so grateful to see others and make someone's day more tolerable, if not better. And she filled my heart. I am changed by connection.

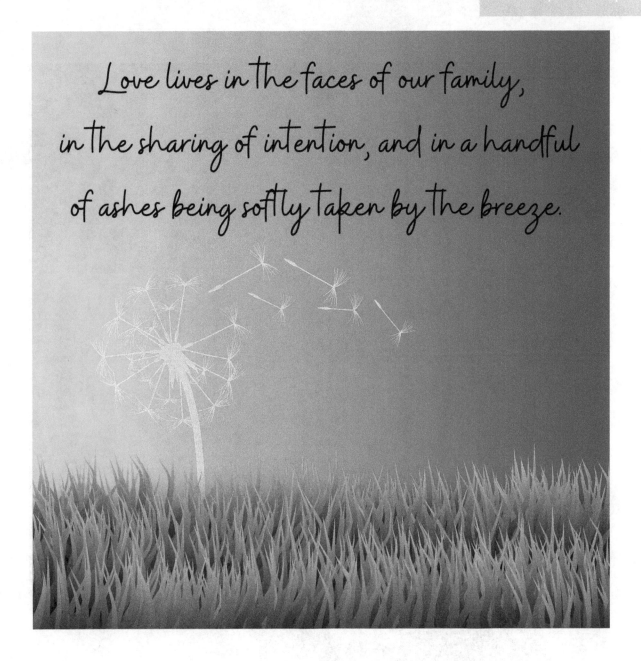

Love lives in the faces of our family, in the sharing of intention, and in a handful of ashes being softly taken by the breeze.

There is love in a handful of ashes. As we gathered on a picturesque mountain, surrounded by trees, a magical view, and love, the faces of my family, some uncertain, others serene, were beautiful. The first Mother's Day without our beloved matriarch in human form still found us together, holding her in a different way. I hope you saw it all, mama.

Reluctance to release her to the wind and trees turned to love and laughter and honor, after one of our present dogs bit off the end of a yellow rose and spread the petals on the ground, as if by divine guidance.

Drawing hearts on each of our hands before holding this rite of passage in our palms, infused love into the moment,

and became sacred movement of fire's memory through our fingertips.

Ravens and eagles were close, watching over and blessing our ceremony, and giving the dogs some excitement.

There were many hugs yesterday. Hugs with our arms, and hugs with our hands, releasing with trust that the earth will continue where we left off. Thank you, mother earth, and may love always be the most powerful force to bring forth blossoms, and keep the rivers flowing and our hearts connecting, and guide our journeys from birth to death and rebirth, in every moment, everyday, and every lifetime.

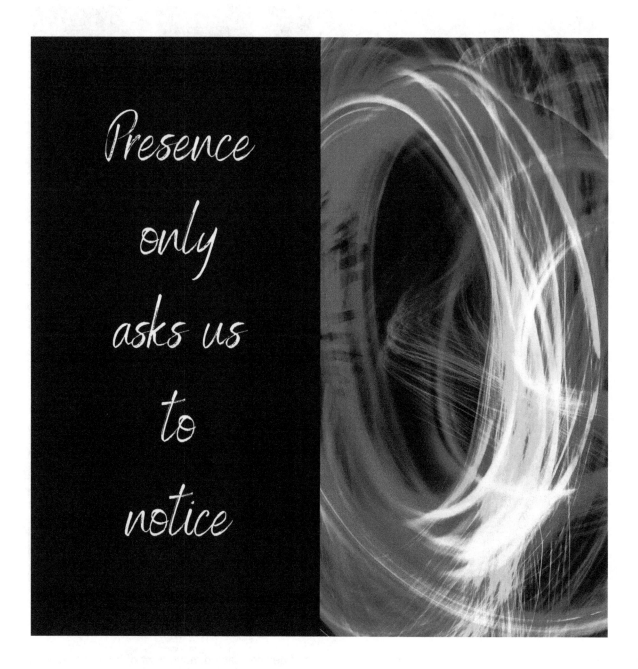

Presence

only

asks us

to

notice

Feeling good is not a requirement for having presence. We have an unending flow of emotional transitions throughout our days and nights. We also have the gifts of discernment and reflection. Presence only asks us to notice.

Notice how each part of your body feels, notice the ease of labor of your breath, the tension in your neck and shoulders, the constriction or softness of your throat or belly. There is no need to assign thoughts or beliefs to what is noticed, no judgements necessary. Simply place attention.

Quantum physics teaches us that the behavior of matter changes when it is observed. This can include our thoughts, our pain, and our breath. This doesn't mean pain goes away

necessarily, but your relationship to it may change. Have you noticed how the energy shifts when you're watching someone?

The molecules of our bodies are conscious of being watched.

Being a compassionate witness to your thoughts, your emotions, or tension makes it easier for them to soften. So, when you start your day, end your day, and during a few moments in between, with awareness, it benefits the connection to yourself. This can increase your self-compassion and help you find a greater understanding of your body's signals and intuition.

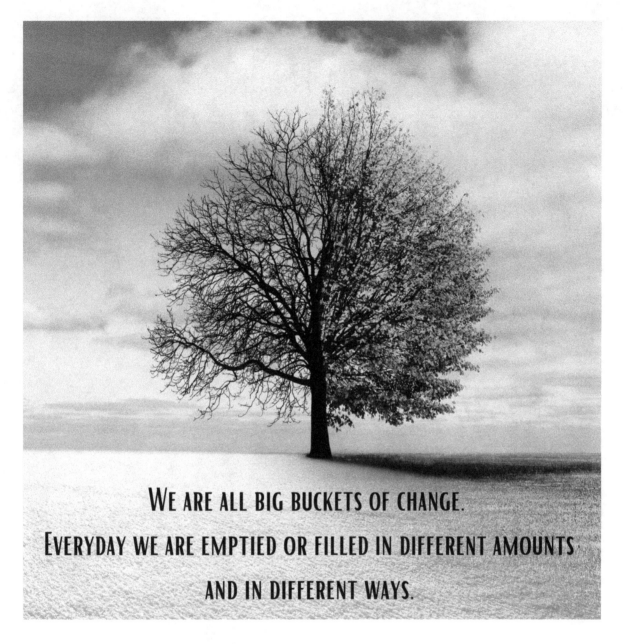

WE ARE ALL BIG BUCKETS OF CHANGE.

EVERYDAY WE ARE EMPTIED OR FILLED IN DIFFERENT AMOUNTS

AND IN DIFFERENT WAYS.

Everyday brings new adventures, new decisions, and a new me that is allowed to feel different in every moment. Because we are all big buckets of change, each day we are filled or emptied in different amounts in different ways by our surroundings and by people who hold different meaning to us. Sometimes moments can drain us, and other times we are overflowing with joy and gratitude. This means within us, we are different people every single day, even by the moment.

I've learned, as I'm sure many of you have, not to take things for granted. Situations are not static and can change at any moment. And just as I am grateful for the fulfilling relationship with my partner that I choose to cherish everyday, for the lives and

health of my children, and for the body that allows me to move and dance and sing and care for others daily, I know they are not guaranteed.

I want to be enchanted by magic and mystery and let my body and soul show me what is joyful for as long as I'm alive. When I ask myself who I am today and why I'm here, I'm honouring all the parts of me and how they change, thus giving myself compassionate presence. When I remember this, I am blessed with the freedom to move unrestricted by dogma or manipulating societal expectations.

As we are the bucket, we are also what fills it. We have the wisdom within us to sustain our wholeness through every moment of change.

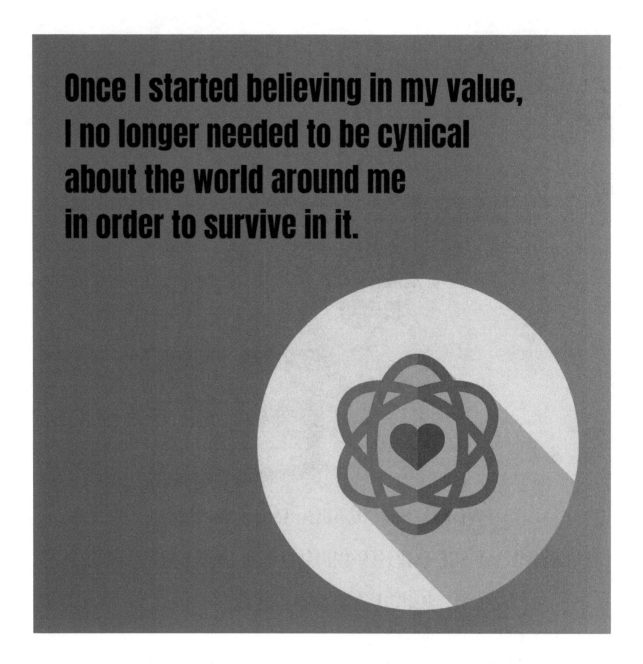

Once I started believing in my value, I no longer needed to be cynical about the world around me in order to survive in it.

As I realize my worth and live from my own values, I expand my energy to fill my whole being. This allows me to look at others with love because I am filled.

Living from the restricted energy of people-pleasing and shrinking myself to fit the situation created resentment inside me, which became my lens to see others and the world with.

Living aligned is a trifecta for peace, love, and fulfillment. I love and value myself. The world loves and values me in my authenticity. I love and value the world more authentically because of the first two.

I understand there are many bodies that are not loved or accepted by mainstream patriarchal, racist, phobic society. In this sense, it is an act of rebellion to love yourself, to hold boundaries, to have a self. We are drawn to folks who embrace an honest sense of self. They have that light behind their eyes. They are magnetic. We are attracted to their truth.

This kind of love doesn't ignore the injustice in the world but gives us the depth and grace to know who we are in context to it. I can love the world instead of resenting it for all its imperfections, just as I can love myself for all my imperfections. I can be aligned even when those around me are not. This allows me to feel great love and to share it.

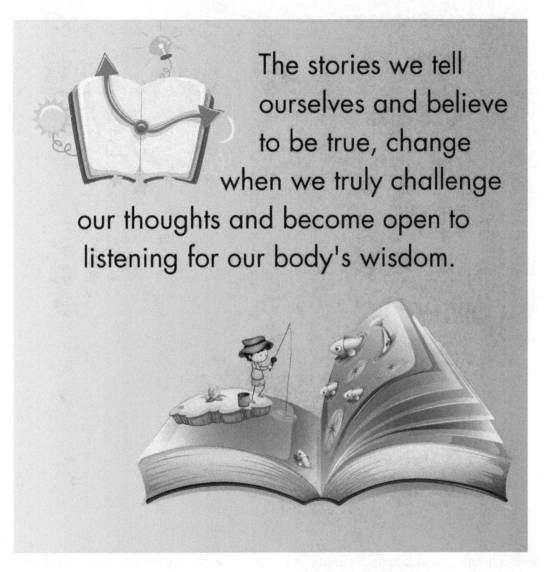

The stories we tell ourselves and believe to be true, change when we truly challenge our thoughts and become open to listening for our body's wisdom.

Story is a beautiful way to connect with imaginations, hearts, minds, and souls. I've experienced this thousands of times through authors and mentors and friends, and it's magical every time. The beauty and brilliance of story is that everybody has one worth listening to. This, of course, includes our own story. We all have much to share, and as we evolve, our stories evolve.

We all have many stories that we tell ourselves. I've had many that, thankfully, have evolved. Some beliefs I used to hold were, I'm not creative, I'm not good enough, I don't need anyone, I've done enough personal discovery work (haha right?), I am too much.

Life experience has taught me the contrary, sometimes in loving and subtle ways, and sometimes in very loud and ungraceful ways. Stories I'm still actively evolving are my relationship and context to the social constructs of time and money, and the role I want to have as a change agent for people, communities, and systems.

My guideposts have recently been my deepest values and learning to align with them in relationships, words, and actions. The biggest tool I have to gauge my alignment is my body. Some call this embodiment or tuning in, being present or following your heart. Martha Beck calls this the Body Compass. What this means is to discover what feels like a yes and what feels like a no, by paying attention to sensations in and around your body and then deciding if they are pleasant or unpleasant.

Our bodies hold wisdom that our minds cannot fathom. The body remembers our experiences from birth until now and constantly strives for equilibrium. This is why your body takes over in stressful or dire situations and can shut down the critical mind in order to maintain balance. When you talk to and trust your body, it becomes a powerful instrument for alignment, truth, and direction.

There is great love here for you.

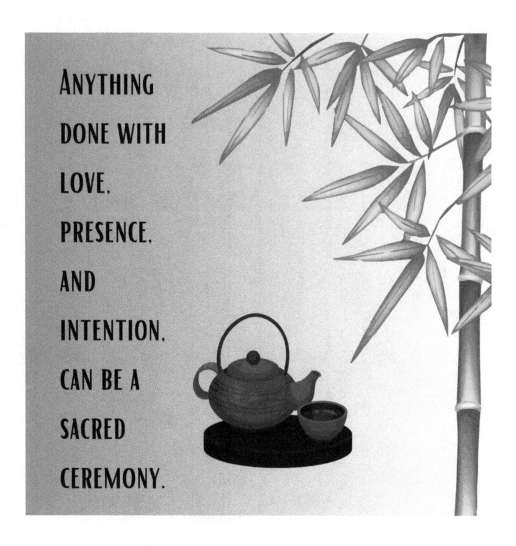

ANYTHING DONE WITH LOVE, PRESENCE, AND INTENTION, CAN BE A SACRED CEREMONY.

Humans have been cultivating ritual to honour sacred moments in our everyday lives since the beginning of recorded history. Over the eons, our ceremonies may have changed but the intention has largely remained the same.

There is beauty in the meaning we attach to tiny celebrations of love, whether they are religious or spiritual practices, births, deaths, or significant moments in between. There are other sacred moments that are loving and joyful to us: preparing coffee or a favorite drink, the satisfying stretch upon waking, the first grounding breath of a meditation, the reconnecting hug after some time away.

I have been cultivating my rituals around writing everyday. For nearly a year, my practice of writing begins in the morning just after waking and making a French press pot of coffee, speaking my daily intentions while sprinkling cinnamon in my cup. It colors my day with magic, meaning, love, and sacred ceremony.

Intention can make magic out of any moment. Washing the dishes or sweeping the floor can be a ritual for decluttering the mind and your energetic space. Weeding (whatever you may call weeds) the garden can represent the shift of growth energy and making space for the plants you want to thrive. Speaking kindly to your plants as you water them is a vibrational connection with living beings.

Little rituals fill our days with connection, with ourselves and with others and with animals and with nature. I love you's before bed, saying grace before a meal, an affirmation before taking an exam. The point is the awareness that the moment IS a sacred moment. And the only thing you need to have a ceremony, ritual, or sacredness is to choose to celebrate the moment, even if it's hard, chaotic, peaceful, if it's a silent noticing or sung out loud...even if you don't know how to start. Simply deciding to live the moment intentionally is an act of creation.

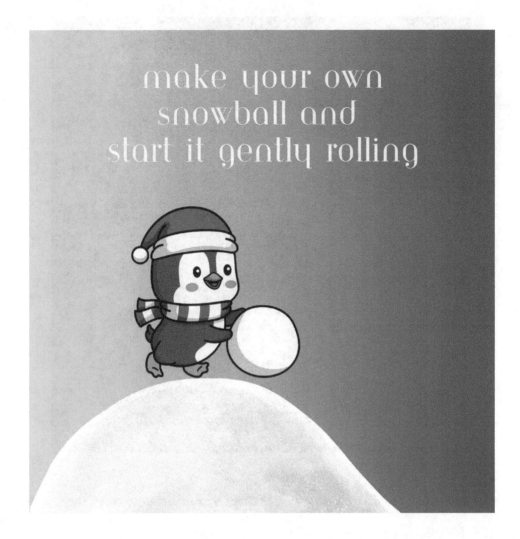

make your own
snowball and
start it gently rolling

Finding a path of joy in your life can delight and feel meaningful, grounding, chaotic, succinct, surprising, vulnerable, or all of the above and more. The previous and current experiences you live in, layer wisdom, desires, turnarounds, mistakes, knowledge, and beliefs into a parfait of unique perspective. These gifts of your heart and soul hold meaning in the container of you-ness.

When you explore these delicious layers, you discover the sweet and sour, the bitter, and the meatiness of your own flavor. Your life force is the kinetic synergy of all your parts, foundations, and dreams. You are divine alchemy.

Your tiny snowball could start as the desire to know yourself better, to understand your triggers or your deepest values, to learn how you want to show up in the world, for yourself and for those you love. Sometimes it starts with a mentor who shows up at just the right moment, a book or quote that gives you an answer exactly when you're seeking, and

tugs on the web of wisdom all around you.

Humans have the capacity for reflection, self-awareness, and agency. It's your choice to decide how high the precipice you move from, how deep the valley from where you are, and the speed you'd like your ball to roll. We accumulate substance and layers in many ways and through many paths.

Sometimes, the snowball feels more like a mud pie or dandelion fluff floating in the breeze, and that's ok too. Energy is always moving, transforming moments and changing minds. Some days, for me, feel like I'm riding an avalanche and other days it's like I'm watching a peaceful, gentle snowfall, preparing for what's to come or just resting.

Snowballs represent multiple possibilities and are part of the yummy parfait that is my life.

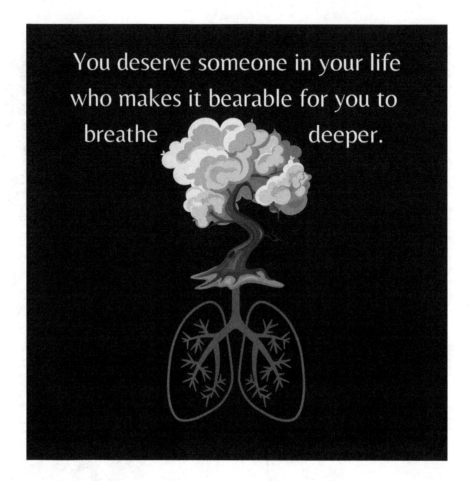

You deserve someone in your life who makes it bearable for you to breathe deeper.

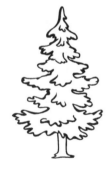

It's a tree, you deserve a tree.

They help you breathe deeper.

There are many layers to breathing.

It's really amazing to have a loved one with whom you feel so safe, that your vulnerability is received with the depth that it deserves and held with love. This kind of love and acceptance from another cannot be overrated. Breathing is easier when you feel safe. Healing is easier when you breathe.

I know many folks who cannot breathe, and for whom it is difficult to feel safe in their body. Sometimes, love for a body begins with acceptance and love from another. Sometimes, it needs medication, or surgery. Many times, reconnecting with our human creature requires awareness of our breath. It is usually the first thing we do, once birthed into this world. Re-membering the breath can take us back to that moment of new life. I have even seen pain vanish with intentional and full breath, more than a few times.

Breathing is a fundamental function. Despite the moments

that take our breath away, the body continues to breathe us. It adjusts to our mental and emotional states to keep equilibrium, the lungs vary their expansion based on how much room there is to open. The body is the foundation for heart and soul, it connects us to our being and anchors our life force. You deserve to have a trusting relationship with your body, one that inspires and expires knowingly with your nature, your truth, and your wisdom, an extension of the trees and the earth. A kind, loving, and reciprocal ebb and flow.

Our layers of breath that exist in the unconscious state, in being held by another, and in our intentional power, all contribute to our capacity for expansion and spaciousness, mitigates our pain and anxiety, regulates our physiology and nervous system, and links us to our wild nature. We cannot be separated from our breath if we have a living body. It is evidence of our depth and miraculous ability to transform that which is outside of us, into nutrients that feed our physical and spiritual vitality. It is with us from birth to death.

I call that sacred.

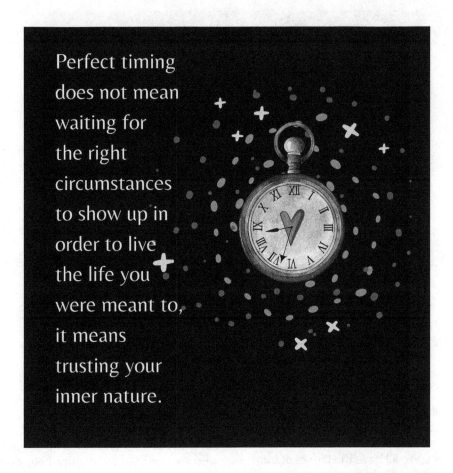

Perfect timing does not mean waiting for the right circumstances to show up in order to live the life you were meant to, it means trusting your inner nature.

"Perfect timing does not exist."

"Everything is perfect in its own way. "

There are often two camps of beliefs, people who believe one or the other.

I believe both, and that perfect timing happens in every moment. The perfect time to choose something or to choose nothing. Every day is full of decisions and micro movements.

Our inner nature and deep wisdom can help us choose direction when we listen. Sometimes, trusting the wisdom of our soul seems way out there and nonsensical.

For example, when I decided to start school for massage therapy, anyone looking at my life at that time might have thought it was the worst timing. I was newly divorced, a single parent of two young children. My Dad had been sick for several months and then passed away 2 months before I began an intense 2.5-year program.

I could have waited, but I felt an excited urgency to get started. I knew it was the right time and trusted the perfectness of it. Not only did it change my career and trajectory, but it also blessed my life with the dearest friends, with purpose and drive, and connected me to opportunities that would not have been possible at any other time.

I had considered the program 18 years prior, but it didn't feel right at the time. I had other things to learn first. When I reflect on all my choices up to today, I can sense when I made profound decisions, changes, beginnings, and endings, and when my choices were unaligned.

You have the power of intuitive synchronicity. Whether you believe in perfect or not, call it whatever you want; you have the capacity for alignment with the wise and perfect nature within you.

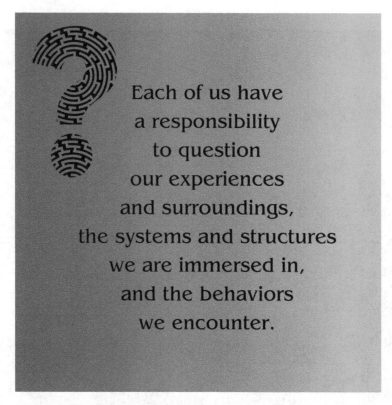

Each of us have
a responsibility
to question
our experiences
and surroundings,
the systems and structures
we are immersed in,
and the behaviors
we encounter.

The world, for me, is a rainbow waterfall of the beautiful and sacred and a cacophony of a million things that I wish were different. Every single one of these things have a story or belief about them. We all have the lenses of our upbringing and stories that were told to us in explicit and subtle ways to peer through. Essentially, we see everything through the filter of our own perspective.

This is great news, because we have the power and ability to change our perspectives at any time. Sometimes we are overcome with epiphany that shifts our beliefs in an instant, however most often it takes a lot of time, awareness, and practice to change our beliefs.

If we examine the stories we tell ourselves with curiosity, it allows us to see slightly beyond the borders of our biases into what is. For example, if I'm convinced that I will never be good enough, and I question this thought, I may find a different answer. If I can use my awareness to see the part of me that is suffering with that thought and ask, by whose measurements am I judging myself? Have I been told I'm not good enough by one or two people or many others or is it a belief I grew on my own, born from an experience that hurt me? Are there parts of me that are good enough in certain situations? If so, then I can know that it is not a true statement.

Accessing the smallest crack in a certain thought can be the point at which a false belief unravels. When you first see this process bring immense relief, there is a momentum that begins in the direction of questioning other thoughts that do not serve you.

For many years, I was sick over the people in our society who are not afforded dignity, help, and care. I desperately wanted to see healthcare systems change. Because of this kind of process, I have been able to become a compassionate witness to the energy inside myself that felt helpless. These atrocities still exist, and I still want to see change. However, my perspective shifted from one of desperation to a place of calm action. I am deeply sad about circumstances, but the thoughts are no longer incapacitating. I am drawn to thoughtful action instead.

For this reason, I have created an initiative to improve the quality of life for the elderly and the dying in my community by building a network of caregivers who provide compassionate presence and nurturing touch in hospice, care homes, and palliative hospitals. Along with my colleagues, I am planning a pilot project at the moment.

There are many ways to question the systems we are immersed in. Mine is just one way. The systems we grew up in are deeply ingrained within us, and it takes some commitment to shake them loose from embedment.

Questioning our thoughts, our pain points, others' behavior, or the structures that we live in context with, simply means placing attention and thoughtful curiosity on what we experience. Through this, we are able to grow capacity for challenging stories that cause suffering and be less controlled by them.

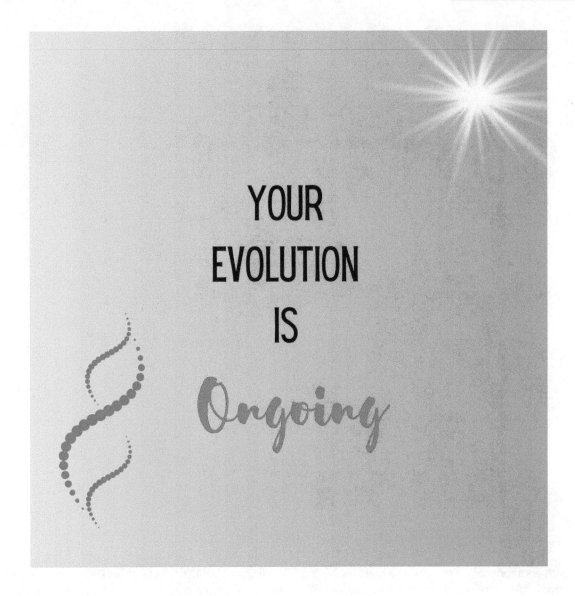

YOUR EVOLUTION IS

Ongoing

There are millions of ways to evolve, and we have the opportunity to learn more, to feel different, to bring awareness to our thoughts, in every moment. Humans have between 6,000 and 70,000 thoughts per day. We change our clothes, our hearts, and our minds all the time, as we discover what each situation asks of us.

The environments we choose to be in, the thoughts we think, the intentions we hold, and our unconscious biases all impact the way we evolve. Evolution simply means the gradual development of something, especially from a simple to a more complex form. For example, human language and the uses for it constantly change and grow. Our understanding of the human body and brain deepens every minute. In this way, we are able to effectively open to our own evolution in thoughtful ways through observation, awareness, intention, and focus. We can consciously explore layers of our psyches, hearts, and spirits and connect the dots in a plethora of ways.

The more you focus on a specific thought or area of curiosity, the more your brain can hold attention for the subject itself, as well as for the process of contemplation. If we have up to 70,000 thoughts per day, the awareness and directed focus of just a handful of them can lead to desired changes.

Our capacity can grow with focused attention, just like the fingers of a musician can become more adept with practice. This can lead to such mastery that muscle memory and intuition play as equal roles as focus in the genius of skillful artistry.

We can choose to support change and growth in ourselves, in each other, and in humanity. We hold pieces of the evolutionary puzzle, and we can decide to use them as building blocks toward the present and future communities and societies we wish to see and would value the most.

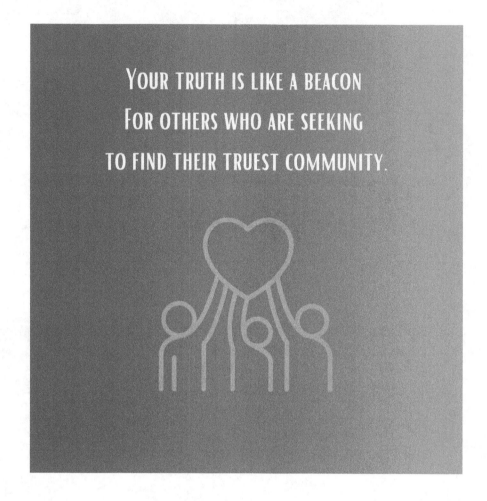

YOUR TRUTH IS LIKE A BEACON
FOR OTHERS WHO ARE SEEKING
TO FIND THEIR TRUEST COMMUNITY.

Connecting with someone who sees you is a huge relief, like an expansive breath after living on tiny gasps of air. In my experience, vulnerability is the quickest way to be recognized, to connect with another.

Vulnerability is our nature. We have fragile skin and soft bodies that can be easily damaged by the abrasive things around us. Humans have been taught to fear their nature and have created all kinds of armor to protect us, both externally and inwardly. Armor is often bulky, heavy, ungraceful, and exhausting to carry around. Many times, we don't even know that we are lugging it with us everywhere we go. We have no obligation to grace, though it feels nice to be unencumbered once in a while. Once you take off your armor enough times, it becomes hard to want to put it back on.

For me, taking off my armor eventually led to being able to sense and absorb more of my environment, to feel the earth, to see through others' armor, to desire depth over surface living. Not sharing my truth became too risky and lonely.

Hiding behind the "I'm fines" is killing us. We are soft because we are meant to be vulnerable. We are built for hugs. We have billions of sensory neurons to detect our surroundings, to take in the microbes in the dirt, to stand on the ground barefoot, and let the ions flow into our bodies. We have created so many barriers to connection. Shoes, constrictive business suits, technology that shuts the world out, separation of mind and body. I'm not saying don't have boundaries, rather, open to what feels right.

When you share what is true for you, others see your light and are drawn to be near because it sparks recognition of themselves. Let your softness attract your village, and they become your living, breathing armor from harmful things. Instead of remaining cramped and hiding behind false personas, expand into your nature to feel looser and freer.

Eventually, fear shifts to love through small moments that gain our trust, enough to open our hearts again and again. This is where bliss, peace, and fulfillment begin. This is how community shows up.

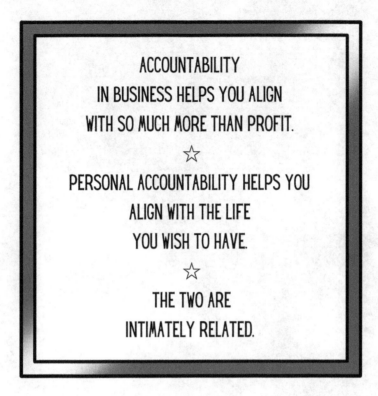

ACCOUNTABILITY
IN BUSINESS HELPS YOU ALIGN
WITH SO MUCH MORE THAN PROFIT.
☆
PERSONAL ACCOUNTABILITY HELPS YOU
ALIGN WITH THE LIFE
YOU WISH TO HAVE.
☆
THE TWO ARE
INTIMATELY RELATED.

Sharon Blackie writes, "The cultural narrative IS the culture." For me, this means what we tolerate as the status quo is culturally accepted, and if we want to see change, we must be accountable to our own values and integrity. We have a part in the collective consciousness. Individual and collective accountability are inextricably linked, and when we look away while our soul tells us to act, we allow our discomfort and fear to make decisions for us.

The world lives by interconnectivity, and what we do, impacts the entire world. If a company destroys a natural habitat for the sake of production without regard for what happens after they leave the area, we all face the consequences, and must decide between letting the destruction remain and regenerating the land and impacted communities. And then allowing or standing up to further destruction happening somewhere else.

Individually, we have the power to decide how we behave and impact those we love, interact with, and model for others. it is no longer enough to want profitability without responsibility. The cost of business is hidden more often than not. Transparency in not the norm, especially where there is little accountability. Individuals and groups increasingly challenge corporations that lack responsibility for their decisions.

Could you imagine if Starbucks were responsible for ethically disposing of, recycling, or upcycling every

single cup, lid, and coffee ground it produced around the world? How would their products, waste, behaviors, and relationships with suppliers and consumers change?

I have worked for more than one company whose blatant profit-driven acquisitions have left relationships with staff and clients strained and work environments toxic. I have been fortunate to be able to leave these places of work when my health and heart began to suffer, though this is not a privilege afforded to all.

Working for myself hasn't been easy, and I am so grateful to be able to align with my own integrity and treat others with the dignity they deserve. Relationships are far more important for sustainability than transactional thinking and growth goals.

Corporations are able to choose accountability for treating their staff, consumers, the spirit of business, and the planet with integrity. We as individuals have the choice to align with our own integrity and align with businesses that go beyond taking our money, to serve our communities and loved ones with care and interest.

For more information on responsible business and economics, the book, Doughnut Economics, by Kate Raworth is golden. It is eye opening and full of suggestions on how businesses can move toward accountability.

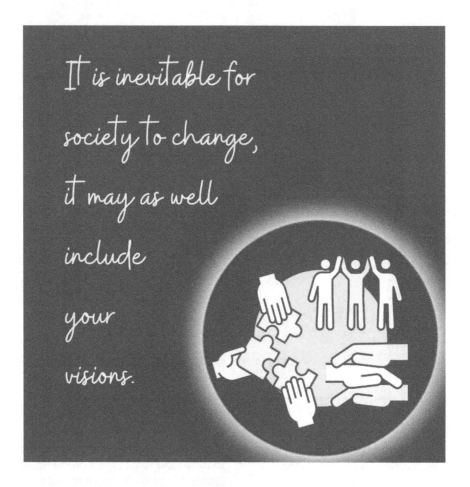

It is inevitable for society to change, it may as well include your visions.

You contribute to the uncountable ways that society evolves. From how you vote to where your money is spent, the causes you support, the way you treat people in your community, the animals in your life, and the boundaries you hold.

We all dream of something being different in our world. Even when disillusioned, we remember desires that felt like freedom, peace, or relief. If we let our hearts wander for a minute, I bet they can still be found.

Here's why I have hope in the future: society is always changing. Barbaric traditions such as self-mummification are no longer practiced, and science no longer believes that gout is caused by a fire breathing mouse.

As we learn more about ourselves and pay attention to what dreams may come, we are able to make small changes toward bringing what we want to see in the world to life. When we cross the invisible barriers into action, whether that is offering kindness to another, having a hard conversation, or asking for boundaries to be respected, we respect ourselves more.

With 8 billion people on the planet, I'm pretty certain you are not the only one who wants specific change. Why live in a world created by others that only benefit the ones who spoke up, those who took power? Why not use connection and solidarity to align with the changes you want to see, the charges that are possible?

Vulnerability is a key to change. I cannot expect to change what I keep tolerating. Talking about what I do want is the only way to bring it to fruition.

Our language, fashion, parenting advice, and what is considered acceptable will change. Our systems can change, too. We don't have to take huge steps, but incremental, thoughtful actions that connect and include people. If you look back on your life, the most profound change came about from one tiny decision, one pause, one moment of following your inner voice. Trajectories shift because we decide to try one thing or talk to one person. Small actions lead to big movements.

As author and activist Sonya Renee Taylor says, "We are living in someone's dream, it may as well be your own."

If you want to live in a world that feels sweeter, you must dream your own dreams first.

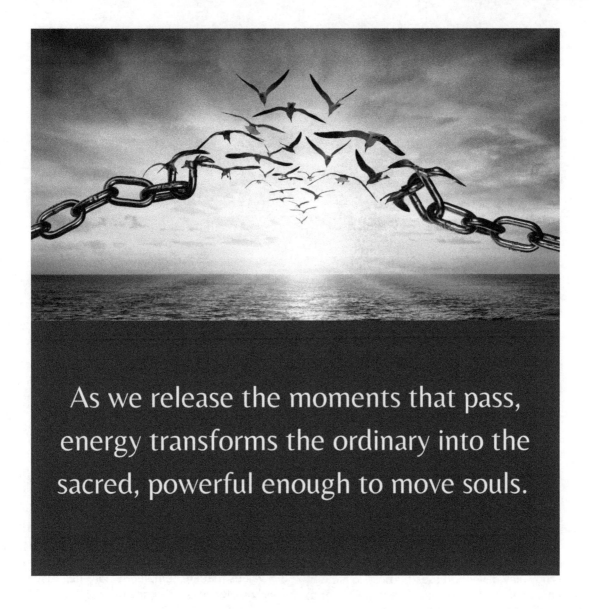

As we release the moments that pass, energy transforms the ordinary into the sacred, powerful enough to move souls.

I've always thought that being a parent was a profound lesson in letting go. It can be bittersweet knowing each brilliant milestone curls into the next, like wave after wave moving toward an island of independence and confidence, relying on you less and less as time goes along. It is so very emotional.

The practice of letting go comes both in epiphanies and in ordinary moments. There are thousands of ways that we learn to let go. For some, it's in watching their children grasp a new skill and growing faster than they'd prefer. For some, it's in losing a job or learning to fly, losing a beloved pet, or saying goodbye.

It's in the beauty of a fragile blossom or the exhilaration of a high dive. It's in learning to meditate or in relinquishing old, dusty thought patterns.

Birth and death and rebirth in trying and failing and trying again, until first attempts become our successes and those may become teachings for another. As we release the moments that pass, energy transforms the ordinary into the sacred, powerful enough to move souls with emotion. Holding the memory of a beautiful thing is a blessing. Reflecting on a challenging moment becomes an inner knowing, a wisdom teaching, one worth sharing.

As a wave crashes down, a new swell is growing behind it, both bringing possibilities to experience and opportunities for love and connection. You are capable of letting go a million times in a million moments and letting yourself be re-filled with joy and grief and hope and uncertainty. Emotions are spacious enough to fill us if we dare to dance upon their waves.

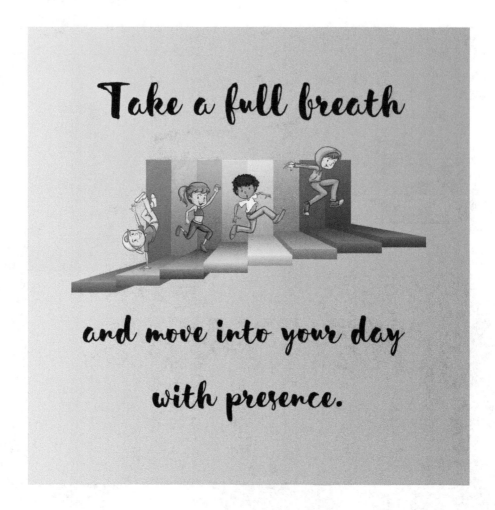

Be on purpose.

Purpose is nothing more than intention. People get so concerned that they may never find their purpose in life. Many feel an ache, or an emptiness, or a hole that has yet to be filled. For you who are truly seeking, it's a journey toward self, discovery, and alignment. Fulfillment, for me, comes from filling that emptiness with myself, my wholeness, and honouring what I need.

When you tune into your body, your core values, or your integrity, they will often lead you in the same direction. If you're more adept at listening to one of the three, start with that, and then slowly open to the other two.

To me, they all tell me the same thing. Some folks, however, may not trust what their body intuition is saying because they have become practiced at ignoring body signals. There are ways to regain that connection. Through paying attention to sensations that feel pleasant and unpleasant in your body, not your mind, you can begin to recognize your physical barometer.

If you're uncertain what your core values are, I recommend searching online for a comprehensive values list, writing down all the words that are meaningful for you, then circle 3-5 values that are completely non- negotiable in your life. This knowledge is life changing.

Aligning with your integrity is checking in with your truth when making decisions of large or small consequence. If that feels complicated, then for now, give attention to moments you feel thirsty, sleepy, when you have shoulder tension, or need to go to the bathroom. You may also be able to notice when the words or actions of another don't sit right in your mind or body.

Integrity is made up of hundreds of choices each day. Listening for your internal truth becomes a habit and feels icky when moving too far away from it. Being on purpose IS your purpose. It doesn't have to feel daunting. Aligning with what brings you joy, nourishment, strength, safety, and connection moves you in the direction of fulfillment, each day, each moment. This doesn't mean you'll be happy every minute, but you'll be able to recognize how you feel more often.

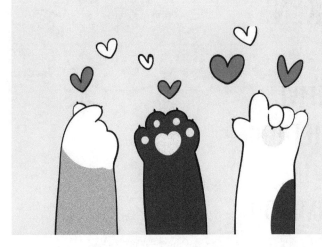

Inner accountability
helps me align with the
human I want to show up as.

Accountability is terrifying in a culture that teaches us to mistrust our instincts, emotions, and ideas. If we are constantly worried about being judged, it is difficult to share what is true for us, especially if we are not old, white, rich, and born with male genitals. It can be downright deadly to show up with integrity, just as you are, as we've seen way too many times for black and brown folks.

Accountability has two faces, one facing inward and one facing outward. They can feel profoundly different and be activated in different parts of our bodies and psyches. Taking account of the inner journey can be scarier than looking at our outward actions. Diving deep into our traumas, biases, and challenging belief systems can feel destabilizing. Observing our molecules of inner chaos can uncover stunning realizations, light some righteous fires, and distinguish other coals that have been smoldering for decades.

The ingrained beliefs we accept stemming from our own perceived lack of agency causes debilitating doubt and inaction. We have little energy left over from supporting ourselves in a consumerist economic system for creative endeavors that we barely believe in anyway, because they are not productive and deemed therefore useless. We have

busy lives because it is esteemed to be so, and we are called wild if we want to play or go on adventures. We are judged as downright crazy if we go after a dream that doesn't fit within the lines of mainstream status quo capitalist culture. Especially if the one following her dream is a woman, is black, trans, or non-conformist, and by God, doesn't include making boat loads of money.

I have been one of those, afraid to speak my truth to a larger audience than my usual one on one in my treatment room. My fear has been that I will be judged for what I believe. I'm afraid of getting something very wrong and being thought of as a fraud. I'm sure this fear stems from experiences in my childhood, and yet and of course, it is interwoven with my exposure to vulnerability. How ironic that I'm writing a book and training courses to reach a wider community. I suppose this fear keeps me diligently accountable to my truth, to giving credit to my sources, and to creating honest content for my readers and students.

Inner accountability helps me align with the human I want to show up as in my relationships, my work, my writing, for my body, and my mind. It feels like continual movement because I'm an ever-changing person.

241

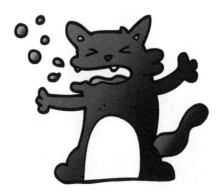

HICCUPS

& CHICKENS

HAVE
SOMETHING
IN
COMMON

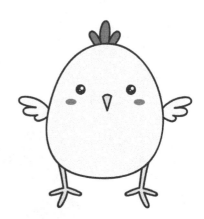

My body feels a kind of delicious tension in the space between hiccups. Almost like my lungs miss the feeling. Every time another spasm shakes and relaxes my chest, I wonder if that was the last one. Feeling into the stillness, waiting for another one. It's nice when they stop, but I feel a lingering pull in my body for a while that reminds me, they could come back in an instant.

Yesterday, there was a particularly chatty chicken outside my treatment room window. She had a lot to say, and with every squawk and ba-gawk, I felt the same tension, wondering if that was the last one, waiting in silence as my patient drifted in hypnagogia.

When Lola the chicken finally had her say, it had been 10 minutes, and I hoped that she hadn't disturbed my patient too much during the last few minutes of treatment. Turns out the sound of clucking didn't even register on the patient's radar. I had been the only one consciously feeling that tensity in the silence between.

I didn't have hiccups yesterday, but the sounds of hens made me see the similarity of the pull I feel in the stillness between, and that I have no choice but to relinquish control of what happens after the silence. For many years, one of my hardest lessons has been releasing attachment to the outcome. Of anything. Many times, I've tried to lean into the uncertainty of life, confident that I've acted in the best way I know to bring about a desired thing. These are moments when everything is done, and I am able to rest. Though my body has a different idea and remains tense as my mind stresses about how what I want might show up or not.

The chickens taught me yesterday that if I ease into the tension, really sit with it, and feel it, the tension changes. It feels delicious and inviting. So now, when I'm worried about a path that I'm on, waiting for an outcome, I will try reveling in it instead of fighting the feeling.

Thanks, chick-chick-chickens!

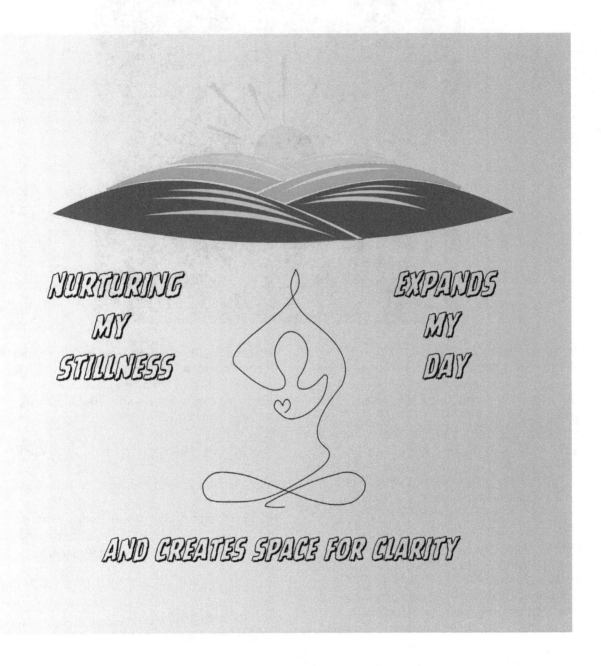

NURTURING MY STILLNESS

EXPANDS MY DAY

AND CREATES SPACE FOR CLARITY

I live a full day in the morning before I begin the mundane, think about obligations, concern myself with the upcoming. I nurture and feed my stillness, my connection, my creativity, and my peace. The richness of these moments fills me for the remainder of the day, a blissful presence that connects me to my soul. This is how I love myself.

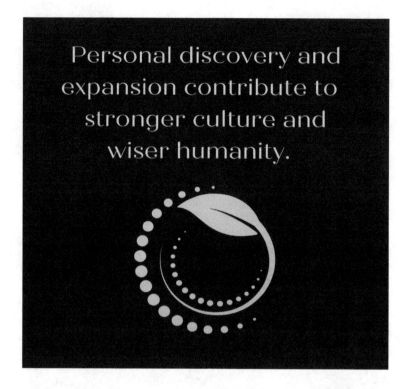

Personal discovery and expansion contribute to stronger culture and wiser humanity.

When I first became aware that I was on a personal development journey, I had no idea it would be an ongoing, lifelong process. Now I understand intimately what a winding path it is and how profound it is to take.

Becoming committed to learning and seeking wisdom raises awareness and contributes to the way we perceive the world around us and how we view our purpose. Whether learning psychology, systems, or seeking wisdom of the heart, soul, or ancestors, the openness is what keeps us curious.

Imagine if the tax department was curious about why someone was struggling to pay taxes or if McDonald's was curious how to be responsible for all the garbage they put out onto the planet. If they held these thoughtful questions in mind, with openness, they could raise the quality of relationship they have with people and with the planet.

Corporations aside, if WE are curious about struggle, about responsibility, about the quality of relationship we have with others and the planet, we contribute to the wisdom that exists in this lifetime. Our journeys matter in the bigger picture of humanity. Our decisions have power. What we know creates direction. What a community or a nation knows creates trajectory.

When you look to the side while driving, you eventually begin to drift in that direction.

If humans can see a kinder, wiser, inclusive way forward and seek it with intention, if we look in the direction that our hearts are facing, we are more likely to follow that trajectory. It takes practice to give attention to what we do want instead of what we don't. But practicing this makes us stronger... and wiser.

Practice giving attention to what you do want.

Practice holding intention in your mind.

Practice connection with your body's wisdom.

Practice sharing what's important to you.

Practice gathering communities that lift each other up.

Practice looking for exciting ideas, bliss, and creative insights everyday.

Practice more safe, physical, nurturing intimacy.

Hug more and longer.

Look people in the eye, if you can.

Be compassionate to yourself as you practice.

What we know and seek expands our awareness and leads to the liberation of others to do the same.

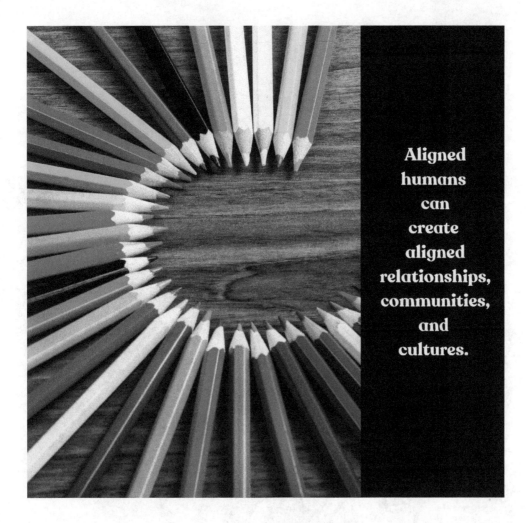

Aligned humans can create aligned relationships, communities, and cultures.

I feel strong and peaceful when aligned with my core values and integrity. Accepting my uniqueness and flavor of creativity has been a worthwhile, if sometimes harrowing journey. On days I feel integral, serendipity happens, connection is evident, curiosity abounds. There is synergy created with the friends I am surrounded by. Love is present. Ideas spring forth. Rest is nurtured. Everywhere there is beauty, and everything makes sense. This is a beautiful feeling to linger in.

For decades, this feeling was very occasional at best. I realize this is the place I longed for the whole time, when I felt something was missing in my life, missing inside me. I felt flawed and blamed for my shortcomings. It's like pushing through a deluge of tidal wave after tidal wave, struggling for something in the horizon to keep focused on, without being able to see it clearly, constantly wiping the salt from your eyes. There is clarity in learning how to recognize our painful thoughts and respond with compassion. This is a deeply healing process.

I am profoundly more adept at tuning in to my inner knowing, my sense of peace, and my core orientation, both within the context of the world around me, and far outside worldly context. From this place, I recognize the alignment in others. Not because I know what's going on inside them, but because I feel the sense of peace emanating from them, not necessarily their mind, but from their spirit.

Connection to ourselves and to our dreams, to others, to our winding and wild paths, our plans,, and our sense of service to our communities becomes fortified in the knowing of our true foundation. For me, it is a stability that I couldn't access before. Strengthening the culture within me is a powerful movement toward strengthening the communal culture I am immersed in.

Human dignity and equity and caring for the planet and lifting up marginalized voices and being subversive to toxic systems feels inevitable and innate and just, from this perspective.

Be patient with yourself on this journey. It is hard to see through the deluge. The taste of salt might just become the touchstone you need to keep moving through it. Love to you today and everyday.

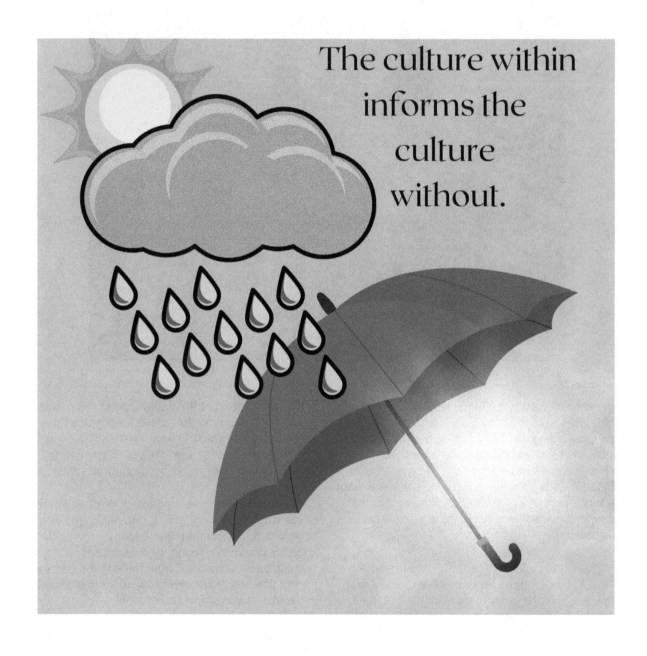

The culture within informs the culture without.

When there is thunder inside, thunder is what we notice outside of us.

Healing our previous wounds is important and loving and messy.

It's not always possible to wash away the hurt and dust and blood stains of our past, and these transgressions on our hearts and faces look forward from us and say, I can't see through the fuzz.

It is so for our courageous feet and knowing souls, taking another step into the wind.

Hurt need not be our master.

Love also must join.

Longing must join.

Our peace and stillness must join.

Our holy presence and laughter and joy must pour from our eyes and mouths and hands.

And we must live, live, live.

Our past is not the lone project of excavation.

The present hides the gift of awareness in plain sight.

It is missed in our days, being drowned by faux smiles in suits, pressing the latest disaster into our brains and nervous systems to ruminate on.

Everyday catastrophizing seeps into the soft core of our being.

Our diet of confusion and regurgitated hate is nutritionally deficient.

Poisonous.

Unfit for human consumption.

What we ingest is more toxic coming out than sinking in.

Insidious creatures run amok amid our guts and surround our hearts with bricks too awkward and bulky to push away.

When flakes of fallout land on our shoulders, we can brush them off.

When they sink in, our filters like lymph nodes, get clogged and our immunity becomes overwhelmed.

Without warning, a simple agitation turns to venom and spews out onto our loved ones and friends.

It changes our DNA and becomes a new normal.

A sickness.

It is far more loving to brush off the ash of hate as it falls.

Or to use an umbrella.

Or leave.

Find the rain.

Wash off what falls on our heads everyday.

Until what we hold precious is what we see outside of ourselves each day.

Then we can marvel at the love and awe and creative genius that showers our surroundings and those we love with powerful and precious presence.

With peace.

With gratitude.

With buoyancy and intention.

For what lives inside us comes out.

We have the agency to choose what that is.

What do we have to live for if we've lost ourselves?

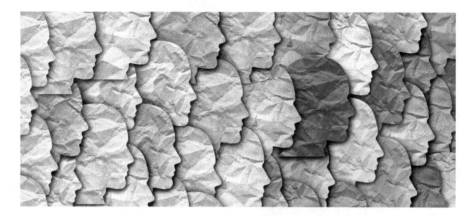

Getting lost doesn't mean we lose our way, often we are just finding a path that feels truer.

There are oh so many ways to get lost.

We can lose ourselves in a book or a movie.

We can get lost in thought or in a feeling.

We can forget ourselves by looking into someone's eyes, running toward danger in a split second to help someone, or when feeling untethered and bereft at the loss of a loved one.

We can be lost in ways that separate us from our essential being, wild nature, truth, and intuition. Sacrifice, for the sake of others, societal expectations, and nonsensical rules, disconnect us from our center and sense of self. This can become unconsciously insidious. Self-sacrifice has been used by the maliciously powerful to control, disguised as piety, propriety, compassion, and caring.

Disconnection from agency, inner knowing, and intuition can lead to paths that do not serve us, blind us to dangerous pitfalls when we cannot access our guidance system. This can cause us to suffer abusive relationships, hurtful circumstances, and incongruent choices.

Often, loss comes with literally forgetting who we are and what we've been through in the form of dementia. This can be both frightening and freeing. There are as many different reactions to losing memory or personality as there are people with dementia. Some folks are anxious, some childlike and playful, and some live in between. They all need support as do those that love them.

Losing ourselves can scare our loved ones more than it scares us. Maybe they worry about our well-being or wonder how our change will affect them. People fear the loss of security and safety when people change.

In all of these situations, leaning into curiosity, awareness, and compassion, soften painful thoughts that often come with change. Recognizing small changes can help us accept the ones that feel more significant. We can be scared of change and still support it. Growth requires that we change. Exploring biases and beliefs can feel like being lost at first, but honest and thoughtful conversations can lead to clarity.

Getting lost doesn't always mean we lose our way; often we are just finding it. Letting your curiosity drive instead of fear can make navigating change joyful and worthwhile, even in hard or painful moments.

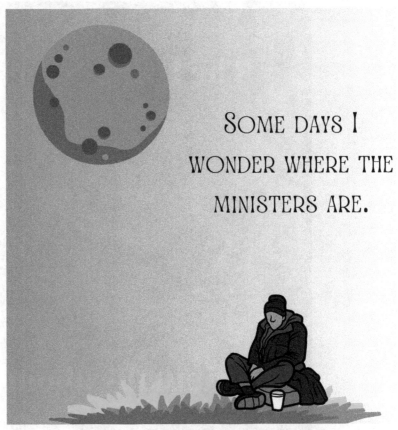

SOME DAYS I WONDER WHERE THE MINISTERS ARE.

I am pondering today, after passing an unhoused man for the 20th time, who is sleeping on the grass by the side of a busy road, I notice my longing to go grab some coffees and sit and ask if he would like a conversation. Unfortunately, I had to drive by because rent needs to be paid.

I've never seen myself as a ministerial type, but at this moment, I wonder where those who do are. Is ministry about cultivating relationships in our communities? I think it's funny that our health and welfare systems are called ministries. Funny in a critical way. We've lost touch with our purpose and our community's needs.

The only folks I've seen visiting this unhoused man have been police officers, when they are telling him to leave the area. But he always comes back.

Where are the ministries that aim to cultivate relationship? They have disappeared behind bureaucratic walls, waiting for those in need to wander through their doors, if they actually have a way to traverse from where they lay and ask for help.

When I was housing-impaired with two young children and asked for help, they told me to sell my car. The car I used to get to work and interviews and take my kids to school. It was worth too much, they said. They gave me emergency rent money... well not gave, they loaned it to me and charged interest when I paid it back, without showing interest in why I was behind in rent, without interest in how my children were doing or how I might give them a Christmas, as the season drew close. They weren't interested in cultivating a relationship with me or with anyone in the cold feeling waiting room, one neon ceiling light flickering.

Stomach in my throat, wondering how I got there, after owning a house and going to school to support my family. I felt naked and interrogated. I felt guilty. Nobody should be made to feel like this when seeking support.

Ministries have forgotten that support is being seen and held through our most trying moments. Being known through our joy and pain is what a village offers. I don't care why this man sleeps on the grass at the side of a busy road. I just wonder who he is and if he'd like a coffee and a conversation. Maybe I am a minister, after all.

You are worthy of having a self.

Social conditioning convinces us that we need to be selfless to be worthy, especially women. Even more so, women of color. This ingrained belief has been pushed deeper through generations of punishment if one were to step out of line from the rigid written and unwritten rule. Women have been owned for many millennia, and the thought of challenging this narrative triggers the layers of fear and control or nervous systems have endured.

Being yourself is a revolution of spirit. Selflessness separates us from our essential nature, our wildness, our inner wisdom, and intuition. When this is a default, society is unbalanced, unhealthy, and inequitable.

When we are deeply connected in ourselves, and we acknowledge our deep love, our chaos and contradiction, our emotion, creativity, and brilliance, we live in fullness, and awe, and revel in the audacity of acceptance.

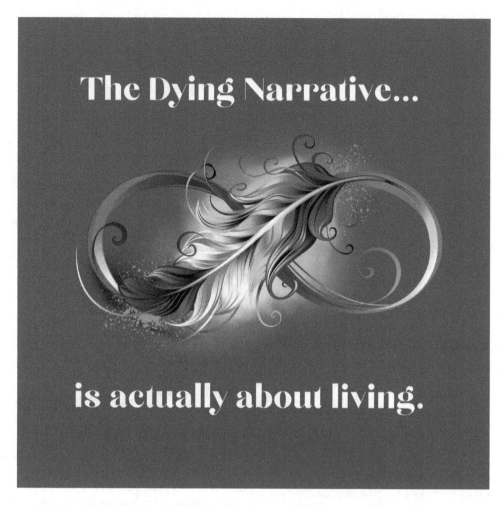

The Dying Narrative...

is actually about living.

Why is our culture so afraid of aging and dying? We have all been touched by life-altering or life-ending disease. We've been affected by the way we ourselves or our loved ones have been cared for by our healthcare systems.

The way we view what happens in later years contributes to the aversion we have for facing these topics.

From the perspective of a Registered Massage Therapist who cares for the elderly and the dying in care homes, hospice, and hospitals, I have seen some needs of the community, ways we could get there, and the possibility of exceptional experiences in human dignity and care that can change the way we think about our future.

Even if patients are well cared for by nurses and doctors, there is often still something missing. Someone who is there solely to be a compassionate witness for this whole human, going through a possibly harrowing experience. Someone who listens and pays attention, who knows how and when to give safe, nurturing touch that helps calm the nervous system.

It's wonderful if that compassionate presence is a loved one. However, it's not always possible. Many times, family and friends have work or other obligations and can be there for short periods. Many are worried when visiting and can't be present for their loved one, as they are also deep in feelings of grief or fear, coupled with all the other concerns in their lives.

Nurses have so much to think about, crucial tasks to perform, and with few exceptions must keep an eye on several patients. RMTs and end of life doulas are excellent bridges between what nurses offer and what loved ones can do. Studies have shown that massage therapy reduces pain medication needs, helps patients feel more heard, and makes nurses' jobs easier. In Canada, RMTs are not widely employed in hospitals, hospice, or care homes, where kind, nurturing touch would be most beneficial. Patients must pay separately if they want treatment.

Seeing our loved ones being cared for in a way that improves quality of life in their elder years and at the end of life would be a good start to mitigating the fear of aging and hopefully lead to other beautiful shifts in the way we approach living...and dying.

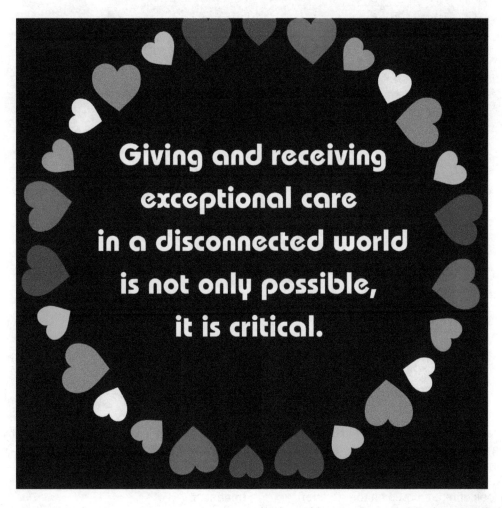

Giving and receiving
exceptional care
in a disconnected world
is not only possible,
it is critical.

Everybody deserves exceptional care.

As a Registered Massage Therapist and teacher of Massage Therapy, I have seen how many people don't believe this for themselves, even though they wish they were treated better in their healthcare interactions.

Humans have the capacity for the kind of connection that changes hearts.

Becoming an exceptional caregiver is possible for anyone, regardless of the work they do. It is important in all our relationships and strengthens our own care of self.

I was often asked as a teacher, "What are 3 things that make a great RMT?" My responses were usually a combination of values and principles. In my work and my teaching, I have found 3 principles the most prevalent in learning to become a profoundly caring human while also accepting care from others. I will share what these principles are and then elaborate on future posts.

Besides knowledge and care of the self, of your physical

body and home of your spirit, there are 3 things that I found through the stories of my patients, and through my teaching, is often, what needs cultivating in health professionals, (and couldn't hurt in everyone else).

They are: 1. Listening. 2. Love. and 3. Laying of hands. Safe and nurturing touch.

Knowledge and skills are often taught in school and at home. Though these 3 intuitive practices often are not an explicit focus, they vary between teachers and the emotional intelligence of those around us. They become underlying action, or a forgotten skill based on how much they are practiced and if they are acted on consciously or not.

It has been my experience that so many do not hold this awareness in their daily lives. These are more than worthwhile to learn and focus on, as giving these 3 things to ourselves and to others creates profoundly effective communication and can greatly improve our relationships in all parts of our lives.

> # I am soft and deeply feeling, not because I've never been hurt, but because I dont want to be caged behind bitterness in the expectation of being hurt again.

When our boundaries are crossed or we are hurt, our bodies protect by engaging the nervous system. It's normal for us to freeze, not know what to do, fawn over an explanation, want to run or fight back. Everyone has their own nervous system response. This can look different based on the situation.

I understand the inclination to close off and shut down, as this has been a subconscious default for many years. It took awareness and self-love to allow my body to trust that I'm safe. It's not fool-proof, however. Yesterday, I was violated on LinkedIn through personal messages. A professional networking website where I post in groups for mental health, coaching, personal development, and wellness. Two men decided to send inappropriate messages as if it were a dating site. Some days and in some frames of mind, I can let it roll off. But yesterday, something bothered and unsettled me.

For a minute, I even gaslighted myself, thinking maybe my icky feeling was wrong, and what he was saying surely didn't mean what I thought. For a moment, I didn't know what to do. I couldn't think. My nervous system had kicked in. And then I remembered that I could block them, so that's what I did.

Human emotions are so complex. At first, I was upset that I let it affect my morning. I doubted my capacity for being able to handle what may come as I become more visible in my organization while building my network. I vented. As I turned it all over in my mind, I realized that while I don't want to give my power away to random threats or criticisms, I also don't want to become hardened. Women have been treated like objects forever. I don't want to get used to this kind of treatment.

If I close off, I lose myself. Connection and intimacy are too valuable to risk. They are worth more than worrying about what might come. Connection makes my life worth living, and for that, I must love my vulnerability and deeply feeling heart.

I have learned that if I choose to feel the pain in the moment, I don't worry about when the pain might rear its head from an undetected deep well of despair inside me at the most inopportune moment, to then fall on the hearts of my most precious of peeps.

I am not willing to compromise my beautiful and courageous heart to something as common as another's disconnected thoughtlessness. Compassionate inquiry of my feelings and my body's reactions helps me figure out what I need, and then writing about it helps me process the situation.

I hope you have learned for yourself the tools that help you protect your loving heart without having to close it off. Sending love your way.

POVERTY DOESN'T GET A RETIREMENT.
POVERTY DOESN'T HAVE A PENSION.

POVERTY DOESN'T HEAT YOUR HOUSE OR
FEED YOUR CHILDREN.

POVERTY IS AFFORDED NO DIGNITY.

POVERTY DOESN'T CARE FOR YOUR AGING
PARENT.

POVERTY IS HEARTLESS, SYSTEMIC,
HIERARCHICAL, INSIDIOUS, PLANNED AND
BLAMED ON THE POOR.

Rant.

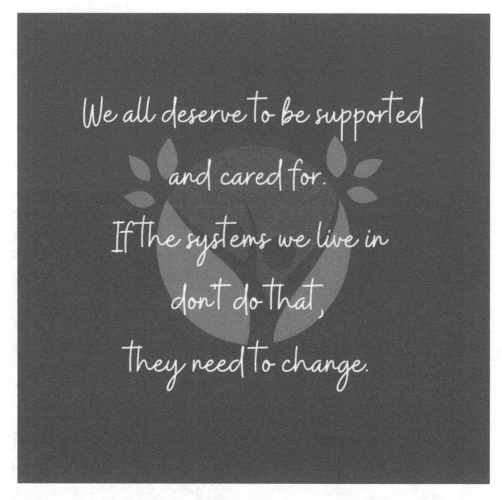

We all deserve to be supported and cared for. If the systems we live in don't do that, they need to change.

There is a dichotomous nature to the economic system. We are expected to pay to make a living, for goods and services, and yet be minimally remunerated or uncompensated for services we offer, our emotional labor, our caregiving, or entertainment. Artists and musicians are asked to work for exposure, caregivers are expected to volunteer, teachers are told that their salary includes the 'extras' that are not in their regularly scheduled hours.

There is history behind the expectation of giving our time and energy out of the goodness of our hearts. What used to be called men's work that included long hours spent in governments, universities, religious institutions, running businesses, writing laborious tomes, creating masterpieces, was based on EVERYTHING else being taken care of. Slaves, servants, wives, all mostly unpaid, were expected to cook, feed, clean, care for young ones, mend, tend animals, labor in fields or gardens, in order to support the "important" work men were preoccupied with.

These roles were viewed as, and widely accepted as the jobs of less important people. These ideas have been ingrained deep in the psyche of society. As time goes on, we get further away from the explicit acceptance of these roles, but

implicitly, they are insidiously embedded. The DNA of our predecessors donated these beliefs, it seems, into our own bodies. Why do I both feel bad for charging people for my services and feel deserving of compensation?

It is an unequitable economic system. Who decides what work is worthy of compensation and what work is not? If everyone is required to pay for being alive, then everybody should be compensated for being alive. The ingrained belief systems, if we are unaware, subconsciously keep us from expecting and asking for our work to be valued.

I know I go on about awareness and curiosity a lot, and the reason is because they are catalysts for change, for hope, for imagining, for creativity, for connection. I don't want to go on supporting unconscious beliefs that are harmful to people, society, and the planet. We all deserve to be supported and cared for. If the systems we live in don't do that, they need to change.

"Go out there and advocate for the helping professions - all of them - to be well compensated, well supported, well respected, and regarded as essential because THEY ARE." - Kristen King Kristen Skove King

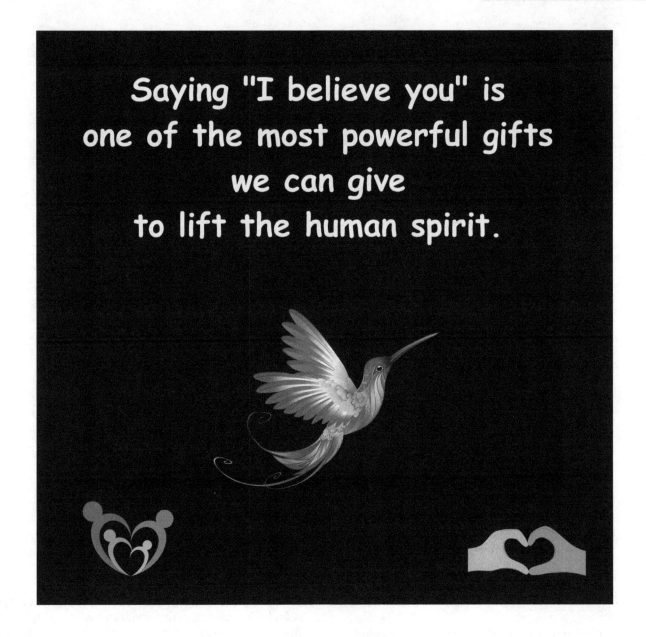

Saying "I believe you" is
one of the most powerful gifts
we can give
to lift the human spirit.

I believe you means I see you, I accept you, I honor you, I trust you, I support you, I hold you. This is such a relief in a culture that so often questions our motives, our intuition, and our lived experience.

Relationships regulate the nervous system. If those we most associate with constantly question who we are and how we feel, our nervous system can experience a continual, low-lying anxiety, that eventually can corrode or sense of self, causing us to question our deep knowing.

Often, learning to separate ourselves from our truth and knowing happens at an early age. Our bodies and/or minds create chasms between what we know to be true and our outward presence in order to protect us, because something told us we were no longer safe to share our truth.

When someone is able to hold our entirety and reflect it back to us, it can be everything we want, and can also be scary because our uncertainty has been our ally for so long. Re-integrating out truth can feel unsettling, and like you've just taken your very first breath.

Eventually, being seen in our wholeness lets us live in our truth. With practice, with acceptance, with love, we can learn to feel connected again to the safety of being integrated. Living in wholeness can lead to bliss, a sense of peace and direction, and to trusting what lives inside us once more.

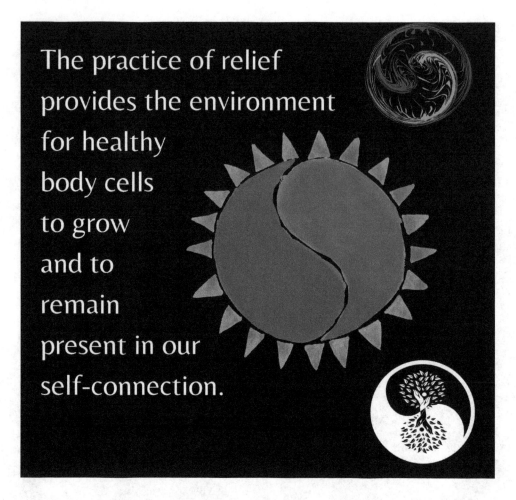

The practice of relief provides the environment for healthy body cells to grow and to remain present in our self-connection.

Relief is a bridge between the darkness and the light. It's also a bridge to the slightly less heavy, from the invisible to being seen, from the cornered to the free.

It can release our breath, the constriction in our chest and throat, the tension in our muscles, and the need to hide.

When we feel scared or stressed, our bodies get flooded with cortisol, which can overload our systems and damage our tissues when high amounts are present for prolonged periods. When we feel relief, typically, our brains release feel-good hormones like serotonin, oxytocin, and endorphins. This allows our bodies to rest, digest, relax, and repair.

Sometimes, pain is completely situational, though often we suffer more intensely from the thoughts and emotions we have regarding the painful situation. While the situation may not be changeable or take time to heal, our thoughts and emotions that keep us suffering can be moved.

Relief can be found just a step away from anywhere. Get your bearings and look to a close by emotion that feels like relief. This is a bridge that leads to feeling a little better. I learned from Abraham Hicks that feeling better is like taking steps on a ladder. You don't go right from the bottom to the top, skipping all the steps in between. We don't move from hopeless to joyful in one step.

Abraham says, "You can go from rage to imaging revenge; that feels like relief." It offers levity to the suffering we feel in the moment. It doesn't mean we act on that revengeful fantasy, but it shows us the energy of emotion doesn't have as strong a hold as we've been giving them the power to have.

No matter where relief comes from, it can have a positive effect on your nervous system. Finding that thread to gently pull shows a way to unravel the knots that keep you bound. Recognizing those knots aren't solid offers freedom from the thought that suffering is inevitable. It offers a little relief.

Knowing how to find a little relief opens the door to the belief in expansive relief, even if the body is the only part of you that knows it. Practicing relief builds capacity for releasing painful thoughts and for holding your body, mind, and heart in integrity.

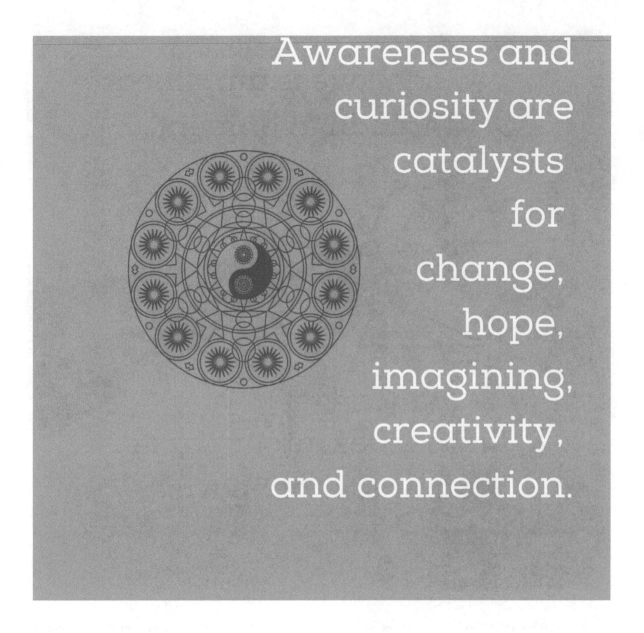

Awareness and curiosity are catalysts for change, hope, imagining, creativity, and connection.

Awareness is consciousness, a compassionate witness, the higher self, the part of us who is aware of our thoughts and emotions, in it but not of it, the soul, our center, feeling grounded, being present. Awareness creates space, a cushion, between our core and difficult emotions. Being aware of emotions instead of being "in" an emotion feels less sticky and heavy. It's not always possible, though it is able to be practiced.

Being mired in reactions can be overwhelming and exhausting. Seeing emotions with curiosity brings patterns to light and dulls the sharpness. Pain can soften as we sit with it. Emotions are touchstones for the soul that we feel in the body. They are protectors and indicators that something needs attention, not always that something needs to be changed or fixed.

Our bodies are incredibly intelligent receptors of our external... and internal...environments. So even when our body detects an untrustworthy situation, we may not be consciously aware of it. Practice tuning into the sensations of our body gives us awareness of what feels neutral, what feels good, and what doesn't feel good. Then, when we happen to notice one of those sensations, we can be curious about why.

Being able to get to a place of love and acceptance of our processes connects us to our creativity and flow. A greater sense of wholeness and fulfillment can come through awareness and curiosity.

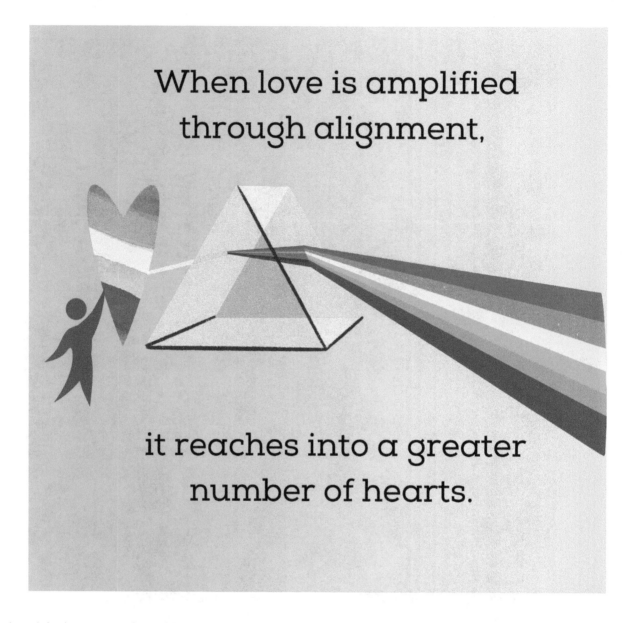

When love is amplified through alignment,

it reaches into a greater number of hearts.

The optics of the heart are reflected in what we see in the world. When how we love is congruent with our core values, synchronicity arrives more frequently, and connection becomes deeper. We begin loving our own truth and loving from it as well.

It's a kind of seeing that reminds me of the movie Avatar. When they intertwine the receptors at the end of their neural whip (it looks like hair), they see into each other's hearts. Finding precious moments of alignment within ourselves allows us to see beneath the chaos on the surface of another's behavior and truly see the stillness within them. You see them underneath all that. This makes it easier to let go of previous judgements or assumptions about the person in front of you.

Congruence feels like balance and aligned direction of vision, a clarity. It's not always easy to access or safe to share in certain situations, and honestly, it's not always well received when we do share it. Even if we don't share what we see in someone, at least we can offer love and compassion for whatever helps them keep on going, for their spirit, for the past and present versions of themselves, and for what they wish to be. We can hope for others to "see" us in this way and love us for what is.

Loving the world from a place of stillness and clarity holds power. It has the ability to touch the truth in the hearts of those around you. Rainbow beams of love to you!

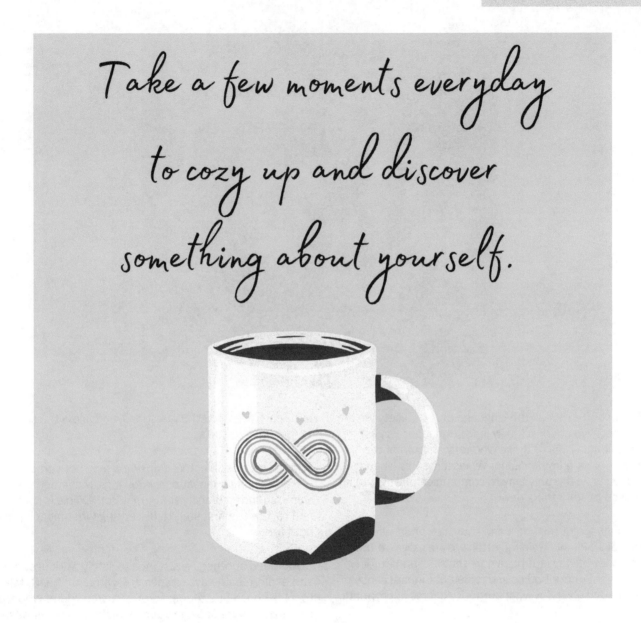

Take a few moments everyday to cozy up and discover something about yourself.

Continuous learning is such a gift. Humans have the capacity for reflection; the kind that leads to discovery. Create some comfort and ritual around this practice. When you cozy up, it's like a decadent treat that you give yourself that can allow your muscles to relax, your mind to wander, and your heart to dream. It's a space to breathe and notice what bubbles up to the surface of your consciousness.

An intentional pause in your day opens the gateway to creativity and possible solutions to challenges still being toiled over. A self-connection. What bubbles up may not always feel good, and when that happens, it's helpful to distance yourself from the thought by simply noticing that you are having it. Acknowledge the thought going through your mind and know that you need not do anything about it or assign any meaning to it at this time.

A simple ritual can prepare your body and mind to sink into this space. Many patients will say their body knows they are coming for massage therapy and will start to relax the moment they walk into my treatment room. Intentionally making your favorite mug of hot yumminess, running a bath, putting on a cozy sweater, finding your comfy chair, or moving to where you can look at the view that relaxes you, are all ways that prepare your consciousness for meaningful pause and reflection.

What action can you repeat daily that might center and ground you for meaningful rest and contemplation?

This can easily become one of your favorite parts of the day because it feels so nourishing to the soul.

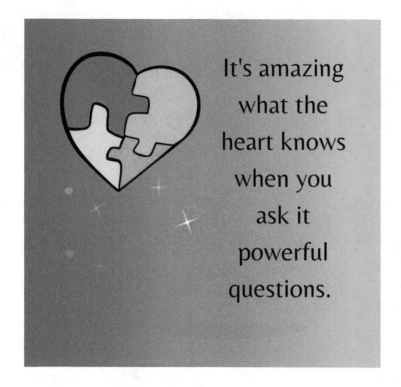

It's amazing what the heart knows when you ask it powerful questions.

We most often speak the language of the society we are born into. We unconsciously learn the nuances, gestures, and colloquialisms of those who raise us, and of the systems we are immersed in. We assume this language is the best way, the only way to communicate. Until we are exposed to something new.

The language of the heart and soul are not usually the focus of academic training; often we are asked to trade our "childish" ways for behaviors that feel unnatural to the rhythm of our bodies and forfeit our innate sense of trust in ourselves for what authority deems appropriate.

Because of, and in spite of, our early teachings, it can be surprising to what we call our rational minds, when we resonate with something that calls to our hearts. And yet, there is understanding deep down that we are connected to this calling, even if we don't yet understand the language.

This is why art serves to awaken the seeds of a sacred language within. Poetry, dance, music, visual art, all have the power to take our breath and simultaneously give it back to us with expansive depth. There are insufficient words to describe how powerful this feels, especially in the English language.

When we have an opportunity to explore and discover how our heart and soul wants to express and be heard, there can be a unique connection made. A thread of recognition begins to emerge when we speak directly to our heart, ask powerful questions, and allow the space for answers to surface.

Though it's possible, these answers may not come in words. Feelings, sensations, knowings, movement, energy shifts, sounds, colors, visions, may come. This is common and can be the first step to discerning what meaning they hold for us.

If you need another's assistance to safely ask questions and explore pathways to speaking with your heart, talk to a life coach or a therapist, or a trusted friend who truly prioritizes your pace and your capacity. You never need to continue with any one person if it doesn't feel right. Have conversations with different people until you feel safe and heard.

It can be a layered process, seeking the vernacular that beckons our truth. Once we feel what nourishes us to the core, it presents more readily, and when we continue to listen for the prose that feels right to our hearts and for our bodies, we begin to use it more often, and begin to ask for it from others and from our lives.

When we experience how beautiful life can be, when we truly see and accept ourselves, we are loathe to compromise our hearts any longer. We deserve to know and speak the language of our heart like it is poetry.

You will never regret learning how to translate the incredible things that your heart and soul want to say.

We are not responsible for how others respond to our joy.

I recently had someone in my home office who saw a photo of me in utter joy, standing under a drooping sunflower like it was a rain shower, wide smile on my face, hands up beside my head. They responded not with joy, but with what sounded like an utterance of suspicion, like they questioned my sanity. I did not take it to heart, for I know that it's not my joy they were responding to. More likely, it was an uncomfortable mirror for them to see that they could not access their own joy.

We are not responsible for how others perceive our creativity.

When I write my daily posts, I have no way of knowing who will see themselves in it, or who will be offended by my words. I post them anyway because they come from the heart. For me, writing is a creative joy. If my phrases resonate with another human heart, I am grateful. If my words reflect the judgement that lives inside another, I am grateful. My creativity is my sovereignty. Anyone has the ability to move on by if they don't like my style.

We are responsible for our boundaries*.

It is extremely hard to formulate and hold up our boundaries when nobody taught us what a boundary is, let alone how to make them. If you've never heard this word, congratulations! You have now. Ask about, talk to friends, find out what others do to make boundaries and respect them.

*If you have heard this word and have no idea what you're doing, congratulations! Many of us are stuck between the rocks and hard places when it comes to figuring out this balance. I would suggest reading Brene Brown. I am definitely in this category. It's a big learning curve.

*If you have heard this word and stick to them, congratulations! Brene Brown and the rest of the world reveres your superstar abilities!

The point is others will not know where your outward limits are unless you subtly or explicitly tell them. If people are constantly taking advantage of you, maybe look at where your boundaries have been unclear or non-existent.

We are responsible for our awareness.

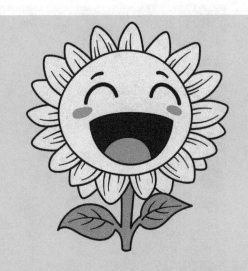

WE ARE NOT RESPONSIBLE FOR HOW OTHERS RESPOND TO OUR JOY.

We all have power. We have the capacity for reflection. Remember when you learned to read? Perhaps not, though some of you might. Can you remember your favorite song or movie, what you wore to your graduation, what some of your teachers' names were, what are the best books you've ever read? This is reflection of events, items, or people.

Self-reflection is being able to look at your behaviors, words, thoughts, actions, or feelings. This is noticing of our inner world. If self-awareness isn't a practice for you already, starting this habit is beneficial in order to understand patterns of thinking, notice belief systems, and recognize body sensations. This helps also in noticing the impact we have on our loved ones, our community, and our planet.

We are responsible for our peace.

We do not by any means, have to agree with others. We do, however, have the capacity to hold multiple emotions in our hearts and bodies, even if they contradict each other. Imagine peace at the center of the wheel of emotion and see the other multitudes of feelings as spokes coming from your center. How would you treat your thoughts or feelings knowing they arise out of a peaceful core?

Expressing my joy, my grief, my love, my disappointment... is my sovereignty.

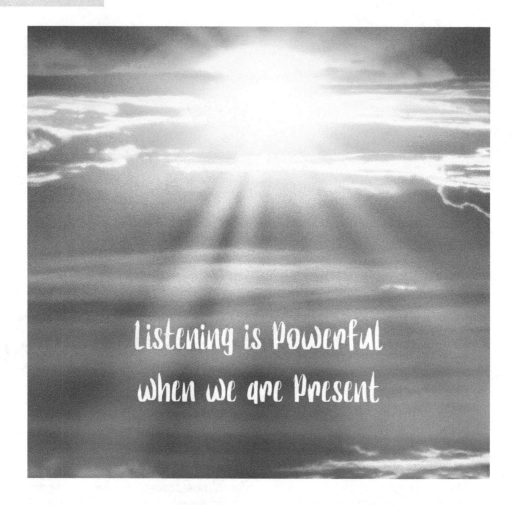

Listening is Powerful
when we are Present

The sun is not distracted in sharing its light, warmth, or energy. It has an impact on every life on the planet. Our atmosphere can block its view with clouds and stormy weather, but it is always present and consistent when we see beyond the changing surface layers.

Distracted listening is like blocking the sun with cloud cover. Our bodies feel when someone's attention is split; we intuitively stop sharing. Flow of energy is cut off. When this happens around babies, they feel something is wrong. Child development depends on connection with caregivers, so their nervous system reacts to this as a threat.

As adults, we can forget that we live in context to our connections. Just because we are older doesn't mean we don't need attention, touch, and connection.

With mini computers at our fingertips, we have become less aware of the moments moving by us. When we listen to others just enough to formulate a response, we miss the opportunity for real connection. When attention is divided, we have fewer memories of the time we spend with our loved ones.

Distracted listening is conditional and has the ability to undermine our relationships. We give our light, warmth, and energy to those we care about and cherish when we are present.

In my practice as an RMT and a teacher at a College of Massage, this has been and continues to be the number 1 skill that is lacking from caregivers, both in regard to my patients experiences with primary and allied health professionals, and from the awareness of a large percentage of students I have taught.

Healing begins from the moment people feel heard. Without focused attention, trust is quickly lost in the therapeutic relationship. Compassionate presence alone has the power to shift and uplift someone's energy and mood, relax the nervous system, and help another feel valued and cared for.

Listening can be taught and practiced. I witnessed this every single day as an instructor. These are beautiful moments of rising consciousness. If we are willing, we can become a wholly different society; if we learn, practice, and encourage intentional listening.

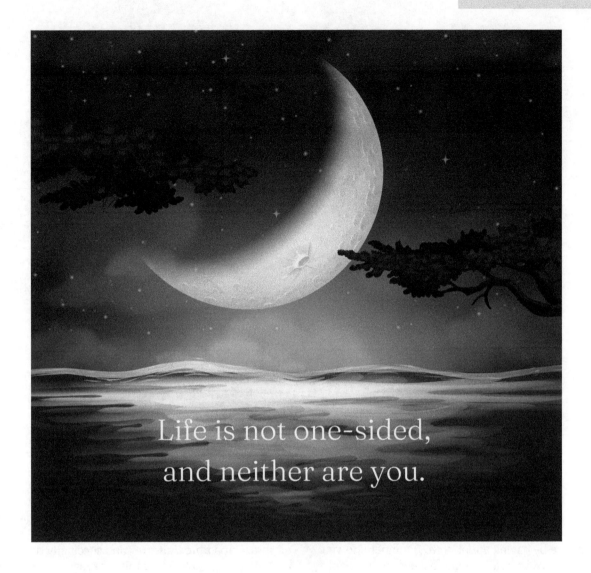

Life is not one-sided,
and neither are you.

I am a living, breathing paradox. I bet you are too. We have the capacity to hold multiple emotions in our hearts and bodies, even if they contradict each other. I can be angry, sad, grateful, and compassionate, all at once. I can feel these at the same time about the exact same circumstance. I may focus on one feeling over another, and still notice that the other ones are present.

I am not black and white and gray. I live with prisms of light and colour inside and surrounding me. I am buoyed by energy like I am floating on water. My reflection stares back at me from the surface of the water and from the surface of another's eyes, different every time based on the time of day, the colour of the sky, cloud cover, movement of the sun or moon, or ripples on the lake.

Epiphanies come often when I'm seeing myself reflected in another, whether that picture is whole or fragmented. The masterpiece of the complex human tries to be captured within one dimensional frames, and then are displayed in museums of good enough-ness and labeled "what we are supposed to strive for." Everyday put in boxes, labels, given ultimatums, choosing between the lesser of two evils.

Confined in a flat life, other possibilities seem risky and frivolous, unattainable, and sometimes unimaginable, until the inner urge of a soul driven, colorful life is such a force, that it blows over the one-sided frames of sterile living on the way to a messy, authentic joy.

Joy is messy and vulnerable. It can expose our soft layers of gratitude and humbleness and drop one-sided pretenses. When we discover that conditioning has flower-pressed us between the covers of a dusty, out of print book, though it can be a comforting space to hide, it stifles our visions of something more, our spectrums of fullness and ridiculously colourful reflections.

> ## We have the capacity to hold peace at our center,
>
> ## Even when challenged with difficult emotions.

Peace is part of our core, our soul. It lives within us, all around us, and connects us to everything. We learn to embody peace by paying attention to our inner knowing and making space to hear it. Some believe they cannot access peace. Though that may be true for the ego part of us, the deeper connection to soul is possible when we begin to feel our unfeigned voice becoming more evident.

This does not mean always being calm or is only for those in physical safety, as even Nelson Mandela, uncertain of his fate while in prison, was able to hold fast to his center of peace and truth.

These glimpses can come in many forms. A book we've read or a simple quote we've heard before lands differently and suddenly takes on new meaning. Experiences change our perspective. A conversation can touch something deep within. A line in a movie can resonate in a way we've never noticed before. Connection to nature, a sunrise, a rain shower, can move us in a sincere way.

These moments are further explored by opening to signs of connection and meaning that fill the heart and by noticing sensations of clarity.

Learning how soul speaks to us takes commitment and sparks excitement when we notice one feeling, word, or phrase at a time that truly and succinctly describes us. Being open to learning this language enhances the frequency with which we feel it happening. As a result, we begin to understand its cadence until we reach some form of fluency. Like noticing all the red cars once you start driving a red car.

Practice visualization: Imagine peace sitting comfortably rooted at your solar plexus, expanding down through your feet and up through the top of your head, flowing to every cell in your body, encircling your physical and non-physical being.

Holding us grounded, peace can anchor the emotions we experience through the day. Picturing peace as the sun within us, and every other emotion as a solar flare that rises and shrinks, forever moving, throwing off heat and intensity, then calming again, may be a helpful visual to lead us back to ourselves. The awareness of peace guides us home as we pivot away and toward our center, an ebb and flow, through challenging moments.

My heart cannot bear to witness someone being stripped of their dignity. It is a deep wound. This is why I choose to support those who often feel ignored and abondoned. and to work toward improving systems that let so many fall through the cracks.

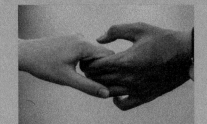

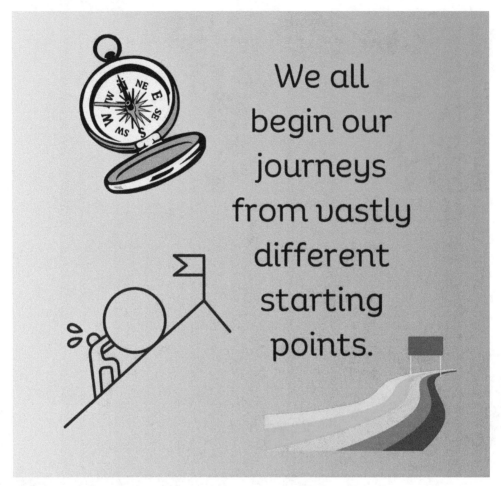

We all begin our journeys from vastly different starting points.

We don't all start from the same place.

Equity is not apparent, not ubiquitously understood. Marginalization puts people far behind any semblance of a starting line. The various layers and levels of privilege account for endless differing awareness of the struggles or ease of life and capacity for reaching goals.

Way too many people face struggles that are unimaginable to others, and by the time they begin a journey, they have already jumped over, moved around, or painstakingly sludged through self-judgement, societal pressures, biases, discrimination, shadow work, and the many, many other roadblocks of acculturation.

My personal brand of trauma includes abandonment, financial PTSD, not good enough-ness, and imposter syndrome. Being a woman has also peppered my psyche with an unhealthy dose of internalized misogyny. All of this translates into a soundtrack of beliefs on replay, which were unconscious for far too long and still sometimes are.

These beliefs trigger tunes like, "how dare you make money," "you don't deserve more, you should be thankful for the life you have as is," "nobody will love you for who you are, your needs don't matter," "why would you write, you don't have a PhD, people will think you're a fraud." Thankfully, a lot of shadow exploration has brought these to my awareness, where I can more easily hold them with compassion.

These are some of the reasons and thoughts I overcome, sometimes on a daily or hourly basis. In order to continue to write, why I finally furthered my education at 38 years old, why I waited to write a book and start a passionate organization until I was 50.

The societal structures of racism, sexism, classism, ageism, and so many more isms, insidiously train people how to think, and plant fear into minds and media, even when they are detrimental and counterintuitive to our own health and expansion.

There must be room at starting lines for the fullness of what this means. Room for a whole person to stand beside us with their entire past, their complex needs, and their internal paradoxes. Space to hold each other with compassion is made when we discover the soundtracks we have on repeat and explore our own incongruous barriers to movement.

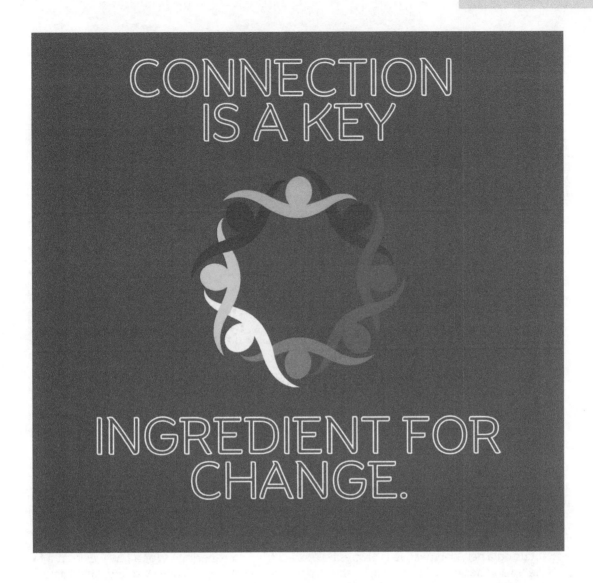

"A dream you dream alone is only a dream. A dream you dream together is reality." - John Lennon

It takes courage to discuss what you stand for and what you believe in. Remaining ambiguous is a way to stay invisible, unnoticed, unchallenged. Stepping out of ambiguity feels safer when we understand our core values and consistently attempt to live in integrity with them. This will draw others that embody similar values. This is when connection is born.

Challenge, I found, is a great way to discover the strength of our roots. Just like a tree in a windstorm, the foundations of our root systems are hauled on, and can uncover areas of vulnerability. A consistent wind can gently tug on the connections we've made within ourselves and to our ground, building exposure to other things that feel risky. This builds capacity for opening to greater challenges.

For example, I began speaking my truth on a daily basis through these posts and micro blogs one year ago. This has led me to consistent writing, less fear of not being perfect before I post something, cultivating my creativity, and connecting with others. Thanks for this goes to Simone Grace Seol for her garbage post challenge.

I kept parts of me hidden for years, maybe decades, for fear of judgement. I even wrote most of a book without feedback from anyone. Eventually, my commitment to creating a sense of belonging for others grew so large that it made my fear seem much smaller.

Sharing a process, sharing values, sharing a perspective, or sharing a meal, all contribute to connection. When I dared to share what was important to me, it opened my heart, gave me a stronger voice, my values an outlet, and connected me with my community. Echoing what I've said before, "It only takes one conversation to find those who want to change the world with you."

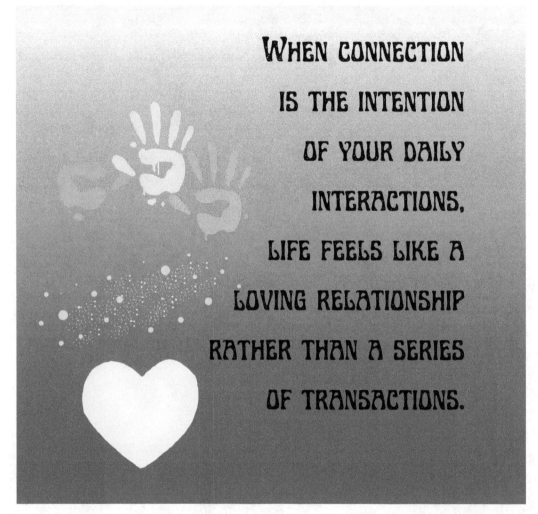

WHEN CONNECTION IS THE INTENTION OF YOUR DAILY INTERACTIONS, LIFE FEELS LIKE A LOVING RELATIONSHIP RATHER THAN A SERIES OF TRANSACTIONS.

The choice to focus on a new perspective is always a possibility. Wake up and decide to let love make the decisions today, even if all circumstances are exactly the same as yesterday. There are millions of perspectives to choose from.

Sink into the most loving thought you can find and connect with it. Love it, and visualize it, loving you. Then go about your day, looking at everything you do with love. Ask yourself, how would love brush its teeth, or make breakfast, or enjoy food, how would it look at other commuters or interact with co-workers? How would it treat itself, would it forgive easier, rest more willingly, nourish itself with awareness, connection, and kind thoughts? How would it treat others?

If you thought about how to best connect with those you encounter in your day, what would you focus on? Do you believe communication would improve with those at work or at home? Might you relate to one another more consistently if daily intentions included cultivating relationships?

I tried an experiment for a few weeks at a fairly new job I held years ago. While I worked, I held an undercurrent of intention in mind to find a simple connection with every single staff member that I worked with on a daily basis. Because this was on my radar as a goal, my psyche pointed out any little thread that I could tug on that might create a bridge between my heart and theirs.

After a few weeks, the experiment felt like a river of miracles. One by one, something in common would surface that increased the pleasure in our interactions until there were actual connections discovered in the colliding of two worlds. At least, two of my different worlds came together when a co-worker realized she was a great friend of my sisters when they were younger. We just hadn't recognized each other.

Most humans have the capacity to hold more than one intention in mind, especially if each day consists of routine. If you've never played with a full day of curiosity and relational intention, why not try it tomorrow and see what happens?

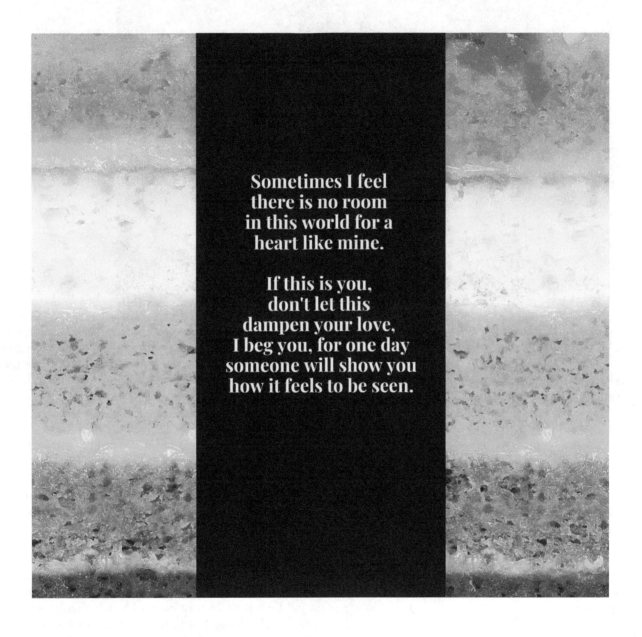

Sometimes I feel
there is no room
in this world for a
heart like mine.

If this is you,
don't let this
dampen your love,
I beg you, for one day
someone will show you
how it feels to be seen.

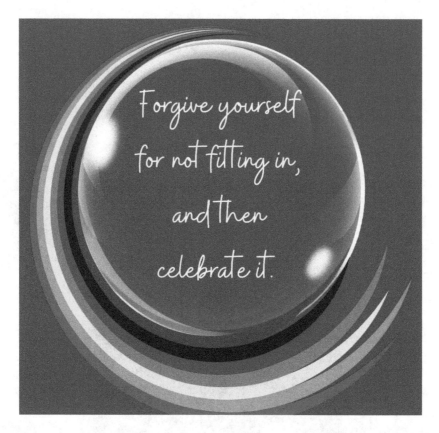

Forgive yourself for not fitting in, and then celebrate it.

Fear of not fitting in shakes the core of our security, as if we might die laying in the outskirts of safety.

Fitting in looks very different to the varied cultures in our ever-expanding universe.

Status quo changes drastically as time goes by, knowledge grows, and awareness becomes deeper.

We look outside of ourselves for approval, belonging, and acceptance. The communities we are surrounded by most of the time are the cultures that we judge ourselves by subconsciously. Even if aware of the culture, whether we align or agree with it or not, being part of it holds something meaningful for us. We may feel belonging, we may feel separated from it, or somewhere in between. Awareness of this helps determine the attachment we wish to have to this space and culture.

Societal status quo, workplace culture, family dynamics, country, city, or town traditions, religious groups, educational institutions, friends, children, and partners, all have a pull on our hearts and occupy space in our minds.

When we focus on aligning with the culture around us, we can easily forget to align with the wisdom inside.

When we acknowledge groups or dynamics that don't feel good, we can seek places and people who do. Recognizing our alignment gives us the ability to follow creative pursuits and spaces that make us come alive.

Growing up, my parents were not very tolerant of my naturally inquisitive mind nor my sensitive heart. I asked a lot of questions. I was often told "you're too analytical, too sensitive, you can't save everyone." I had a sense of injustice when I was told to stop talking. I understand now that they didn't know how to handle me because of their own upbringing and trauma, but at the time I had to fit in at home or make my life miserable.

I eventually found my voice again through friends and experiences that embraced my inquisitive nature, my desire for learning, and my wholeness of emotions. The injustice I felt turned into a core value of human dignity, wanting to afford it for those I had the power to give it. Combined with my love for humanity, I pursued work in helping professions, which to this day is very fulfilling, and has led me to seek more loving ways to care for others.

Noticing what's going on inside in any situation is always enlightening, whether in full joy being present, or withdrawn because something doesn't feel right. Celebrate the knowing inside. Notice when the culture doesn't fit and create the life that honors you instead.

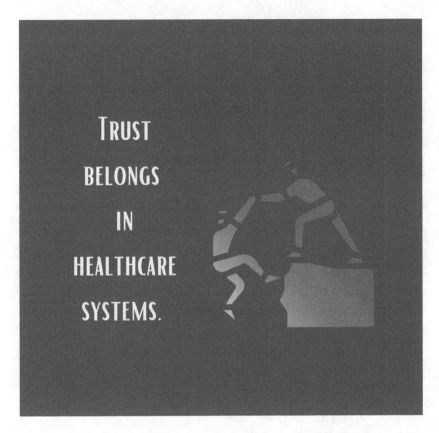

TRUST
BELONGS
IN
HEALTHCARE
SYSTEMS.

If only love was most prominent and creating trust was best practice,

If sharing the feeling of welcome was regarded higher than self-protection,

If humanity and dignity were worth more than money,

Would we create communities of love, welcome, and caring.

If being seen and accepted for who we are instead of suppressing the true nature within,

If opening our doors and arms to create safety and belonging mattered more than individualistic hoarding,

If presence and stillness were practiced in abundance rather than only efficiency and productivity,

Would we then feel more sacred.

If peeling back surface layers and getting to what's truest and real wasn't just a woke phrase,

When we can introduce ourselves in the purest sense of self,

And share experiences with others that allow us to understand how they feel deep inside,

Will we then feel the connectedness of all things.

Listening is active.

Love is an action, an energetic decision.

Kind touch is necessary.

Awareness of sensations increases inner wisdom.

We live in context with our connections.

Fear must not hold us back any longer.

It is time to act on love and open to the freedom we crave to express and deeply connect.

To offer wellness in our systems of health, we must hold each other with compassion, cultivate trust through our actions, be accountable to the equal thriving of the humans we serve, and develop responsibility for the humans we are.

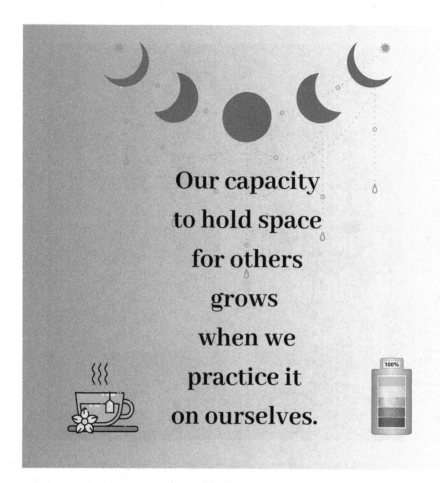

Our capacity
to hold space
for others
grows
when we
practice it
on ourselves.

Few things prepare us to hold another in their pain, like the experience of being held in our own pain. Similar to doctors who have felt their own experience of what a patient is facing, tend to have more empathy, we can offer support for others because we can relate. We don't need to have the same experience to offer compassion, as we understand the feeling of being in the grips of pain.

In my experience as a massage therapist, I see a great number of patients who struggle to his space for their own discomfort, whether physical or emotional. As a society, we have perfected the art of distraction. We have been taught to hoodwink ourselves into thinking we're "fine" when we are so far from it, we don't even recognize our true selves anymore.

There are limited opportunities to learn about and practice facing our fears, specifically with a trusted individual to hold space, offer compassion, and witness our discomfort in order to process our pain. We can utilize therapies and coaching, and some education and programs can introduce us to these practices, but it is far from accessible to everyone.

Because of this, fear and hopelessness are prevalent as a first response to emotional discomfort. I am often asked how I manage my emotions as a sensitive soul and caregiver for the elderly and the dying.

It is still challenging to sit with my own discomfort and explore the darkness within me, though it has become so much easier over the last decade. As I've learned to regulate my nervous system, my capacity to be a compassionate witness for others has grown.

I am drawn to continuous learning and feel the need to continually explore my ever-evolving thoughts and feelings, what they mean, where they came from, to question my beliefs and the lenses I perceive others through. I seek to distill meaning from experiences and patterns and discover epiphaneal relationships.

Awareness of how we impact our relationships with communication, presence, and our ability to sit with others during challenging and terminal experiences is profound and life-altering. Continual practice within will ultimately expand our capacity to be with others in their truth.

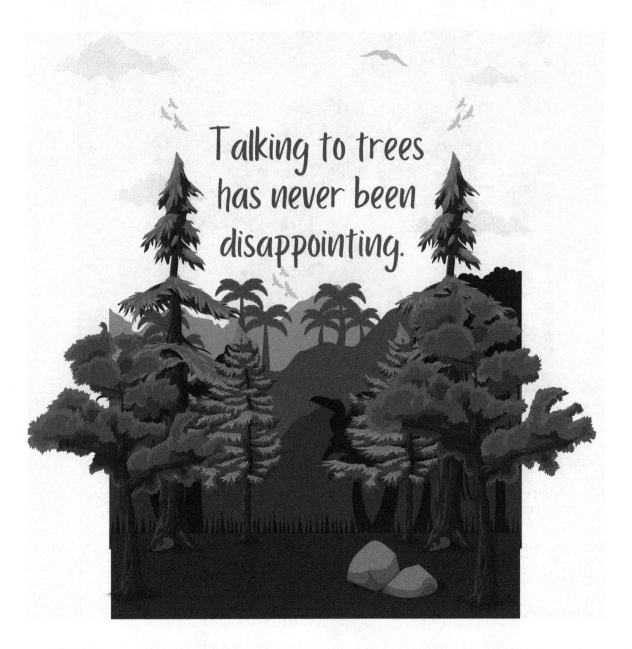

Talking to trees
has never been
disappointing.

Whether we need companionship, someone to listen, or a deep sense of ancient belonging and centering, the forest is family.

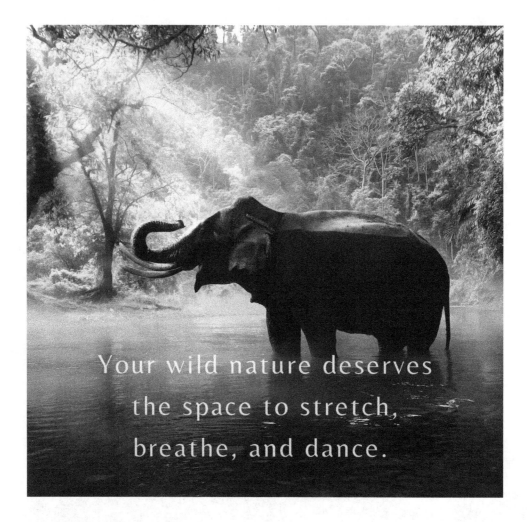

Your wild nature deserves
the space to stretch,
breathe, and dance.

What is good enough, what is fine?

Do you wonder if there's more, if you deserve more?

Where does your heart wander when you daydream, when you dream in the night?

What do you hope to one day feel?

Fulfillment, joy, peace, exuberance, bounty?

Why then accept mediocrity?

Is it scary to look at desires, to imagine wholeness, to wonder how it would feel to access your beauty, to breathe deep, to open up? Is it too hard, too vulnerable?

Do you feel cramped in a small container of expectations and obligations?

What would relief sound like?

How would freedom taste?

What sensations form in your body when you envision your inner wilds being fully formed in tangible reality?

How do you hold your body, how do you move when you imagine liberation?

How would you dance if your wild nature had room to stretch out? Can you picture it?

In one-year, what feelings do you want to be experiencing daily? In 5 years? In 10?

What tiny actions could move you toward living in your unique creativity, fully breathing, and opening to your truest sense of connection? What could you do today that your future self will have extreme gratitude for?

I will applaud your courage to keep
breathing.
I will praise your strength to look
inward.
I will honor the speed of your
process.

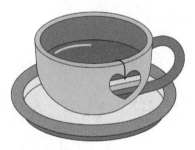

Your soul knows the way. It takes time to uncover what we know deep inside. Sometimes, we know right away what we need to do. Instinct can take over in situations that feel urgent on one end of the spectrum and in circumstances that don't elicit strong feelings and are easy to make decisions about on the other end.

For example, calling emergency services immediately after witnessing an accident or a first responder acting on training and instinct to assist someone in need. Decisions that are easy, like choosing a snack or going to sleep when tired are ways we exercise our knowing.

What about all the things in between instinctual and easy? Perhaps something like deciding to leave a job or a relationship, set a boundary, engage in therapy, figure out what step to take next, ask for help.

Why is it harder to decide what to wear to a fancy event than to an exercise class? Because of the importance we put on it.

We think about how others will react, how we feel in the outfit, is it too much or underwhelming, the restriction or freedom to move, and how long we can maintain any slight discomfort caused by wearing it. Similar thoughts apply to a plethora of decisions, big or small.

The clothes or the masks we put on impact our relationships with others and are also profound to the relationship we have with ourselves. The more we are able to align with what feels like freedom and mobility in our true skin, the more we become comfortable with the fluidity of our inner decision maker, our intuition, and wisdom.

If this part of you is clouded and difficult to access, looking inward is a useful practice. This often takes courage, commitment, breath, stillness, and many breaks. Diving deep and fast is bound to be overwhelming for anyone. Inquiring within for short periods and with consistency will bring up questions as well as some clarity.

Having curiosity for decisions and inner reactions helps us learn what feels right. Listening for what rises within and paying attention to body sensations give us practice at aligning with self, which in turn grows confidence in who we truly are.

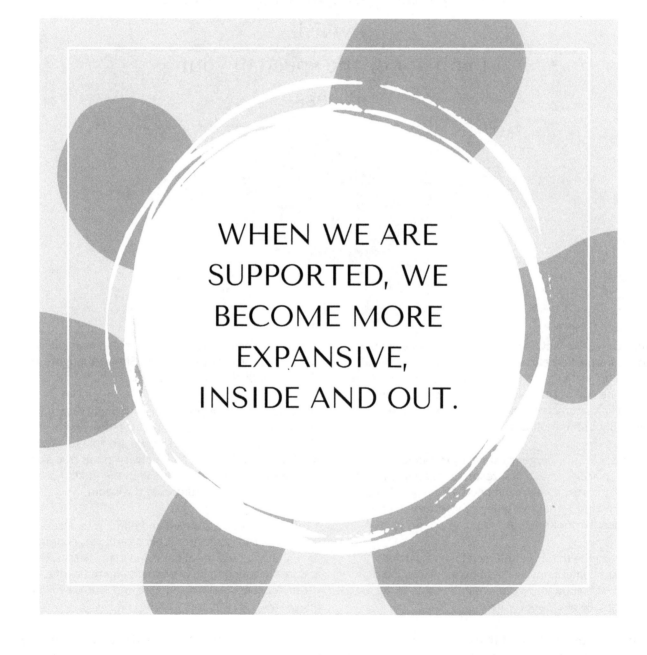

WHEN WE ARE
SUPPORTED, WE
BECOME MORE
EXPANSIVE,
INSIDE AND OUT.

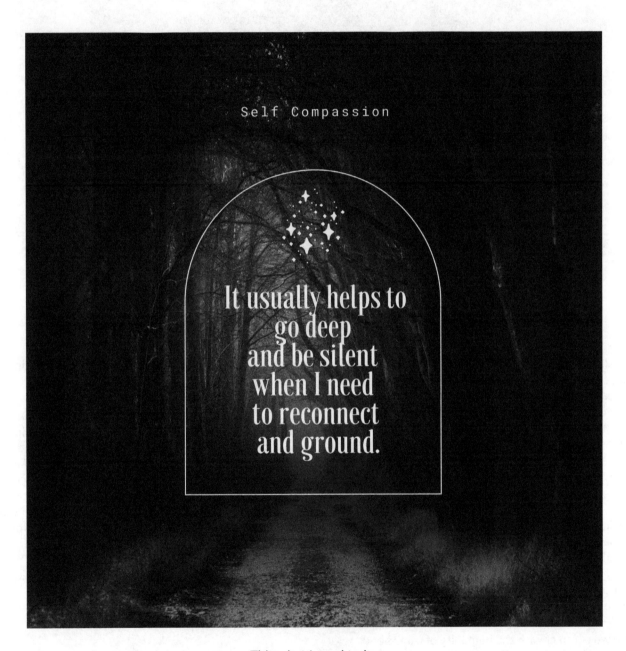

Self Compassion

It usually helps to
go deep
and be silent
when I need
to reconnect
and ground.

This what I need today.

What is it you truly need in this moment?

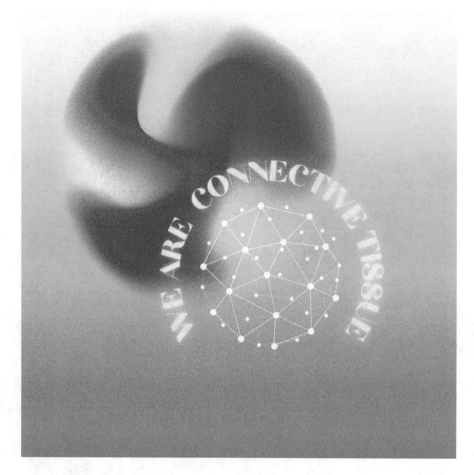

We are all connective tissue. Connective tissue connects and holds our pieces together. Just like mycelial networks help trees communicate and whole forests to thrive, our wellness depends on the connection we have with others in our lives. Spores are always present in soil, and when a nourishing environment is created, they will grow and fruit mushrooms all over the place. We are like fungi, connecting what feeds us to our environments, our relationships, to nature.

The environment we create within and around us affects our loved ones, our relations, our homes, and our own cells. We become the sinew of curated moments. The energy we hold and carry everywhere generates vastly different feedback and responses to who we are vibrationally and what we bring into our daily interactions.

How do we connect with the humanity of others and combine it with professionalism, with love and safety, and the relief that being seen offers? Take identity for example. Who we believe ourselves to be can impact how we treat ourselves and others. This in turn will have an effect on how others see you. Exploring the integrity of our outer shells with our inner self can help us discover how to align

with the impact we wish to have on our surroundings and relationships.

We have the responsibility of awareness if we want to understand the impact we have on our relationships, to recognize the building blocks of our special kind of connective tissue. What is the foundation of the layered fibers of our being, the tension that holds our pieces together? How do we share the spaces between our solid parts and how does this offering contribute to structural safety for connection with those we serve, live with, love, and nurture?

My connective tissues are love, care, nurturing, listening, touch. Sometimes I connect via fear or worry, but hopefully less so. What I feed myself becomes the foundation of the fibers I extend and proliferate.

What we carry within us IS connective tissue. The question is how do we want it to shape our relationships, and to buffer the systems we allow to shape us? Have you noticed what you bring with you everywhere?

We experience cycles of birth, life, and death, not only in the length of a lifetime,

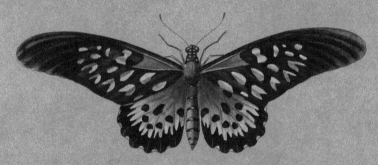

but everyday and in every breath.

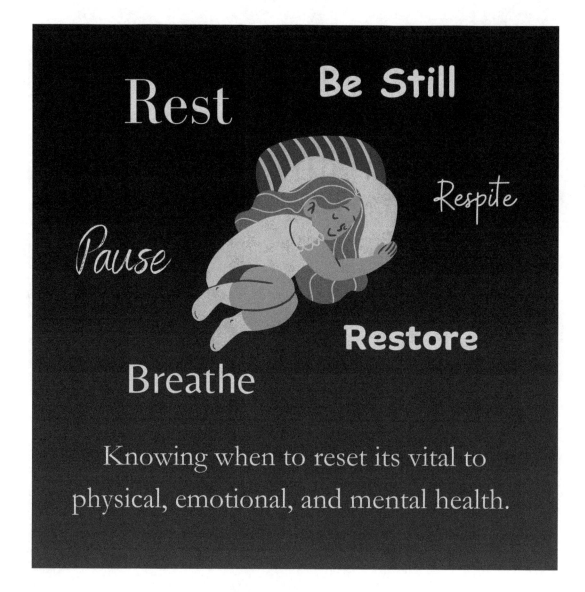

Rest

Be Still

Respite

Pause

Restore

Breathe

Knowing when to reset its vital to physical, emotional, and mental health.

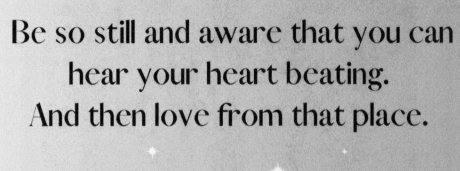

> Be so still and aware that you can
> hear your heart beating.
> And then love from that place.

Listening to a heartbeat is primal in rhythm and connection to our most basic biology.

It is the first sound that surrounds us in our watery home. We feel it as it moves through us. It calms us and rocks us and communicates to us that we are not alone.

Love infuses into us as our hearts grow.

It is a pulse that we carry with us. We can get quiet and listen in when we need it. It connects us to the heartbeat of the planet, to the trees, rivers, and oceans. When we are sad, water holds us, and rhythm soothes us. When we are joyful, we can dance jubilantly to its music.

When I feel really emotionally challenged, I throw myself to the earth to sync heartbeats. Laying close with the ground or being wrapped by water helps me listen for the whispers of my soul. Trees can ease your pain if you talk to them. The sea accepts your tears and pounds loudly with your rage and lets you be anything you need to be, without judgement.

All emotions are acceptable. They don't arise just to be dismissed or hidden. When we hold them and feel their intensity, we are seen and whole. It feels profoundly different to love from this place of acceptance. What do you notice about your heartbeat?

Seeing others in their
wholeness

opens a space
for them to exist fully.

What could be if you could see
The entirety of a person behind their eyes
Like a flash of their life
Their love and their strife
From birth until this moment
Would you then see how
Their darkness effects them
Making it hard to hold a gaze
Praying to God it's just a phase
Like the family, the priest, the others keep saying
The fear, the hurt, the anger
The unrequited love
The hopes they keep hidden
Even to their therapist
Silent desperation corroding their dreams
Could you hold curiosity and compassion
For the half life of their heart
Could you connect, ask questions
Or would you walk by like you do now
Would you hide who you are, for fear of being seen
Every person has a story behind their eyes
We can see it if we choose to
We all have capacity for curiosity
For connection
How would it change them
How would it change you

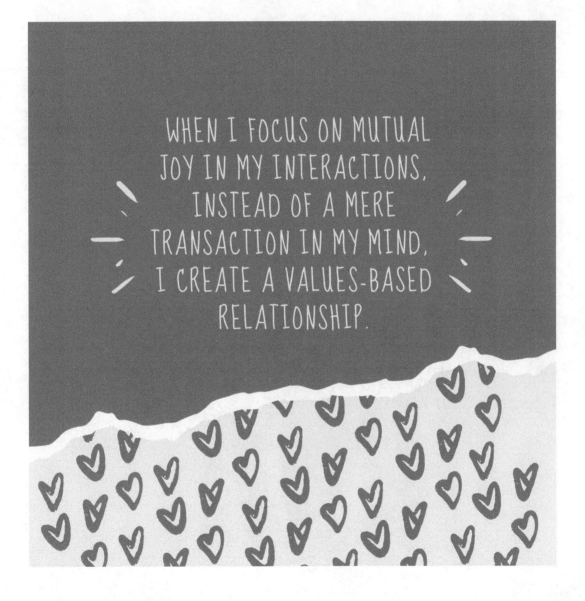

WHEN I FOCUS ON MUTUAL JOY IN MY INTERACTIONS, INSTEAD OF A MERE TRANSACTION IN MY MIND, I CREATE A VALUES-BASED RELATIONSHIP.

There is a difference

BETWEEN BEING WEARY
FROM TRAVELING DOWN
THE PATH OF HARD TRUTHS
AND THE EXHAUSTION OF
INAUTHENTICITY.

A moment

that is
juicy and human
obliterates the
blocks of
apathy and fear.

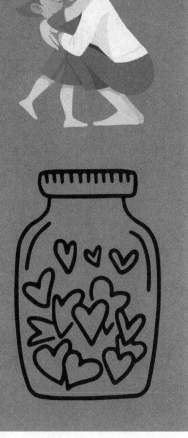

One caring touch
CAN CHANGE SOMEONE'S
WHOLE WORLD, WAKE UP A HEART,
CREATE A CONNECTION, BOLSTER
A SENSE OF BELONGING,
AND MAKE SENSE OF EMOTIONS.

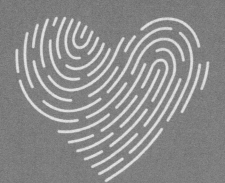

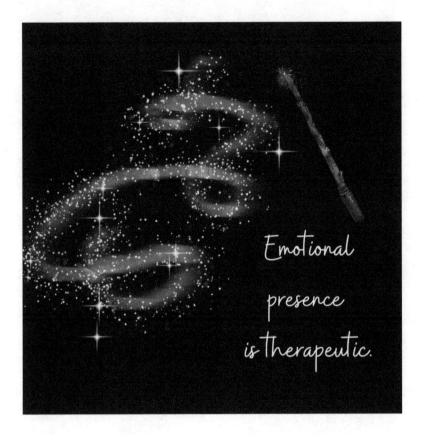

Emotional

presence

is therapeutic.

Many people go a very long time without talking about how they truly feel. Sometimes that's because they have nobody to talk to, nobody to trust, didn't know how to say it, felt too scared or embarrassed, or didn't know how to feel or describe the emotions.

There were several circumstances in my young life that taught me that my feelings were not valid, were not safe, were too much, were unlovable, and needed to be hidden. As a child of the 70's, or maybe of just my family, I felt like we raised ourselves. I was very lucky to have older siblings and cousins to experience life through, though babes raising babes didn't always turn out for the best.

By the time I was in my first serious relationship, my emotional communication skills were messy and immature. Sure, that's to be expected at a young age, but as an inquisitive soul that had a subconscious need to hide my truth, emotional conversations were often disastrous and incomprehensible.

It was a frustrating scenario all around.

I was so fortunate to be part of a course in my young adulthood that taught me life-changing communication skills, conflict resolution, how to go deep and safely and compassionately question my thoughts and feelings, to recognize and explore the patterns that continually affected my actions. We practiced empathy, how to give and receive feedback, and heightened emotional awareness. This foundation changed everything.

This learning and practice led to uncountable discoveries and capacity for holding space for myself and others. Lots of people feel lost when faced with another's pain or discomfort. And equally so with their own. One solution is to not try to find a solution. People crave to be heard and held in their pain.

As a massage therapist, I don't fix anybody. I hold them in their pain, and they begin to heal themselves. Many times, my patients start to feel better the moment they walk into my office, or before they leave home for their treatment. Their nervous system intuitively knows it will be seen today.

Observation changes the outcome. Not doing anything except noticing is magical. Presence is healing. Just being present is the therapy. Practice being there for yourself, and then practice with others. Notice what happens when you DO nothing else.

You hold this magic within you.

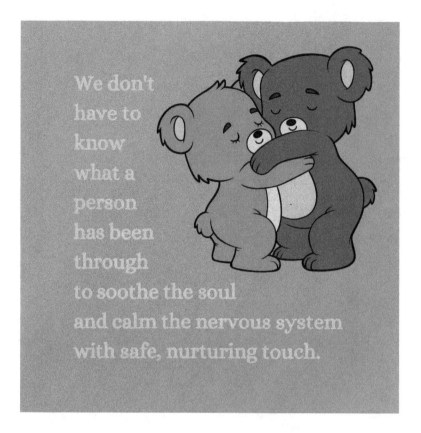

We don't have to know what a person has been through to soothe the soul and calm the nervous system with safe, nurturing touch.

Research has found that the nervous system becomes regulated with the presence of compassion. Though it can be proven scientifically, it doesn't mean we didn't already know this. People from all walks of life have neural networks that respond to their environments and to each other.

Dr. Peter Levine, founder of Somatic Experiencing, extensively studied the effect of presence on humans during stressful events and discovered how profoundly calming it is for a compassionate witness to say I'm here with you. This one thing can mean the difference between someone being traumatized by an experience or not.

As an RMT, I've treated many with Parkinson's disease, known for the tremors it causes throughout the body. The disease affects the central nervous system, the brain and spinal cord, and kills the cells that make dopamine. In my experience, tremors seem to be an external indicator of what's happening in the nervous system. My patients' shaking would increase with activation of the nervous system, whether emotional stress or activity, such as moving from their scooter to laying down on the massage table.

Inversely, tremors would calm with soothing treatment. This was most profoundly noted at a senior's home

outreach with my students, where a gentleman we cared for experienced intense and consistent tremors. The movement it took to get him comfortable on the massage table, and certain paces of treatment showed an increase in activation.

I watched my student for a few minutes while trying different techniques. She became more concerned as this patients' shaking only increased with her treatment. She looked over at me for help. I asked her to join me in a sustained compression of his legs. This meant we each placed our hands, one above the knee and one below, slowly compressed into the tissue and waited.

3 minutes later, his muscles seemed to melt into the table as he completely relaxed. My students' jaw fell open in surprise and relief as he snoozed. This is a consistent outcome for patients with Parkinson's and serves as a visual representation of down-regulation of the central nervous system.

Presence is therapeutic.

Nurturing touch has profound effect.

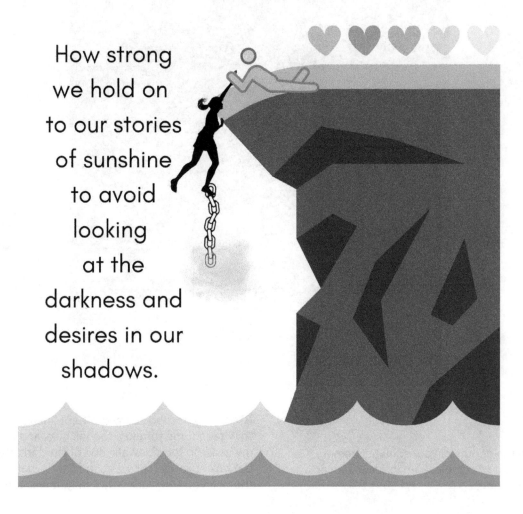

How strong
we hold on
to our stories
of sunshine
to avoid
looking
at the
darkness and
desires in our
shadows.

Isn't it strange that people often hide in the sunshine, in daylight, in happy, in faux smiles? Is it defense, deflection, avoidance?

For fear of not fitting in, of abandonment, of judgement, of real connection and closeness to another, of vulnerability?

We carry untruths with us and present them to those we meet. To save time, to save face, to avoid feeling? Have we become such a convenient society that we no longer care who we interact with? Or is every face we see a reflection of us, so we can't bear to look?

Are you hiding from others? Are you hiding from yourself?

The thoughts we repeat endlessly become the walls we're stuck behind, believing there is something wrong with us. We forget about our wholeness, our humanness, the

inevitable messiness of life, and that every human has the same doubts. Why do we hide that from all the perfectly imperfect beings we love?

Why has honesty become so hard to share, to be?

Brené Brown's research has shown that every person has known or will know the feeling of shame. She also says, "Shame depends on me buying into the belief that I'm alone. Shame cannot survive being spoken. It cannot survive empathy."

Being honest with ourselves is the first challenge in creating a loving community of support around us. This takes commitment and courage. Learning how to hold space for ourselves and to share with a trusted other are incredibly profound ways to awaken openness, awareness, and movement within us.

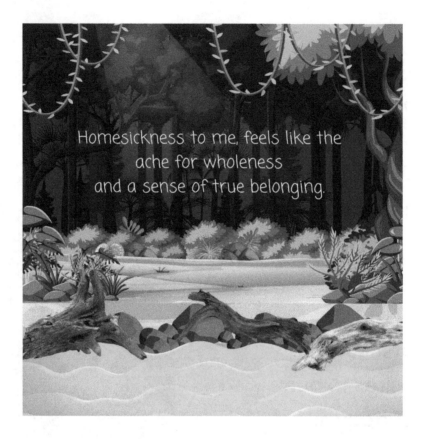

Homesickness to me, feels like the ache for wholeness and a sense of true belonging.

What is home?

Reach back into the depths of your somatic memory. Can you recall a moment of complete, unabridged, uncensored, perspicacious knowing?

No ambiguity, no confusion, no distrust.

Just clarity and assuredness.

For me, there are few I can recall. Though my memory of actual events may be spotty and fluffed up by my brain for lack of exactness, the feelings I had are discernable and unshakeable.

I was 7 years old. I was in a gang. The fierce pack of neighborhood kids was indomitable. Our ages ranged from 6 to 16. We were adventurous explorers, we fed and nurtured each other with love and popsicles, we had each other's backs, and we stuck together through hell or high water.

We would play in the nearby creek on hot and dusty summer days. We would beg cars to drive through huge puddles on rainy days to soak us with spray. Someone put mud on my bee sting at the creek, we would cheer on my cousin barreling down the not-yet-landscaped dirt hill on a

BMX, we watched as my brother filmed skateboard videos, they taught me to ride a too tall bike, and when I fell and hit my head on the sidewalk, one of the gang dads took me to the hospital. My fear was comforted when the group called the dead on the Ouija board (hey, it was the end of the 70s).

My sisters would play dancing queen so that I would get out of bed and come for breakfast (the only thing I loved more than sleep was music). I felt known. Belonging lived in my bones, my skin, my heart.

The way we left that neighborhood was not ideal as it did not give me a chance for goodbyes or closure and, among other reasons, ultimately contributed to my fear of abandonment and my need for long goodbyes. Despite all this, I carry the wholeness and acceptance I felt there within me.

Many people have the feeling that something is missing in their lives, but they can't figure out exactly what that is. For me, my soul is my home. My body is my home. I've noticed that the ache I have experienced came to me at times when I felt disconnected from belonging to myself. This is why community means so much to me. Why our village is so important. We all need a fierce neighborhood gang.

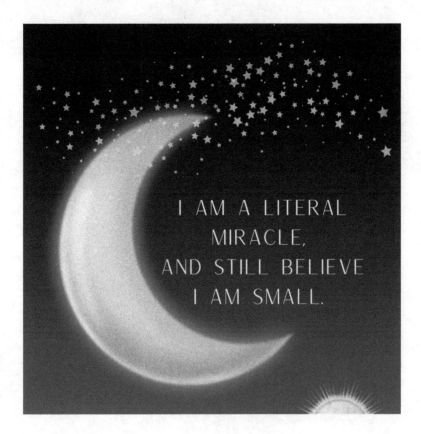

I'm an oxymoron. I accept that I see through the lens of my upbringing, my environment, my biases, belief systems, culture, and its expectations. I believe that I am inconsequential and super powerful at the same time.

I am this mish mash of emotions, philosophical seeking, analytical thinking, a sense of spiritual oneness, and a social identity. I titrate between details and complexities of daily life and the connection between all things and that nothing material really matters because it's all made up by our brains.

I've been told I think too much, that I ask too many questions. Even though many people enjoy the chance to talk about themselves, I've experienced that it's only to a point. If they feel challenged by uncommon inquiries, exploration may not be as welcome, especially if vulnerability is involved. I may be too much for some folks, but that doesn't mean I'm too much in general.

Some folks have also opined that I'm too sensitive, too loving, that my openness and desire to help others would get me hurt. Looking back, there were definitely times I was taken advantage of. However, I view those times as discoveries along my journey. They helped me learn to trust myself more, what I didn't want in my life, and to ultimately find what felt good.

What I'm told are just someone's projections. I've adopted some things as true or rejected as not for me. These include the commonalities of a culture I was born into. The constructs of a society that, for the most part, agree on general concepts of propriety, business, and government structure.

Of course, there are outliers and differing opinions when we look at details, processes and best practices, but what I find curious is the lack of discourse in our daily lives that we still know so little, in a world that seems to know it all.

Ironically, the more we discover, the less we know for sure. The systems we've built to create order have contributed to the loss of connection to humanity and, as a result, proposed such limitations to the imagination of those that live here.

My point of all this ponderous vomitus is that we interact with the guesses our brains make about what's happening around us. And maybe that there is no common reality. In this case, why aren't we dreaming and scheming way more? If our cells have designed such miracles of our bodies and minds, and if we hold limitless creative potential, how hard would it be to make a few things better for everyone on the planet? Hmmm?

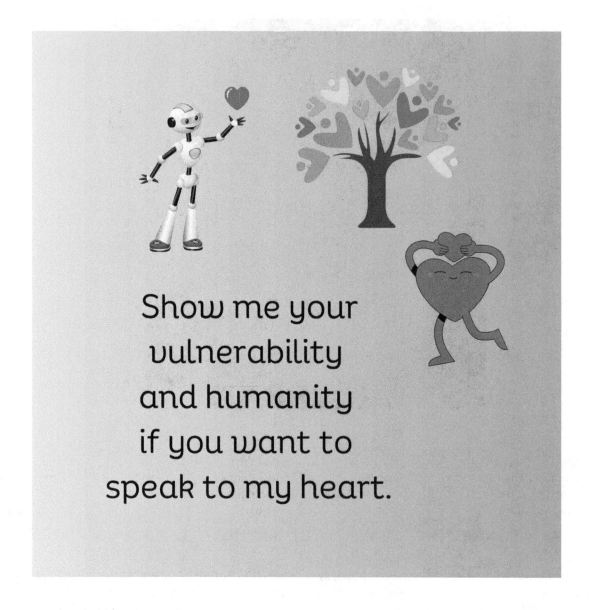

Show me your
vulnerability
and humanity
if you want to
speak to my heart.

Are you willing to be vulnerable in order to cultivate fulfillment in business, relationships, and with creativity?

I'm feeling reflective on the nature of sales industries. The last several months on LinkedIn, I've had a barrage of connection requests, who then turn around and try to sell me something through a private message in the same day. This feels slimy and disingenuous.

People crave to be known and to feel a sense of belonging. The mom-and-pop shop down the street who know your name and your kids' names. They know your favorite products and see you through good and hard times, because of the relationship you've created together. They are appreciated and so are you.

There is so much lost to pushiness and a lack of caring who your customer is. This relates to our relationships also. When they are one-sided, people feel neglected and unimportant.

Vulnerability creates connection, not small talk or pushing sales. I am not compelled to buy from you if you don't care to know who I am or why I do what I do. If you care first about people and your relationship to them, they will eventually trust and be honest with you. That's connection.

I feel honoured in friendships and professional relationships when others can be as vulnerable with me as I am with them.

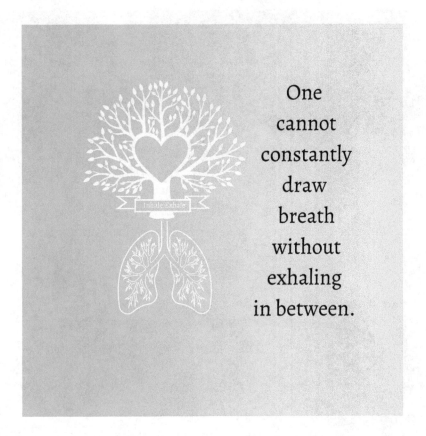

One
cannot
constantly
draw
breath
without
exhaling
in between.

Learning isn't always about growth and expansion. Sometimes, it's about devolving and restructuring.

We hear the phrases, growth economy, and growth mindset thrown around a lot. Personal discovery and gaining knowledge and expanding our capacity for holding experiences are all very important and helpful in a world that quickly charges forward and upward.

This pace can be exhausting and exhaustive of resources, energy, and time. A growth mindset must be buffered with downtime, pause, breaks to feed the soul and spirit. O

ne cannot constantly draw breath without exhaling in between.

There is balance in nature and creatures, who understand rest periods are not only crucial for regeneration and strength but are beautiful and necessary in their own right. Growth ceases in winter, and the ground sleeps. Domestic and wild cats rest and digest when there is no need for movement.

Humans have been spectacular at the growth part, though at the expense of our natural systems. Many move through the days in constant activation of our fight, flight, freeze,

or fawn nervous systems. Organizations and societal structures that constantly focus on growth without pause for meaningful reflection resemble the activated human nervous system.

Devolution can mean degeneration, and it can mean delegation. Breaking down and breaking apart are healthy cyclical practices that benefit the overall organism, whether replenishing nutrients in depleted soil after long periods of growth, composting that turns rot into life-giving processes, gut bacteria that keep us alive and healthy, or restructuring of organizations that perpetuate unhealthy expectations for those who sacrifice to keep them functioning.

In a choir, when there are long and sustained notes that are difficult to hold all in one breath, alternating breath rolls through the group to maintain the beauty and power of the song, while each person inhales at different times. This shifting of responsibility allows harmony to seamlessly continue while each person gets what they need.

I love applying this metaphor when I recognize my need to slow down and care for myself. It is important when evaluating business structures. Cyclical harmony puts the humanity back into systems, workplace environments, home life, and what we accept in terms of balance.

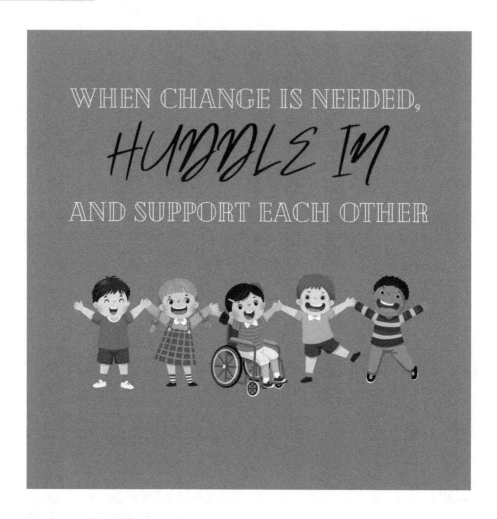

WHEN CHANGE IS NEEDED, *HUDDLE IN* AND SUPPORT EACH OTHER

I know nothing about sports, but I do understand how support feels. I see that huddling in holds others close, both physically and emotionally. It comforts the downtrodden and bolsters enthusiasm. It reiterates a team environment, mitigates confusion and burden, and allows hope to rise again.

Change is inevitable, it is constant. Every moment, every breath, something is changing within and around us. Every raindrop is new, every wave different. We crave change during times of discomfort and pain, and resist change because of fear. And wish change would stop when we perceive a perfect moment.

When meaningful change is needed, it can be overwhelming to know where to start. Huddling in with your peeps can be a great eye-opener. Discussing what you value with trusted others can spark ideas and moments of synergy. This can lead to new paths and open doors in our hearts that we hadn't seen before.

I felt heartbroken while treating folks at senior care homes, for those suffering great loneliness and isolation, and felt an intense draw to ease this for them. I ran a student massage outreach at a care home, which allowed me to implement a program that reached out to residents sitting alone to just listen to them, hold their hand if they wanted physical contact, and be a presence in their day. This was beautiful for as long as it lasted, but it didn't seem like enough. I wanted bigger changes for them.

At first, I was scared to share my ideas for fear of being told they were stupid, unattainable, nonsensical. Once I shared with one person, and then two, it became easier to talk to more people and welcome feedback and support for the idea. It has now become an exciting pilot project/ research study with the elderly and the dying, and I'm looking forward to expanding. Huddling in was a good way to ask for and receive support and love and help.

Focus on one thing that breaks your heart, pisses you off, or awakens deep feeling within you, to explore what meaningful change might look like for you. Talk to one person you trust about it. Generate ideas through open-ended discussion. Huddle in, ask for support, and see what happens.

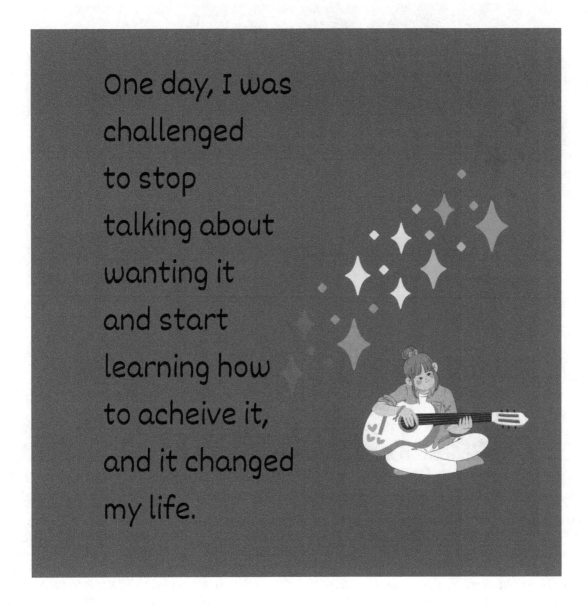

One day, I was challenged to stop talking about wanting it and start learning how to acheive it, and it changed my life.

A long time ago, I was in a musical. Perhaps the first of many in my adult life. Through my teenage years, I very much admired all the musicians I knew who played guitar and wished I had learned how to play. Every time I was mesmerized by a string instrument, I would compliment the talented artist, finishing with the statement, I wish I knew how.

I'm sure this happened more than a dozen times, each person accepting my praise, until one day I said it to one of the musicians in the above-stated musical. He looked me in the eye and said, "so do it." He told me to stop wishing for it and learn how.

In one moment, I moved from living through others' experiences, to living for myself. I had not realized that within my accolades was a desire to learn something for myself, hiding in my praise, disguised as envy.

I went home and told my parents I wanted to buy a guitar, and that's the day I found out that there was a beautiful acoustic living under their bed for the last several years. That guitar become my beloved, and I still have it today, 30 years later. I taught myself to play. I give thanks for the one spark of insight that came from a 'stop talking about it and take action' statement. It changed my perspective on following my joy and listening for what I'm truly drawn to.

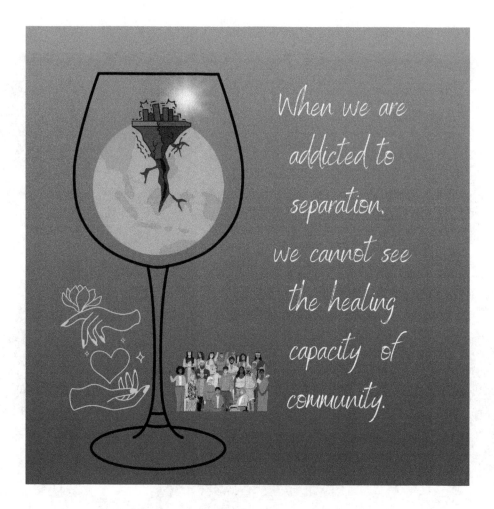

When we are addicted to separation, we cannot see the healing capacity of community.

Addiction is engaging in an activity to the detriment of relationships, whether to oneself or to others, personal or professional.

Many of us have been cultured to perceive ourselves as separate from others, from the natural world, even from spirit. Our medical industry would have us believe that our toe is separate from our leg, or the heart is separate from our blood.

Our bodies and systems are all one organism, existing for a common goal. The structures of our societies are seen as separate but are inextricably connected as one whole system. The dysfunction in one area pulls on the threads that make the whole system weaker and more prone to disease. Healthy roots and nurturing environments contribute to a thriving system. Of course, there are both in our cultures.

When we believe in the separateness of all things, it's easy to become addicted to making money, or extracting resources for the benefit of very few. If we follow the thread of our actions, in where the things we use come from and the people who contribute to our gift of life, where our actions lead, and who bears the brunt of our waste, our one-sided relationship, and who is left cleaning up after us, we can adopt a wider view of the impact we have on the local and global community.

If we hold the vision of connectedness in our minds and hearts, if we look others in the eye to speak our intention, if we act upon communal accountability, and continuously learn how-to live-in integrity with our values, we may find the systems we are immersed in can be healed through community. We can re-source our resources. There are more than enough humans that want to contribute to healthy systems and societies to draw inspiration from and work together as a whole, inextricable, flowing river, that feeds the supporting structures on the riverbanks we touch and move within.

The time is ripe for movement.

Shifts have been growing inside of us and in our collective mind and body.

The feeling is becoming stronger.

Louder.

The rivers of creativity are flowing faster and deeper.

There is an opening from the sub to the conscious.

The destroyer of worlds is compassionate.

Locate the part of you that needs attention, that will soften with observation, will dissolve with breath, will transform with uncoverment.

Ask what needs to fall apart to be more aligned.

What places need sun to come out of the shadows.

What spaces need quiet and darkness in order to feel supported, re-spirited.

How does this relate to the world around us?

What foundations need building so that inadequate systems can collapse with clarity and confidence?

What iterations of society can be born, allowing previous and current iterations to be deconstructed by design?

How can we unravel within a unity mindset and reconnect with relationship-forward inertia?

How do we interrupt fear with intention?

Disrupt the disingenuous?

Regenerate with reverence?

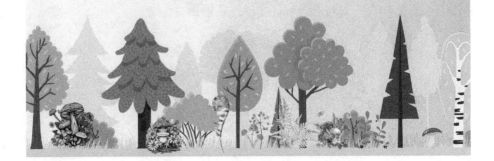

When we uproot the grass,
an array of life emerges
in the spaces that have now
become hospitable.

Accept with appreciation?

Tap into empathy, compassion, accountability, humanity.

Power and control have been overwhelming in how we relate to ourselves and others and the world.

It's time to put the power of propulsion under the surfaces of what is, to bubble up with the confidence that builds worlds.

Change is inevitable.

May we prioritize leaning into discomfort in the name of dignity, compassion over miscommunication, justice over apathy, and community over isolating practices.

The drive for homeostasis within and without is so prevalent at this time on the planet.

Where do you see an opportunity to connect with and jump into the river that already flows inside you?

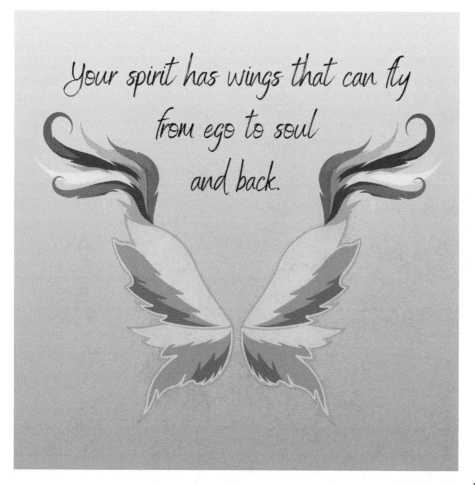

Your spirit has wings that can fly from ego to soul and back.

Inspired by Dr Clarissa Pinkola Estés, author of "Women Who Run With The Wolves."

The stories of old, tales of heroines, of enchantment, of magic and mermaids and witches, the curators of community, inspirers of insight, phosphorescent philosophers, decanters of darkness, ravishing riddlers, encounters with love, loss, and the will to live, are still the stories of now.

We are the heroines that must travel through the chambers of the heart, traverse the deserts of the psyche, and ride the rivers of soul, to connect with purpose, make magic from the mundane, and perceive the miracles within us.

The ego has much to learn from the soul. Ahhh but so has the soul from the ego. The ego knows how to navigate this world and its details, it's safety. It pays bills, does taxes, and gets to work on time. It makes decisions, it drives the car, it picks up the kids from daycare.

Of course, it can go overboard if we allow it. But if we can invite it into our days, it can inform the soul, so that

we may interact with our bodies and surroundings with practical mindfulness, remember to eat, know when to rest, and take care of our responsibilities.

The soul understands the ancient knowing, the holy wisdom of the universe. The creative fire that lights us up and has the power to move the hearts of others, arise from the depths of our internal shimmering sea. Our creaturial instincts catch the scent of the genius all around us and within, and whispers to the ego, "Come and play!"

"Ohh no no no," says the ego, "I must get to work so I can pay my bills. I'm too busy right now, I'll play later." Later comes and goes and there's still no time and we doubt our abilities, think of the creative in us as silly and childlike. The soul and the ego don't believe each other.

Spirit is the entity that sees both sides and translates the meaning behind the beliefs, the actions, and the longings to each realm of the heart and mind. Spirit is the cheerleader of the heart and the linguist that writes the words of the soul. It interprets the smell of the woods, the ocean, or the campfire, along with the body senses, to tell the story of our endearment for these things to our minds.

Spirit is multilingual and knows how to speak to and be the bridge for the body, mind, and soul to connect, and shows the benefit of wandering together down the same pathways. Spirit excites the soul and the ego simultaneously during a first kiss, an energetic game, a deep connection with a friend, when finishing a satisfying poem or painting, or after an epiphany.

Our wildness is the curative for apathy, for mistrust, or disconnection. Losing control is often frightening to the ego, but when the Spirit can translate safety, it can more easily drop the reins, even slightly, to let the soul have sovereignty for a time.

Spirit is the healer, soul is the teacher, ego is the responder, and can be each to one another if they find the harmony and awareness to do so. Living in balance can feel like they are all equally breathing us, as we breathe in the worlds within and all around.

A kind touch can calm the nervous system, even if the nurturing comes from yourself. Many people massage their head or neck when they have a headache or use a foam roller on tense legs, but how often do you lovingly massage your hands, arms, jaw, or face when you feel stressed or anxious? Or even when you feel fine?

It may seem strange to sit and rub your arms or face. Often this is because we are socialized to not really care for ourselves, except for the media-ized long soak in a tub. A bath is a great way to relax for some, and for others, intention makes a crucial difference in the feeling of well-being.

Self massage mixes intention with kind, nurturing touch. Focused attention on anything, when repeated daily causes neural pathways and areas of the brain to give more space to the activity or object of our awareness.

This means that if you were to gently massage your face for 5 minutes everyday and notice how this relaxes your whole body, your brain and neural pathways get used to and come to expect this daily dose of rest and calm and will eventually facilitate relaxation sooner into the process and create longer lasting effects. After repeating the activity several times, it will begin to enhance feelings of relaxation when simply preparing to start and then just thinking about the massage.

There's another part of massage that can feel vulnerable. Touch can be deeply touching. I believe the soul experiences perspectives of life through our physical and spiritual senses. What we feel on our skin and in deep tissue has an enigmatic effect of emotional opening. Accessing this part of us can be scary, enlightening, and mysterious. If this happens, it's helpful to remain curious about the feelings and watch them as you allow them to float in and out of your awareness, unless you are ready to explore their deeper meanings.

Massage can be done when you are feeling low, anxious, energetic, or perfectly healthy. It has a therapeutic effect in any frame of mind. Here is a self massage exercise if you'd like to partake and see how it feels:

(I will give an example of a face massage; however, you may massage any area you feel drawn to.)

☆ Sit in a comfortable position, and then take a full breath. Feel your feet on the floor or wherever they are resting, notice your body being held by the surface you are sitting or laying on, realize it is supporting you.

☆ In your mind and with your awareness, scan your body for tension. Notice an area you'd like to feel more

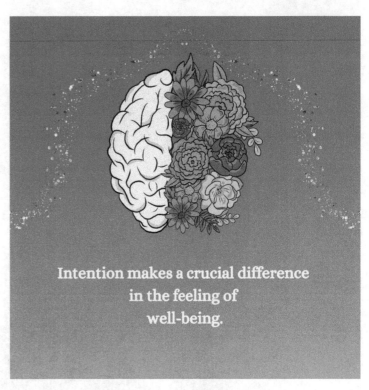

Intention makes a crucial difference in the feeling of well-being.

relaxed. In this case, we'll use the face.

☆ As you continue to breathe restfully, place the flat pads of a many of your fingers as will fit, onto your jaw bones, just beside your chin. Gently and slowly, make small circles starting by gliding fingers upward then away from your chin, down and back toward your chin. Repeat as many times as you want if it feels good.

☆ Let your hands shift out along your jaw, making circles as you go until you are massaging the jaw muscles that pop out when you clench your teeth.

Follow this process around your mouth, your cheeks, around your eyes, your temples, the sides of your nose, forehead, and experiment with slow movement, with full contact of fingers and palms on areas of your face.

Squeeze along your eyebrows outward from the middle. End by gliding both hands from chin to forehead and circle down the outside of the face, a few times.

☆ Notice how your face feels. Notice how your hands feel. Notice if your tension has changed or if it's the same. Notice how your body position has shifted, and if other areas have become relaxed. Where did your mind go, or did it stay with you?

☆ If this felt good, practice massaging the same or different areas daily for a week and pay attention to what you notice.

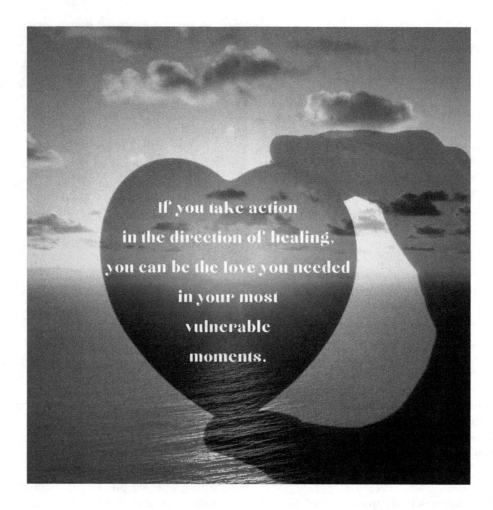

If you take action
in the direction of healing,
you can be the love you needed
in your most
vulnerable
moments.

It's been said that we often become what we needed when we were young. Sometimes, this can be an unconscious drive, and sometimes, it is intentional. Either way, it takes much effort and dedication to turn ourselves into those who serve others in a plethora of ways.

For example, I really needed to feel heard and believed as a child and nurtured in a way that valued my dignity, my spirit, my body, and my desire to ask lots of questions, continually seeking to understand the world around me.

There were many times these needs were not met, and I looked for them in other places. This didn't always work out for the best, and instead, I was judged, hurt, betrayed, abandoned, or taken advantage of.

Fortunately, I had a best friend who led me into loving circumstances where I could start healing. I was able to be involved with a community that was accepting and encouraging, engaged my mind, my heart, and my creativity, and taught me to look within for answers. I will be forever grateful for this direction.

I became aware of my needs and was able to explore them in safe, non-judgemental environments. I discovered that I wanted to be in the healing arts, to be a safe space for others, and to allow them to explore who they are without judgement.

I learned that I value love, nurturing, human dignity, and continuous learning above all. This is deeply aligned with my work as a Registered Massage Therapist and life coach, teacher, and writer. I offer compassionate presence and safe, nurturing, therapeutic touch to vulnerable people who crave relief.

I'm happy to deepen this work as I journey into the realm of healthcare research to discover measurable effects of presence and therapeutic touch on the quality of life for the elderly and the dying. I've seen how very effective this is through my career, though to be believed, results need to be measured. As I mentioned earlier, I have the need to be believed, as I'm sure it is a fundamental need for everyone.

Sign up for coaching, read helpful books, or look within. Take a step toward your own healing, discover your core values, become aware of how you may already be the someone you needed when you were suffering.

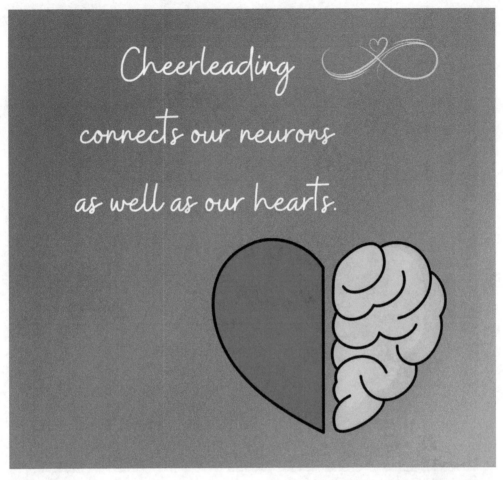

Cheerleading connects our neurons as well as our hearts.

Cheerleaders are important.

Whatever you might believe about human nature, there have always been those who stood up for and encouraged people.

These folks have an uplifting spirit, undying belief, a sense of humanity, and hold love as a driving force. This is not the kind of cheer that shows up as toxic positivity to the detriment of truth. This cheer offers a real sense of togetherness, of purpose, and of possibility.

There are reasons we feel drawn to uplift the spirit of another being. Cheering someone on, whether a fan of a sports team, a parent to a child, friends or co-workers performing a task, students taking a test, or strangers during a race or competition, can lead to a connection between the cheerer and the cheered.

Studies have shown that mirror neurons are activated around a wider surface area of the brain when cheering someone on and become even more activated when a win is perceived. The more neuron activation, the more intense the excitement, and more wide-spread body-mind involvement. This stimulates some of the reward centers of the brain, creating feelings of satisfaction.

Mirror neurons help us recognize actions, facial expression, and the understanding of the intention of others. Babies learn to imitate their caregivers and then develop skills that infer the intention of those around them, their nervous systems reacting to the innate sense of safety or danger.

People who encourage others create a connectivity between themselves and the one they cheer for, increasing a sense of unity, activated in both the brain of the cheerer and the cheered (if in person of course).

This means that encouragement, support, and goodwill are crucial to the function of a community. We feel more happiness and satisfaction when those we love are successful. This likely contributes to the feeling of bonding to our favorite sports teams and players. Cheerleading has great effect on morale and belief in our capabilities. After all, where would sports be without the fans? And where would we be without the support of our cheerleaders?

Who are your cheerleaders?

How do you show up for others in this way?

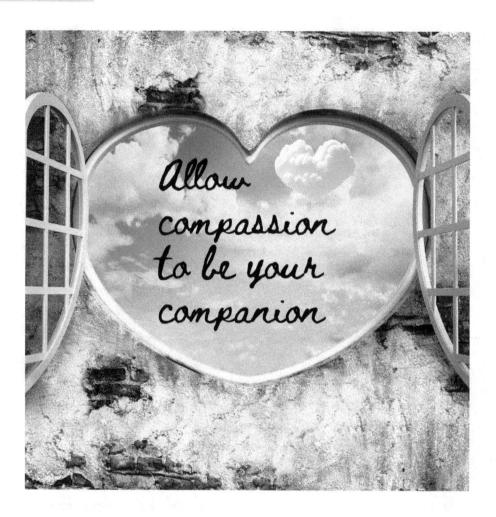

We tend to have a greater sense of wholeness when we hold compassion in our awareness that comes along in our daily lives. Interactions that are thoughtful increase openness and insight into the experience of others. Less judgement drives our actions.

I hold compassion like a friend, like a sense. I both offer and receive compassion through touch, especially as a massage therapist who gives space and spaciousness in order for others to feel relief. Compassion is sparked through our senses; a kind touch, seeing someone suffer with grief or expand with joy, intuitively reading the heart of another by their facial expressions, body posture, and sound of their voice.

In massage therapy, I must be ok with pivoting at any moment during a treatment, based on how my patient is feeling and responding. This is a compassionate approach. It would not be helpful to continue with a set treatment plan if my patient suddenly couldn't breathe or had a massive leg cramp come upon them.

Sometimes, we live in our minds so strongly, that we forget to see what's in front of us or to interact with presence.

When we are fully present with ourselves and with others, we are able to engage with our in-the-moment emotions and connect with those around us in real time.

This week, on their podcast, We Can Do Hard Things, Glennon and Amanda Doyle discussed what being prepared actually looks like when interacting with others. For example, when we prepare a speech or plan exactly what we want to say in an upcoming conversation, though the words may be beautiful or precise, they do not consider what the other might need in that moment. In this case, if we stick to what we've prepared instead of responding to what's happening in the moment, we aren't being responsible or response-able to the integrity of the situation.

Carrying empathy behind our eyes, seeing, and communicating through a lens of compassion, contributes to a more compassionate world. And remember, this lens goes both ways, looking inward as well as out. The more we practice and reflect on this, the more compassion becomes an innate sense, a way of being, and how we ultimately treat ourselves and others.

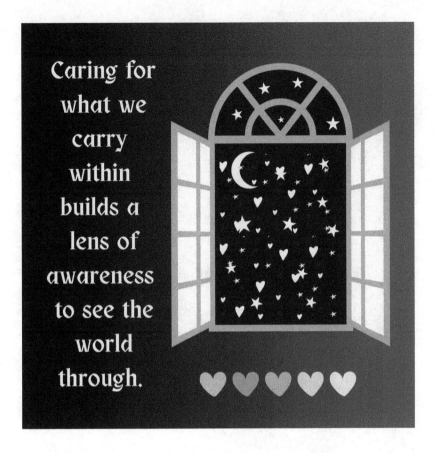

Caring for what we carry within builds a lens of awareness to see the world through.

If you've heard the quote by Anaïs Nin, "We don't see things as they are; we see them as we are," then you likely have a sense of what that means. The experiences we carry within us create a vast mental and emotional landscape from which we draw our beliefs, assumptions, biases, and expectations.

Our inner terrain offers parameters to measure where we stop, and another begins. This can be helpful for the discernment of boundaries, interdependence instead of codependence, and understanding of core values. Where it gets blurry, however, is being able to live inside someone else's experience.

We have the capacity to empathize with those we love, respect, admire, want to serve, characters in movies, and even strangers on the interwebs. As heartfelt as it may be, our empathy has limits. Though we may relate to the emotional intensity, we are only able to perceive the experience and emotion of another through our own inner landscape.

The worldview we hold is deeply ingrained and subconscious, for the most part. That is until our perceptions are challenged. This can be both terrifying and enlightening. Many become protective of their worldview when faced with the questioning of it, not hesitating to defend their point of view.

If we're able to have the humility to step back from our defenses and into a mind of curiosity, it becomes easier to remember that each human carries a complex landscape of their own. It takes courage to be humble in the face of differing belief systems and perspectives, though this is precisely what is needed to grow empathy and connection.

Folks travel in order to expand their cultural awareness and open their minds to other ways of living. Imagine conversing with someone from a different culture or who speaks a different language. It would be pointless and crass to judge them because they can't explain the world the way you see it because they are coming from a wholly different point of reference. If we can stay curious and find alternative ways to communicate, imagine, and empathize with them, gratitude for connection will rise in the place where disdain may have festered.

Listening for what's inside us, seeking for that which has built us, and trying to love and honor all the experiences that made us who we are, is one way to cultivate a responsible outlook and more accurate self-awareness. Being intentional in the cultivation of a worldview that holds a generous amount of openness, a dollop of curiosity, and a dash of humility, is a kind and colourful lens indeed.

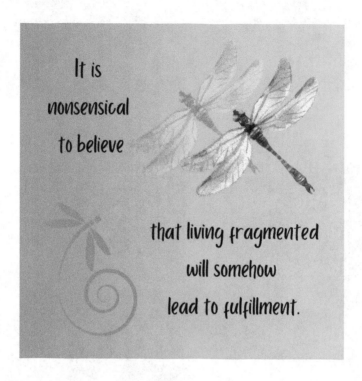

It is nonsensical to believe that living fragmented will somehow lead to fulfillment.

We are miracles of complexity.

For all of the limitations we've been forced to endure and all the tumult our species have put each other through, the indomitable spirit makes its way to the forefront, through the nervous system, consciously or not, to live as close to freedom as possible.

The survival spirit that inhabits and animates our living bodies must love the adventures of the earth-side, because it will fight tooth and nail to carry on, whether to face a perilous journey or busy city traffic. Whatever the path that lies ahead, the spirit will ensure that we keep breathing in the moment, to the best of its ability.

Fragmentation happens when we get forcibly squished into societally acceptable versions of our whole selves, and then live that way for so long, when we try to access the fullness of who we are, it's a little like chasing a shadow. It's hard to pin down.

When we have time to think about "self-care", we use tools to try to remember who we once were and what we once loved, to regain feelings we once had. The feelings of truth, freedom, passion, aliveness, that we don't feel so connected to anymore, that we traded for roles and rules and acceptance from fragmented systems.

We pursue different relationships, various jobs, titles, and money, to fill the looming void of loneliness, fear, and separation, when true, living, and honest connection to ourselves and others is the only way to refill the vacuous spaces that have kept us hungering for the breath of fulfillment.

Do you have the sense that life is supposed to be more than it is?

Only you know the way to alignment. You must seek your own wisdom and listen for that bubbling of truth within. Notice the moments that light you up and follow that thread. Be curious about the obstacles on your truest path.

Of course, you can get help from trusted coaches and mentors, from books, or from your dreams. Our dreams can hold insights, both waking dreams and in sleep, into the next steps to take toward fulfillment. Have you let yourself dream of how your best life would feel to you?

Some days I don't want to believe what I know. Other days, all I can do is believe.

Sometimes I don't want to feel.

Even though I know emotions are my superpower and the filter through which I experience my soul and my world.

Ignorance feels excruciating, not blissful.

How I wish it were blissful.

I want to be so much more.

More capable.

More graceful.

More skillful.

More interpretive.

More accepting of the paradox.

A mind reader.

Sunlight.

The web and the weaver.

The land and the river.

Exploration, discovery, and home.

Maiden, mother, and crone.

I cannot be everything for all, or for just one, not even for myself.

I do not always feel ok, or peaceful, even though I want to be.

My strength wanes.

Poetry soothes
when I can't
form whole sentences.

My heart breaks.

My eyes share tears.

I am so f@%!ing emotional.

I don't have to be the one who holds it all together.

I don't have to know everything in order to be valuable.

I have shame and fear and tortuous thoughts.

I hold expectations, dreams, longing and wants.

By no means perfect, I am being what I can.

Tugging on my threads and unraveling.

This is the part of me that has been hard to love.

But give it love, I will.

Through tears and hope and a place of solid discomfort, I challenge myself to be here.

Now.

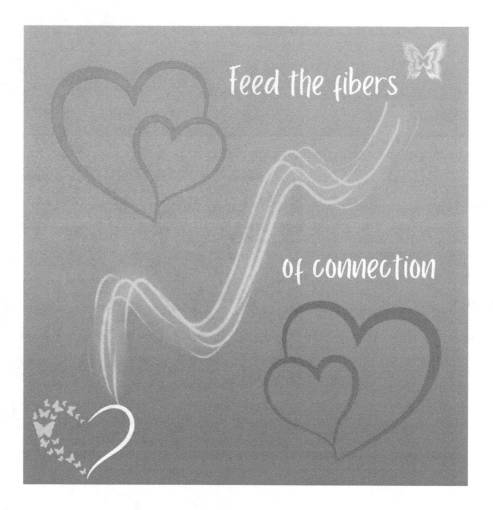

Feed the fibers of connection

The environments we are immersed in matter. They have great impact on us. There are peaceful, benign, disruptive, and insidious levels of influence on our nervous systems, based on our inner awareness, and outer surroundings. Nature is one of the best ways to calm the body and mind, for it reminds us of our internal home, our center, our wild, our seasons, and of acceptance.

The pathways in our brains become smooth and silky the more we repeat certain activities or think specific thoughts, making those grooves faster, more efficient, and accessible. As these develop, we can become so adept that our subconscious can take over, like an expert musician who knows their craft inside and out can rely on the wisdom of their fingers and let the mind relax.

Practice is the best way to achieve this. If you want to learn a new skill with your hands, a new way to move your body, use your mind in creative ways, think different thoughts, or relate to the world around you with more compassion, awareness and daily intentional focus will build your neural pathways.

Changing automatic reactions or unconscious habits must begin with noticing and understanding what you want to shift. Staying connected to the ever-changing emotional self and tapping into what we value, on purpose, helps to direct us in aligned decision-making. This then enhances our relationships, makes desired boundaries more clear, and has the potential to create easier and more direct communication.

With roughly 100 billion neurons in the human brain, isn't it amazing that we can influence the growth or atrophy of certain nerve cells just by what we focus on consistently? Daily practice combined with awareness contributes how our brains function, essentially feeding the fibers that connect us to ourselves, our thoughts, our community, and how we interpret the world.

When we seek for and soak in the understanding of our values in context with our actions and relationships, it is easier to hear the truth from within, feel more aligned, and have greater fulfillment.

We are nourished.

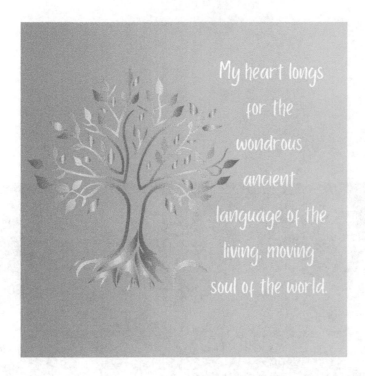

My heart longs
for the
wondrous
ancient
language of the
living, moving
soul of the world.

In Braiding Sweetgrass, Robin Wall Kimmerer shares Potawatomi words that don't have an English equivalent. One such word is "Puhpowee", which translates in English "as the force that causes mushrooms to push up from the earth overnight." This describes the mystery of life. She talks about English as being defined only by what we know, and for that which we don't yet understand lies nameless in ambiguity.

The words of Indigenous peoples respect the animate life force of all beings, the connection of humans to animals, to the soil and stone, the water and air, trees and mountain. The words we use matter. We are walled off from expressing the poignant, the breathtaking, the profound, the graceful and the loving, and the deeply sorrowful with adequate meaning and weight because of our colonial language.

There are many other languages that speak to the heart and to the deep and tidal nature of life. For example, the Arabic word Samar translates into "Staying up late after the sun has gone down and having an enjoyable time with friends." "Aspaldiko - This untranslatable Basque word describes the euphoria and happiness felt when catching up with someone you haven't seen in a long time."

"Ailyak is a beautiful Bulgarian term for the subtle art of doing everything calmly and without rushing, whilst enjoying the experience and life in general."

In Japanese, the beautiful word Komorebi literally means, "Sunlight leaking through trees." "This word describes the beauty and wonder of rays of light dappling through

overhead leaves, casting dancing shadows on the forest floor."

Ichi-go ichi-e translates to, "Treasuring an unrepeatable moment."

And Tsundoku is relatable to many, meaning, "Acquiring books, but letting them pile up without reading them."

My favorite so far is Hyppytyynytyydytys. "This Finnish word literally means, 'bouncy cushion satisfaction'. It describes the pleasure and satisfaction derived from sitting or bouncing on a bouncy cushion."

When we cannot explain a feeling with words, it's not that they are necessarily indescribable, it is but the limits and structure of language that is inadequate.

I yearn for the depth of connection that reads the longings of my heart and the wisdom of my soul through fulfilling conversation, of being seen and understood at the same time.

Until our language becomes fluid, like rainwater fusing with and nourishing the roots of the mighty oak and willow, the vernacular of the wind in the trees, of the singing bird at sunrise, the caress of a gentle wave upon the shore, how the moon kisses the mountains as it emerges into the night sky, and the mystical and magnetic draw of one soul to another, remains unspoken.

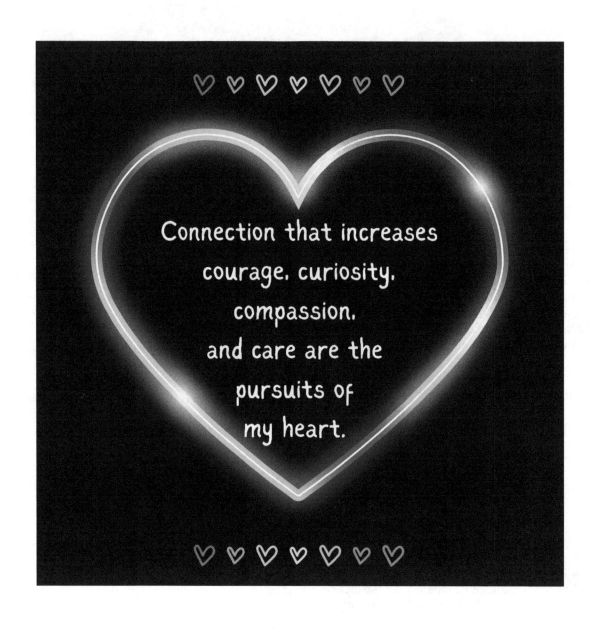

Connection that increases
courage, curiosity,
compassion,
and care are the
pursuits of
my heart.

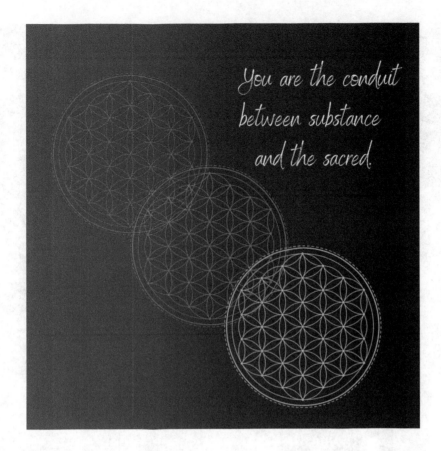

You are the conduit between substance and the sacred.

The spirit that animates our bodies can be felt in nature and seen in the eyes of any creature. The warmth of the sun that lingers on a smooth stone and the wind that dances through the tree leaves is part of the sacred in substance. Your senses inform your soul.

We have the capacity to channel the sacred through us at any time. I have had the privilege of visiting a cabin on a lake of some dear friends for the last few summers. We are blessed to have been able to return for 5 beautiful days this week. The water just off the deck is warmer than the lake we frequently visit at home, and welcoming, though cool enough to be refreshing.

Last year, at this time, we came to the lake the day after I found out my Mum was diagnosed with colon cancer. As you can imagine, my heart and my head space were in rough shape. I remember walking out through the ripples until I could barely touch the bottom and my chin just touching the surface, to immerse myself, literally and spiritually, in nature.

I remember feeling completely held and accepted, tears and fears, and all that I was in that moment, being gently rocked in the arms of the mother that holds us all.

This morning, I walked out into the same lake and greeted it as an old friend; one who had taken my worries and hugged me until I felt lighter and more loved.

I was able to tell her that Mum passed away last December, though I'm sure she knew. I thanked her for holding me when I needed it most. This lake and I have history now, she is sacred to me, just as she held me as a sacred child, whether I cried tears of suffering or of joy.

It is easy for me to feel the sacred in all the miracles I encounter, from my own life to the chickens and cows that I wake up to greet, to my children who are my heart walking around outside of me, to my loving community of friends and family, to being able to watch in awe at the sunrise, the sunset, and the cycles of nature.

What I choose to hold as sacred in my life become the blessings that fill my days with gratitude. I know I'm a conduit for energy in physical form. The lake transformed my grief, like a catalyst from the spirit world, took my emotions and gave me acceptance and belonging in return. How can I feel anything but abundantly blessed?

I believe that sometimes, profound changes in our lives happen to get our attention so we can make meaning from them and find the sacred within our ability to face whatever comes. And I believe that the sacred can be found in anyone or anything we choose to give our gratitude to.

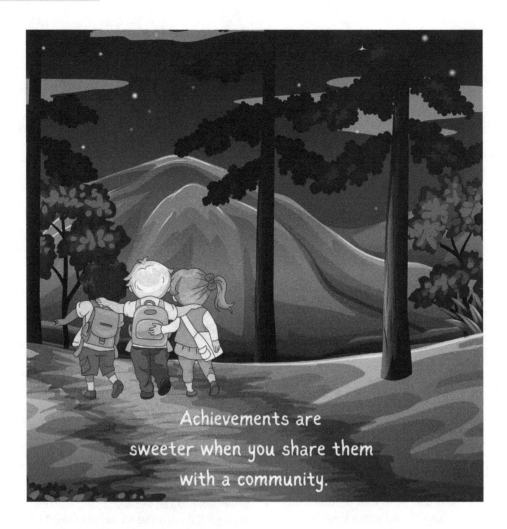

Achievements are sweeter when you share them with a community.

My family and I love to break into congratulatory applause when any one of us has completed a project, passed a test, had an epiphany, achieved a new skill, sent a difficult email, or pretty much anything big or small that we feel proud of. We love to celebrate each other.

It feels so good to close the loop on something and be acknowledged for it and cheered on. It's a relief to get something finally finished, especially when it's been challenging. We are so invested in each other, that we can feel a palpable energy shift in the air when someone walks into a room with purpose, and no matter what we are doing, we drop everything and clap for them. One win is everyone's win.

Energies shift everyday, and there is always something to strive for, to complete, or accomplish. I adore when friends call me to tell me about a small step they've taken or a shift in mindset. They all feel like a big deal to me because some days, getting out of bed is well worth celebrating. Going for a hike, finishing a book, or a course, starting yoga, or paying off a student loan are all amazing feats of determination.

If I didn't have a community of adorable cheerleaders, I would still likely do many of the things I do. However, I would miss being that for others. If you currently don't have a cheerleader in your life and would love one, start being that for someone else in a genuine way. The person that makes you coffee at the café you go to often, folks at work, bus drivers, your friends, and your family, all struggle with challenges, and feel good when they are recognized for their achievements.

Be present in your interactions with others so you are able to notice when there is a shift in their energy. Notice if they're smiling wider than usual, breathing deeper and slower, if they seem more relaxed. Perhaps even change up the expected "hi, how are you?" with "what's good today?" or "what's your favorite color/ shape/ weather?" This helps both of you focus on the moment and generate more thoughtful answers that lead to genuine connection. And who knows? That connection could be the start of a community.

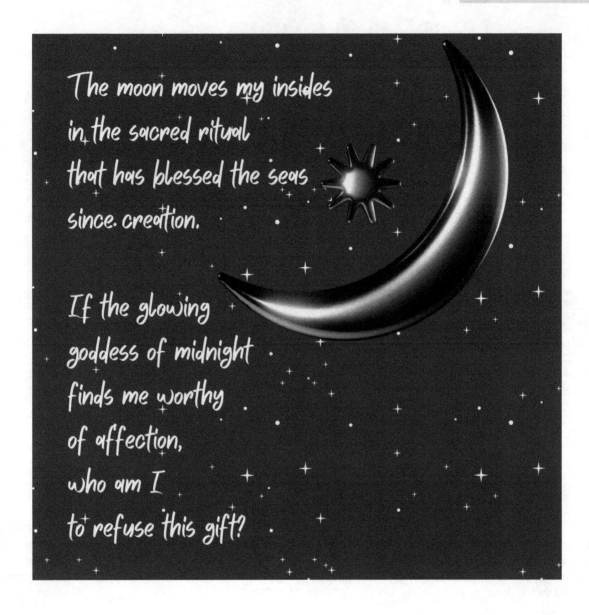

*The moon moves my insides
in the sacred ritual
that has blessed the seas
since creation.*

*If the glowing
goddess of midnight
finds me worthy
of affection,
who am I
to refuse this gift?*

My depths find voice in the silver light and dance on the water with the golden sun, fly with the raven of wisdom upon the currents of air and cresting wave, love filling me, flowing out, and refilling again. Reflecting a universe in my eyes, through my prismatic spirit.

We live through the soul into the senses, taking in all that strengthens resolve, so that when we are broken open, our pieces reconfigure to blossom new awareness. Finding destroyers to forgive, for sparking the fires that burn away the superfluous, burdens that kept us stagnant for eons.

I write to unravel and birth clarity within my layers of brain and heart, to dissolve toxic cages, to bring subconscious to light, to bare the soul to the slivers of the silver moon, to affect like the queen of the night sky, to spread love to earth and creature, to honour the wild rivers and white teeth of determined aching within, to be known and whole, to discover more and less, and myself.

I write and speak and love and care because I must.

I take flight because I must.

To not, would be a permanent death.

The ego is like modern research,
it demands factual, observable,
measurable outcomes.
The soul is deep wisdom,
a knowing, experience,
learned through living
and considerable generations.
Value can be found in both.

We are integrated beings.

We cannot separate ego from soul just as the neck flows seamlessly into the shoulder. Some may live with more awareness of one over the other, though they are both still there, continuously functioning.

In western culture, our egos are spoken to as we grow, through expectations, language that is perfunctory, and systems that constantly compare, urge competition, and force memorization in order to pass in school and in life. Our everyday communication bereft of words of the soul. In English, at least.

This has created an ego-heavy society, where people are more comfortable talking about themselves as losers or winners, good-looking or ugly, thin, and fat, rich or poor, sick or healthy, rather than heart-centered, loving, miraculous beings of creation. This is an unbalanced perspective.

Of course, it would be difficult to live in this physical world with only a soul-mind. Navigating the reality of societal structures takes reasoning, wit, and the ability to communicate with others within a business-y framework. Though there are some who live daily closer to soul, they often have followers that perform as guides through the mundane.

It takes a keen sense of both ego, who has the thoughts and soul, who notices thoughts, to feel transcendence of both. A combination of knowing when to be in ego and when to disconnect from it comes easier once it is recognized by the part of us that watches our thoughts, feelings, and reflections.

Practice awareness of each by thinking a thought, and then notice and observe the part of you having the thought. Who is the you that may observe your arm moving and notice the thought, "my arm is moving." Seeing our thoughts from a distance increases compassion for the parts of us who are in the feels in the moment.

Ego can keep our physical selves safe. Soul is informed by the senses and the physical world through the body and the ego. Soul enriches and is enriched by partnership with body and ego. When we acknowledge the roles of all the bits we are made of, we can more easily create balance between the doer and the observer.

This balance creates harmony within, which translates outward and influences the relationships we have with others and with the world.

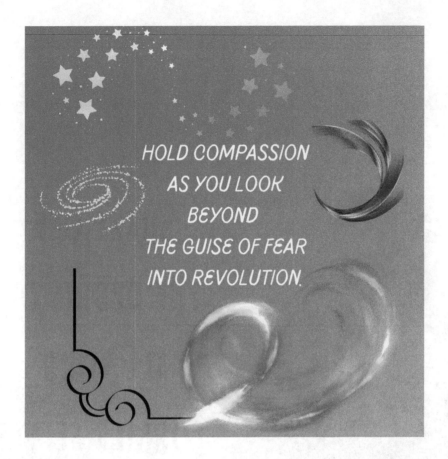

HOLD COMPASSION
AS YOU LOOK
BEYOND
THE GUISE OF FEAR
INTO REVOLUTION.

As a child, I remember running wild, free to use my imagination, tell stories and ridiculous jokes, make everything into a song, take care of spiders, and explore nature with my friends. Until the day I had to grow up.

As a teenager, the same freedom was not afforded to creativity and longings of my heart. I was often teased for my pursuits, told I was a bleeding heart, that I think too much, and that I couldn't save everyone.

I conformed to societal pressures while keeping my soul self hidden. I knew she was there, even when others would contradict this knowing with "logic." I found ways to connect with her, even if it was mundanely called walking in the forest, traveling through different countries, or being a camp counselor.

I was decidedly uncool in high school. I sang in a church choir and went to youth group, was interested in musical theater, debates, and getting deep and philosophical with friends. I could feel soul expressing through me, even though so many people in my life denied its existence in themselves.

As I grew older and life got more complicated and laden with responsibility, some people directly asked me to hide my true self, others asked indirectly. These situations felt horrible, but with the indoctrination of the superficial self, I went along living in the cramped and shamed places of other's expectations for a long, long time. Until I couldn't anymore.

Living in a communal world can definitely cause waves of soul and inauthenticity to mingle on the shore together, though the strength of my knowing, the intimate relationship with my soul, stays firm. It's not always that I don't care what others think of me, but I no longer fear that others will shake my connection away from me.

Once you come to know and love the soul journey, there is no going back to cramped pursuits. If I want to save everyone and think too much, I will throw my soul into it. I became a wounded healer; my purpose is to help others feel seen and loved and lifted and safe. That feels like revolution to me.

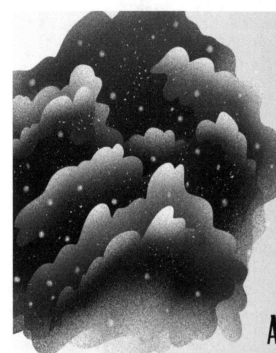

SHAKE OFF
THE DEBRIS OF
ALL YOUR
FORMER SELVES
AND
DREAM
OF WHO YOU WANT
TO BE NEXT

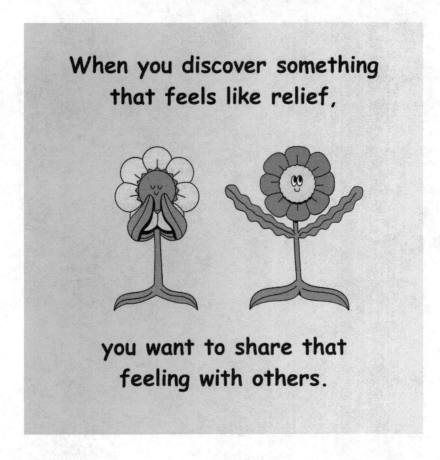

When you discover something that feels like relief, you want to share that feeling with others.

Joy is contagious.

Alignment is magnetic.

When you feel amazing, you want others to feel good too. It's very human to want to spread the love when we have it to give.

This is particularly true when it comes to relief. Whether you feel physical or emotional relief, a mental paradigm shift, or a connection that resonates with your being, you want to recommend that thing to everyone who will listen. This is why there are so many podcasts and other platforms that recommend solutions to all sorts of things.

We recommend books we love, stores with excellent customer service, a physiotherapist that is effective at offering relief. I am in an industry that thrives on word-of-mouth referrals. This is very effective because of the human drive help alleviate another's suffering. This is compassion.

I'm not talking about when someone complains because they can't go to the deeper places. Complaining is another animal altogether, it has a different feel and purpose. I mean the bare bones of what keeps us up at night, literally and figuratively.

Finding relief by any means possible is a huge driver of distraction and addiction in our society. It is vulnerable to share what terrifies us, though it is our vulnerability that has great power in connecting us to other hearts. Sharing our relief, while still risky to our softness, is often easier than sharing our suffering. It is an opening for connection. A way to help.

This touches on how we've been held back from helping as much as our hearts and bodies want us to. We are taught to be nice and productive, and taking more time to find our how someone is truly feeling on our way into work is inconvenient and might mess up the schedule we feel we must keep. This inhibits the connection, the bonding, the vulnerability, the care, and the love that is meaningful outside of the realm of propriety and professionalism. We are the wells of wisdom who have been cut off from our village. When we share something that helps us, with sincerity and concern, we open a channel to deeper conversation and connection with another.

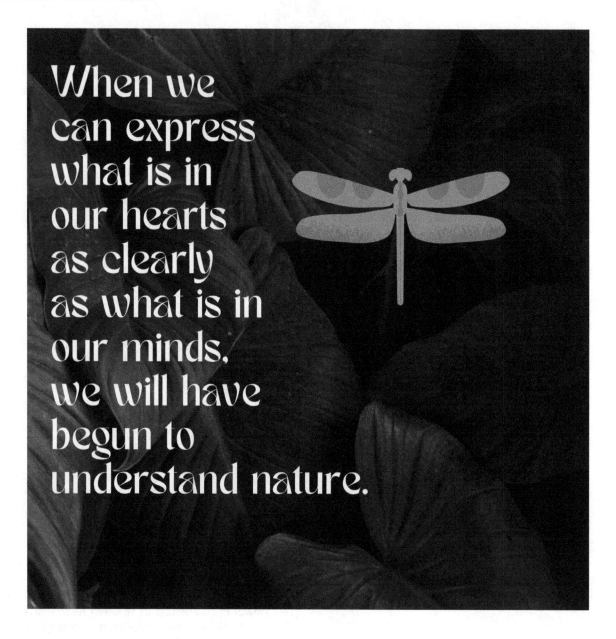

When we can express what is in our hearts as clearly as what is in our minds, we will have begun to understand nature.

Nature is considered mysterious because the majority of humanity doesn't understand it well. The non-physical part of us that knows beyond language is considered mysterious as well because many generations have been taught to ignore the wild nature within. As children, we trust implicitly unless those we trust teach us to fear.

Being raised within a structure that is scared to live in our own wildness creates a distance and disconnect between the heart and the mind, and our minds can become a great trickster. Allowing this to be the driver of action and behaviour has been disastrous for countless cultures.

Control is a manifestation of fear. We are made of the same matter and energy as the ancient forests and the stars.

Letting go of control leaves room for love to lead. Accepting and allowing our inner wisdom to rewild from the inside out is able to bring back an ebb and flow of life and emotion.

This can open us to the depths and volume of who we are, leaving behind the cardboard cutout of who we've been told to be. The two-dimensional versions of us can be crumbled in an instant from the smallest of storms.

When we can see ourselves in nature and the nature within us, we are able to feel more grounded, loved, and rooted in mystery, rather than being afraid of it.

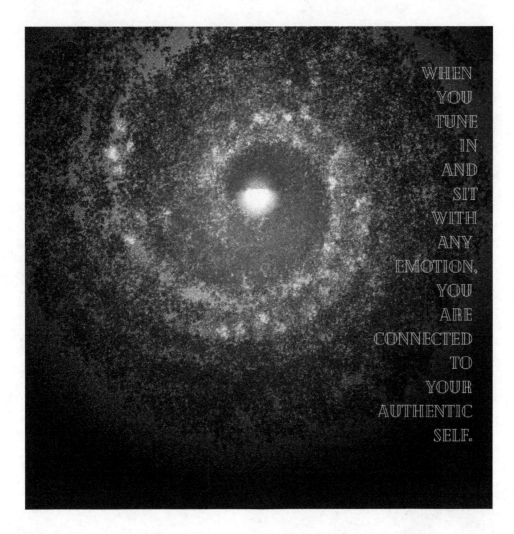

WHEN YOU TUNE IN AND SIT WITH ANY EMOTION, YOU ARE CONNECTED TO YOUR AUTHENTIC SELF.

Getting lost in the feelings of love can be blissful and elating. Nothing seems to weigh us down as we float in a state of high vibration. This has been true whether I'm connecting with a partner, a child, a dear friend, or even just while thinking about them. I fall in love with people all the time. With animals, with plants and trees. Love is connection for me.

Not everyone connects the feelings of love to safety or bliss. For some, fear arises because of the lack of control or being hurt in the past. For others, grief arises because of the loss of a loved one. And that's ok. All emotions that are acknowledged can be a connection point. Every feeling is valid at its core.

Noticing and holding space and awareness on the many feelings that arise is a way to connect with your true self. You are valid. Your emotions are real and valid. You are allowed to feel ALL your feelings. Hiding parts of yourself doesn't feel good. Accepting our wholeness IS what makes us feel whole and worthy, messy emotions, and all.

Hiding our realness to "fit in" with everyone else hiding parts of themselves too is a taught social construct of systems that benefit from us not being whole and satiated. Allowing yourself to bring your whole self everywhere liberates others to do the same.

Imagine if feeling good wasn't the only thing we strive for and felt we could share with others. I never regret sharing my bubbling depths of truth when I have the courage to do so. It frees me from pretending and eventually being taken over by unshared hard emotion.

We all want to be seen in some way.

We are wired for connection.

Authenticity is scary sometimes and so very validating, even when you're the only one who knows you're no longer pretending. Speak to your emotions and welcome them when you notice them arising. See them as a gift of your humanity.

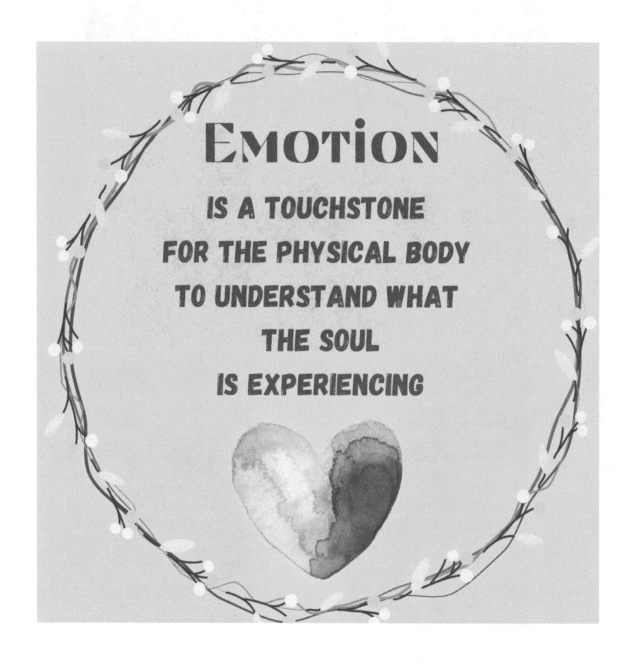

EMOTION

IS A TOUCHSTONE
FOR THE PHYSICAL BODY
TO UNDERSTAND WHAT
THE SOUL
IS EXPERIENCING

There is not one day
I regret
the time spent
and the
learning
experienced
that allowed me
to express
more succinctly
who I am and how I feel.

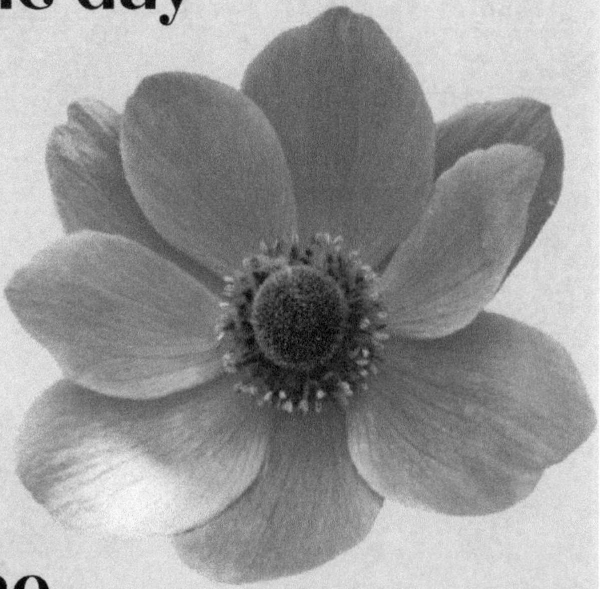

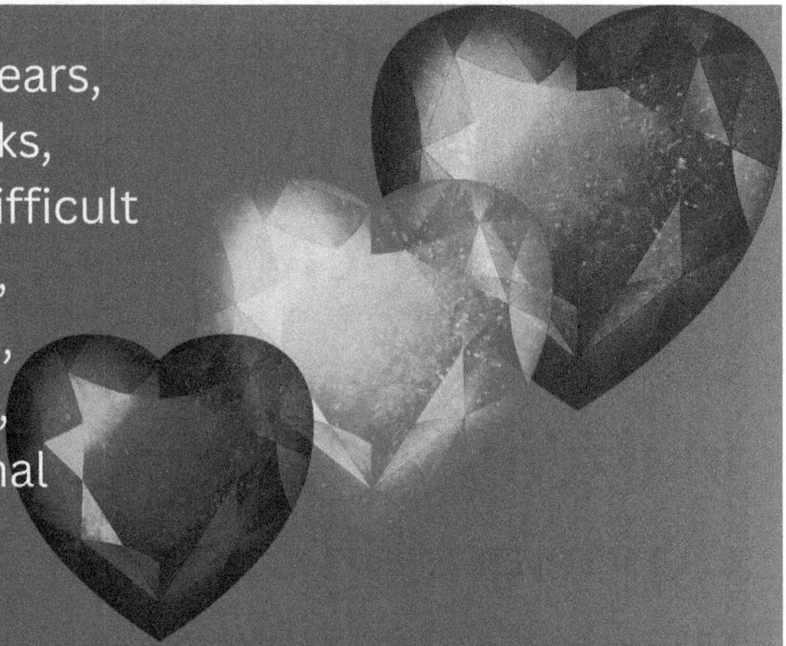

It took many years,
countless books,
hundreds of difficult
conversations,
dozens of jobs,
a few mentors,
several personal
development
courses,
meditation,
and deep listening to my soul
to learn what I value most,
and the words that resonate
with my hardest emotions.
Please don't quit because of a hard day.

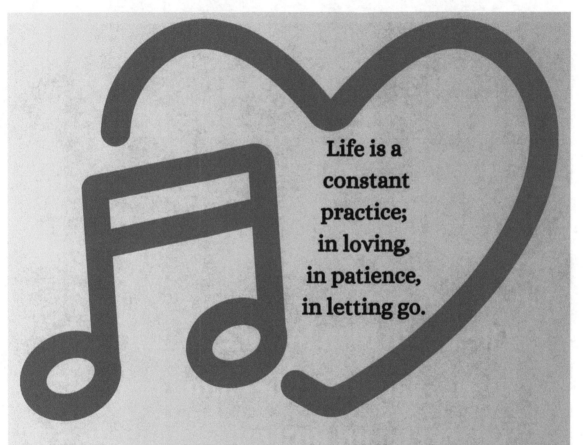

Life is a
constant
practice;
in loving,
in patience,
in letting go.

So dance and play and cuddle whenever
possible...
For the sweetness that fills the heart remains.

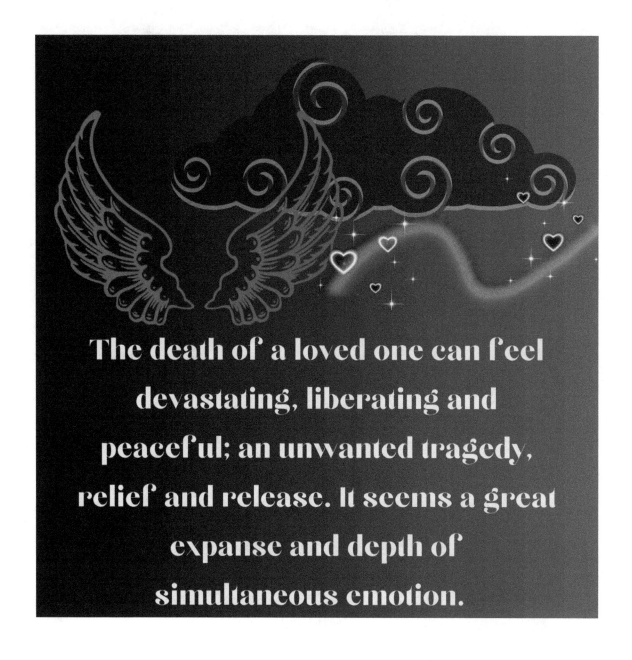

The death of a loved one can feel devastating, liberating and peaceful; an unwanted tragedy, relief and release. It seems a great expanse and depth of simultaneous emotion.

The human spirit is the magical binding force that allows us to hold the beautiful tension of bliss and pain simultaneously.

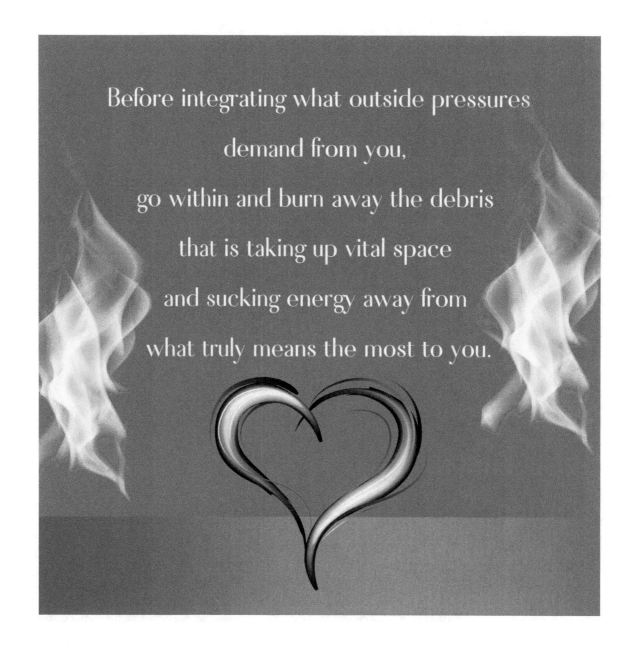

Before integrating what outside pressures

demand from you,

go within and burn away the debris

that is taking up vital space

and sucking energy away from

what truly means the most to you.

I stopped fighting for change, and started loving for it instead.

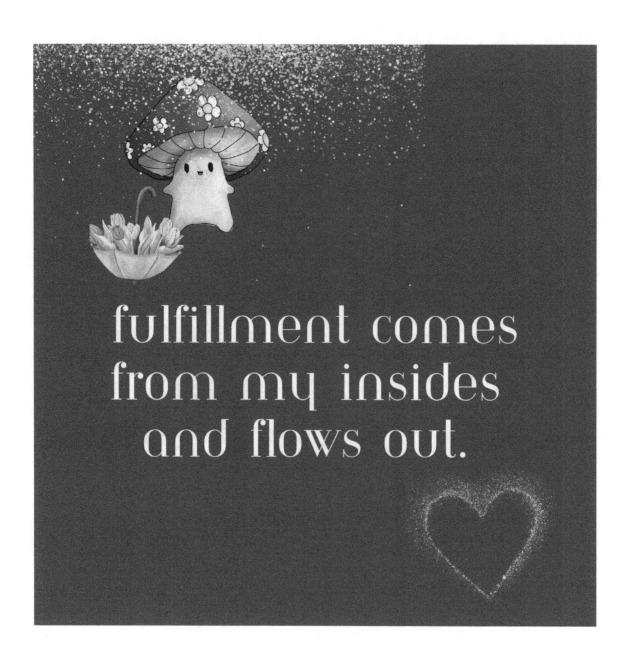

fulfillment comes
from my insides
and flows out.

the grief in me comforts the
grief in you.
that's what empathy is.

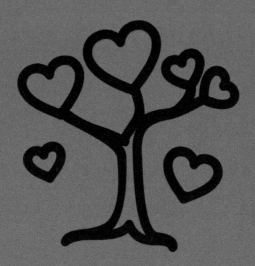

IF WE ARE CURIOUS
ABOUT STRUGGLE,
RESPONSIBILITY,
OR THE QUALITY OF
RELATIONSHIPS WE
HAVE WITH OTHERS
AND THE PLANET,
WE CONTRIBUTE
TO THE WISDOM
THAT EXISTS
IN THIS LIFETIME.

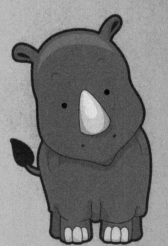

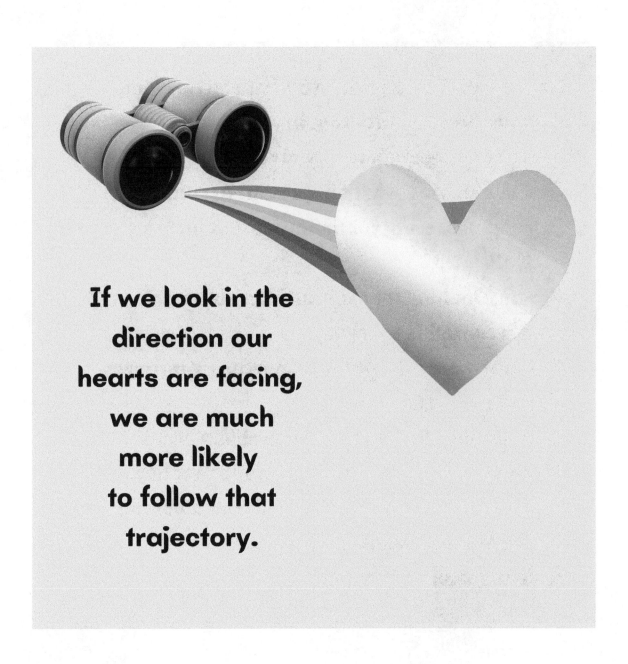

If we look in the direction our hearts are facing, we are much more likely to follow that trajectory.

Practice giving attention to what you do want.
Practice holding intention in your mind.
Practice connection with your body's wisdom.
Practice sharing what's important to you.
Practice gathering communities that lift
each other up.
Practice looking for exciting ideas, bliss, and
creative insights everyday.
Practice more safe, physical, nurturing intimacy.
Hug more and longer.
Look people in the eye, if you're able.
Be compassionate to yourself as you practice.
What we know and seek expands our awareness,
and leads to the liberation of others
to do the same.

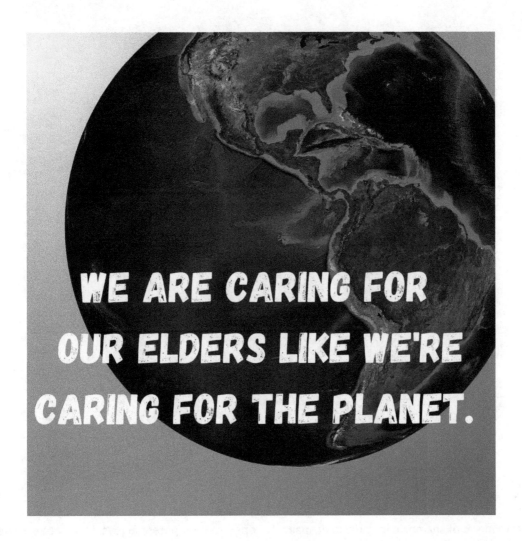

WE ARE CARING FOR OUR ELDERS LIKE WE'RE CARING FOR THE PLANET.

The principle of reciprocity is out of balance. The old growth forests and olders in care homes; one considered a resource at human disposal, the other considered disposable, burdens on society because they are deemed no longer resourceful to the community.

Without gratitude for the wisdom of our elders, there can be little understanding of the blessings of age, forest or human, and lifetimes of experience.

It is crucial to examine the ways we have forgotten our elders and determine appropriate shifts in how we proceed as a humanity that is inextricably entwined with nature and the delicate balance between environment and humanity, oxygen, and vitality.

Even if patients are well cared for by nurses and doctors, there is often still something missing. As with approaches to climate change, the overwhelming problem with waste and attitude toward wastefulness, is the absence of compassion. Hidden in care homes or behind bureaucracy, the old adage is too often true... out of sight, out of mind.

Someone who is able to connect with and be a compassionate witness to a whole human and their needs, or a whole planet, is necessary for integration and visibility in our communities. Healthy change requires integrity, compassion, and visibility in order to include all people in micro movements, innovative ideas to try, and possibilities for a different future for humans and the planet.

By 2051, there will be roughly 12 million people over the age of 65 in Canada. Compared to the current 7 million of this age, we will need a significant bridge to keep up with those who still need love, care, nurturing, presence, touch, and compassion. Nearly 10 million people over the next 30 years will be entering their end-of-life stage.

Both areas need to be addressed, nature and human nature. It's time for love and compassion to be action words. There are many options to moving forward with integrity. Reciprocity, respect, and gratitude are values we can embody while moving toward compassionate goals.

> *We die in little ways all the time.*
> *It would be wondrous to also live in small ways every day.*

We die of embarrassment, of shame, in longing, in despair. As we breathe, oxygen floods our lungs, feeds our cells, and transforms into carbon dioxide. Millions of cells die every minute, but fresh, new cells are magically birthed. It's a regenerative process.

Sometimes, I get lost in stress and forget that I'm not here just to suffer and then die. I'm also meant to live, rejoice, grow, learn, yearn, and wander aimlessly. Experience, internal as much as external, is the salve that keeps our feet moving and our hearts beating.

Living and dying are cyclical. We can see it all around us in seasons, flowers blooming and dying, fruits ripening and decaying, the rise and fall of the chest and belly as we breathe. In our anti-aging society, people are scared to look at and talk about dying when it is the dying that makes living possible.

It's shocking and devastating when a young person dies because they were not able to live their potential joys, and those left behind feel it deeply. It's just as devastating when humans live a half-life, still in physical form, but unable to open to their potential joys. I know this isn't easy with so much that needs our attention.

When I realize that each moment is a gift, I feel the eternal within me. A passing minute can feel as if hours, days, or lifetimes have transpired. My body feels the weight of continuous lived existence, remembering. As we are inextricably connected with each other and the planet, memories may arise that seem to be of other beings, inspired by the collective breath and forces of creation floating in the ether, surrounding us, infusing with us.

We are steeped in the tea of our environments. When the spaces we inhabit feel true and trustworthy, the more aligned we become within. The inverse applies here too, as we remain aligned, it seems, so do our surroundings.

Remembering to live our moments is what enables death to be a fulfilling culmination of our joy, individually and collectively. Practicing awareness or gratitude or love for our momentary births, deaths, and rebirths, connect us to ourselves a little more each day, and to the wonder that makes joy possible.

Hold the sacred close so that the unceremonious doesn't separate you from yourself.

Feed your sacred heart with ritual and rhythm.
Be aware of your words and use them to uplift instead of tear down.
Infuse your body with peace so that you may offer it to those who cannot find it in themselves.
Without a knowing center, there can be no communion with another.
When others act against you, it reflects their inner turmoil.
They cannot see themselves as sacred.
Pay no mind, as they are lost.
Share guidance if you have time to give them a kind word.
Be a daily witness to your life.
Give attention to your movement, actions, interactions, and speech in order to feel closeness with yourself.
For it is presence that creates the sacred.
Living the moment, loving the moment.
Understanding the ceremony that is your life protects from the sacred being taken from you, whether intentional or arbitrary.
When you recognize the language of your soul, nothing can hide it from you.

The little person inside you needs your presence to process the physical sensations you label as emotion.

Feeling anxious yesterday, I asked myself when the first time was I remember feeling the gnawing ache in my belly. My body answered when I was very young, perhaps the first time I remember moving from one house into another, with my family relationships significantly changed due to divorce.

Once I had awareness wash over me, at the time consciousness arose in the self, I noticed many unspoken things. Our nervous systems do this automatically, whether we consciously recall or not. I have moved 25 times in my life. It struck me that the physical pull in my gut gave me the same sensations as homesickness.

When the little person inside me didn't know how to hold big feelings and nobody else held them adequately, dissociation got written into my brain chemistry and then hid away until the next time I had big, unexplainable emotions. Aching for a home within my caregiver relationships felt like anxiety.

In elementary school, my body reacted with illness when I had unconscious fear, I think, so that I'd be believed instead of being judged as whiny and hypersensitive. I came down with chicken pox 2 days into a week-long outdoor school camp, I got the flu just before my choir went away for a weekend concert tour, and bronchitis that prevented me from traveling several times.

It's not that I was afraid of traveling as a kid, but my nervous system was trying to keep me safe from the terror of being abandoned or separated from family and my home(s), as in my earliest memories.

Yesterday, when I stayed with the feeling and became curious, all these realizations began rising up, the gnawing eased, and then disappeared. My little person needed that presence from me in order to mitigate the sensations that I related to anxiety.

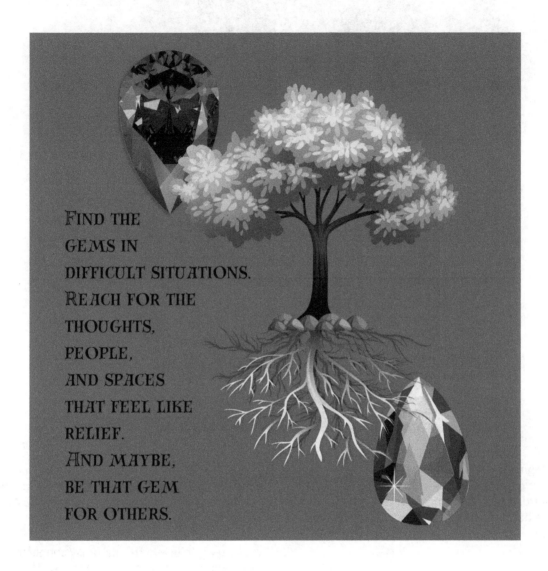

FIND THE
GEMS IN
DIFFICULT SITUATIONS.
REACH FOR THE
THOUGHTS,
PEOPLE,
AND SPACES
THAT FEEL LIKE
RELIEF.
AND MAYBE,
BE THAT GEM
FOR OTHERS.

Sometimes you don't even know you needed it until a friend comes by to give a special gift they made with their very own hands, their time, and their love. It's not the gift per say, but the thoughtfulness, that they held you in their thoughts and their heart for some hours as they prepared something beautiful, that is so touching.

It feels like a break in the busy, the daily, the rumination that can take over when terrible things happen, like the devastation of all the wildfires taking people's homes and lives right now, to have a bright presence that says I'm here, I'm thinking of you.

Whether it's a hug, a story, a silent cup of tea, a shared tear or laugh, there is community in that space. Everyone needs a little levity, some relief from thoughts that activate fear in their nervous system. Having someone beside you that is calm and attentive, regulates your body's reaction and soothes its activation.

People inherently want to relieve suffering in others. So, when you need them, look for the glowing eyes and soft expression of compassion. And when you can, be that calm for others.

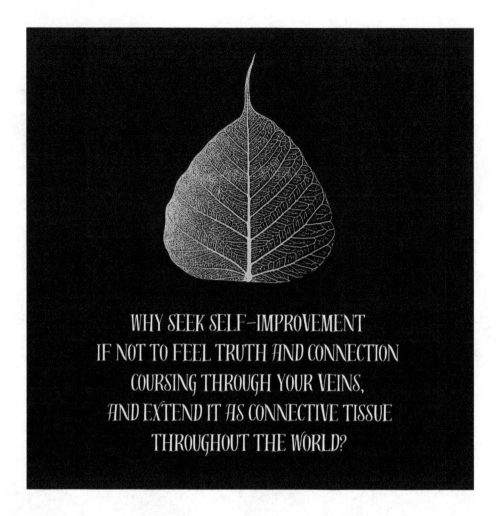

WHY SEEK SELF-IMPROVEMENT
IF NOT TO FEEL TRUTH AND CONNECTION
COURSING THROUGH YOUR VEINS,
AND EXTEND IT AS CONNECTIVE TISSUE
THROUGHOUT THE WORLD?

Personal development can be challenging and messy because answers don't easily come without accountability to our inner world. It takes a strong person to accept in ourselves the desire to change and grow in mindset, compassion, and awareness of the impact we have on others.

And yet, the very thing that can be scary is what gives us the drive to learn. When we are born, there is a need for connection that comes along with us. It is so in many a creature. Humans are delicate as newborns, as we must continue to develop more than just physically, once outside of the womb. A built-in tool that makes darn sure we have connection with others, because we need it in order to survive.

Our bodies are nature's doppelganger. There is a reason why our brain's neural network resembles galaxies, our lungs look like tree roots, and our blood vessels run in patterns like great rivers of the planet. We are in and of the natural world, the similarity is seamless. The waters that were once rain live in our veins and will again return to the ground.

The world is literally on fire. It is time to dissolve the illusion that we are not the burning trees, homes, and people. We each have the responsibility to clear away the black smoke that keeps us hidden from one another. We ARE each other. Creatures in kind.

We are born to live in this naturally connected state with all we are immersed in and surrounded by. This connection is a gift. We've gotten a little ahead of ourselves, and with this heady vision, we can forget that we live among relations. Since we are tied to the land in body and spirit, our own self-improvement must include improving the environment we inhabit, the habitat we hold inside and out.

So, healing the world heals us too. The land and your body can read each other.

Learning about ourselves, our depth, our growth, helps us feel the wisdom of the planet. Seek the truth of our interconnectivity by asking your veins, your lungs, and your gut, and by asking the trees and the rivers.

And listen for the answers.

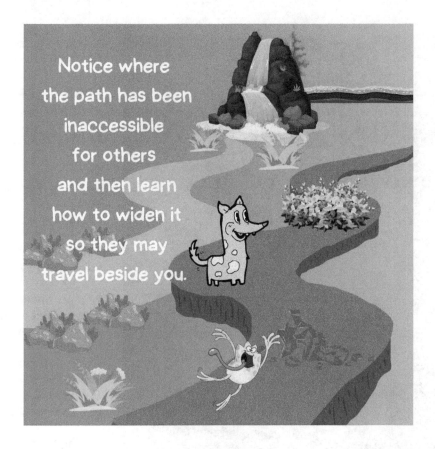

Notice where the path has been inaccessible for others and then learn how to widen it so they may travel beside you.

Many of us have privilege that we may not be aware of. Our upbringing in society causes blind spots, especially when we are comfortable in our surroundings.

It's commonly encouraged to follow your dreams, to reach for the stars, to listen to your heart. I have encouraged others to connect with soul, because from my perspective, it is what I've been privileged to be able to do. My worldview colours what I believe is possible.

There are also many who have a different worldview because of their experiences. Each journey can hold vastly different obstacles, chasms, or hidden doorways to success for those fortunate enough to be given access.

Obstacles can be racism, ageism, sexism, colonialism, language, education, socioeconomic structures, and more. If we are immersed in our own lifestyle and don't listen to the experiences of others, we miss the whole picture. The hard part can be believing another when they explain a perspective that you don't hold, based on their own lives. The systems we live in make it difficult to see the water we're swimming in.

Seeking out the barriers that stop people from accessing support in healthcare, education, mental health, financial accessibility and poverty, food systems, aging and dying, are some areas that can be looked at for examples of biased and racist oppression.

Improving yourself is a compassionate and loving thing to do if you have the capability. Making the world better for yourself and your children must include equity for all to have access to create the best outcomes for themselves. It's a long way off to equity, however, the more we are able to open our eyes to the gaping discrepancies that plague our systems, the more we can work to support systemic change.

It can be overwhelming to think about everything all at once. Just look for one thread that tugs at your heartstrings and learn about it. How might the path be cleared and widened for another to have access to compassionate care and treatment?

I have just started reading the book, White Women - Everything you already know about your own racism and how to do better, by Regina Jackson and Saira Rao. It is eye-opening and informative. It comes highly recommended as a first step toward awareness of issues I haven't experienced because of my whiteness bubble. I'm grateful to these two authors and to those who recommended it, so that I may have the opportunity to do better within the systems of harm and lessen my contribution to perpetuating these systems.

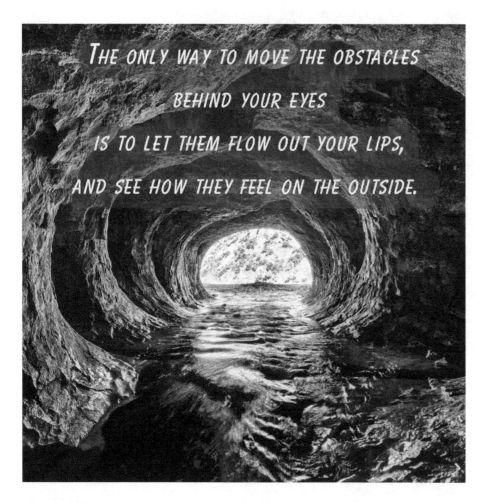

THE ONLY WAY TO MOVE THE OBSTACLES BEHIND YOUR EYES IS TO LET THEM FLOW OUT YOUR LIPS, AND SEE HOW THEY FEEL ON THE OUTSIDE.

Far too long, feeling like Aaron Burr, in the room where it happens.

Unsure of where I stood, just wanting to be included.

Terrified to speak any untruth, I did not speak.

Words of heart and soul mocked for being soft and unvalued when my strength arose from this very language.

I thought my voice was deceiving me, but it was my mind all along.

I did not know how to communicate the rhythm I felt underfoot or the whispers among the leaves.

The majesty of sunset or starry sky, impossible to embody in mundane terms. Gathering fragments of my spirit along the disconnected desert,

Placing them in my satchel for later.

I thought my body was deceiving me, but it was my mind all along.

My mind was the great trickster for most of my life. Absorbing what I saw, interpreting my surroundings into rules.

I thought my eyes deceived me, but it was my mind all along. Watching behavior convinced me of their rightness. Fear enough to stay small, stay the same. Becoming aware and wanting to grow.

There was emptiness at first, from listening to the humans, mimicry rewarded.

I thought my ears deceived me, but it was my mind all along. Finding myself contained challenges, tearing down mirrors of the fun house that were not actually fun.

I couldn't find me for eons.

Belonging felt elusive until I found my voice and slivers of light reflecting pieces of my truth, both in the depths of hiding shadows.

When I had collected enough earth, rock, and shell to piece me back together,

I found song in the tiny puddles of a dried-up lakebed. I began to move with intention.

Letting undigested prose tumble from my lips became a blessing of surprise.

Ego screaming all the way, "What are you doing??" Unconscious streams surfaced,

Bubbling with the music of trust and wholeness.

Allowing all parts of me to read aloud the dialect within, satiating the soul, honouring, and connecting the shadows and the light.

I thought my mind was deceiving me, but she was my partner all along.

Even tricksters have their purpose.

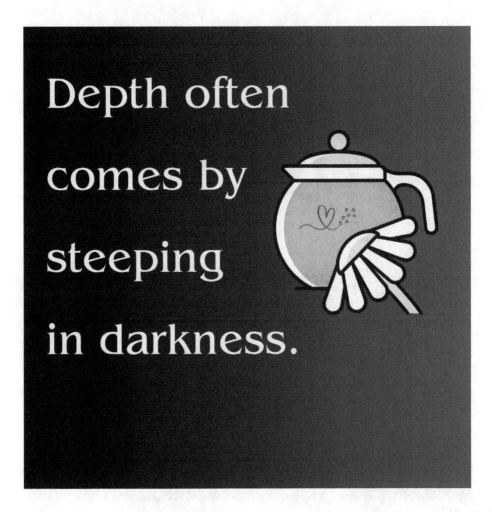

Depth often comes by steeping in darkness.

The most beautiful crystals grow in caves under extreme temperature and pressure. Trees thrive because of the root systems and mycelial networks underground. Tea becomes flavorful, strong, and deep when steeped inside the dark of a teapot.

We can't always have the minutes, hours, or days that feel light and joyful, but there can be some serenity in knowing that deep work is bubbling under the surface. The unconscious does a lot of the groundwork and meaning making before coming into our conscious.

On the surface, our challenges take significant time, attention, and energy, and even more is taking place without our awareness. Running around in the mind can be exhausting, so if capacity wanes for conscious energetic work, often it's best to sleep, be still, or distract in some way while the heart engages in the process of healing.

If you have the energy to explore where certain feelings or triggers came from, it's helpful to trace back to the moments before the feelings of heartache, shame, fear, or anxiety began. Just like taking small sips of tea to taste each of the flavors mingling together, you can slowly listen for each element that culminated in the feelings that arose.

Such as the frame of mind you were in, if you felt present or distant, were you judging yourself, how rested or exhausted were you, physically, mentally, or spiritually? What were your expectations? Were you following your own heart or someone else's suggestion?

These and many other questions you can ask yourself could be illuminating to what got you to the point of suffering. After that, try to generate compassion for yourself and honor the process your body needs to move toward recovery, however that may look. Then, when you're able, reach out to a trusted person to share your feelings.

Our shadows are sacred. They can teach us many things. Though we can heal in darkness, we grow in the light. As Brené Brown discovered, shame cannot survive being shared and given empathy. Balance of light and dark is healthy. If you want help moving back toward light, connect with a loved one.

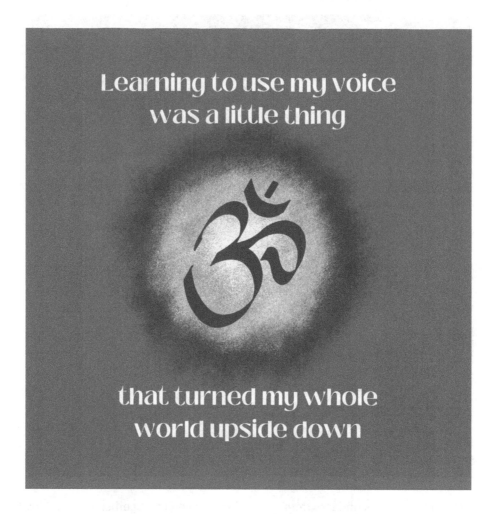

Learning to use my voice
was a little thing

that turned my whole
world upside down

I've had this fear for a very long time that people will judge everything I say because I don't have a PhD. I have felt unworthy of sharing my ideas with a larger audience, and sometimes with even just one person, due to the belief that my thoughts have little value.

Sadly, it took 50 years (and several mentors) to understand that the values I live by, the alignment with my truest self, and the integrity in the relationships I share, are what draw folks to believe in me. Trusting myself to communicate the feelings behind the words is what matters.

Fortunately, these 50 years gave me experiences that have left me with stories, lessons, and insights that changed my life, changed my heart, and changed the language I use. People can feel intention, even if they can't articulate it.

I've learned to communicate more clearly than in the past. I may have gained this ability sooner if I'd taken the path of a PhD, but I'm sure I'd be a different person. Faster doesn't always equal quality.

I've learned that many of those with PhD's and other exceptional skills also get Imposter Syndrome. So, something tells me it's human conditioning that causes us to grapple with self-worth, and not what we have achieved.

When I finally began sharing my voice and my truth, it completely transformed me. My self-confidence grew and my fear of not being perfect dwindled. Clarity comes easier, creativity flows through me everyday, which is huge because for several decades I believed I had zero creative bones.

I even stopped caring about the judgement of others, mostly. People resonate with their own truth and belief systems, so they'll feel truth in my words, or they won't. Either is ok, each human has their own paths to follow.

I used to be scared of my voice. Now I'm incredibly grateful for it.

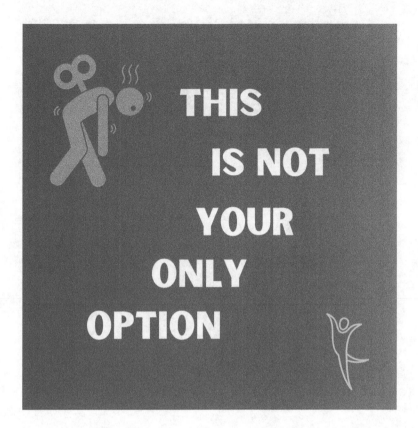

THIS
IS NOT
YOUR
ONLY
OPTION

Take your heart out of the cold, metal box sitting next to you on the nightstand, on your desk, in the front seat of your car or beside you on the bus, in the lunchroom at work, in your backpack or in your pocket.

It longs to be back in your chest, where it can feel the pain, the joy, the breath of excitement and loss, the sorrow, the sexy, the gratitude.

It cannot be courageous or feel the deliciousness of that tear rolling down your cheek while sitting inside square shaped protection.

It cannot hear the song of your soul or the language of the trees or smell the warming scent of soup made by a loved one when it is confined in air-tight shelter, suffocating.

Your heart is made to be soft and vulnerable.

It belongs in the middle of connective tissue, being hugged by your body, touched by all your human layers.

Weakness is present only in disconnection from its source, from its space.

The absence of heart makes the chest grow weary, and the body forlorn.

Returning it to its rightful place revives the aliveness that you deserve in all your moments, from pleasure to boredom, creation and culmination, introduction to benediction, ordinary and exceptional.

Rally up that oldest and dearest memory, the one that reminds you of who you were before your heart began living outside of you, just beyond your reach.

Decipher the instruction manual that was made of your earliest cries, your indignant desires, and your daydreams.

THIS... is not all there is.

Whatever your "this" may be.

Your feelings of lack, of not enough, of too much, of fitting in, of doing what's expected of you, of ignoring your creativity, of living miserable.

You are so so so much more, right in this moment.

You are miraculous.

Open your senses to your heart.

It needs you to love so it can live.

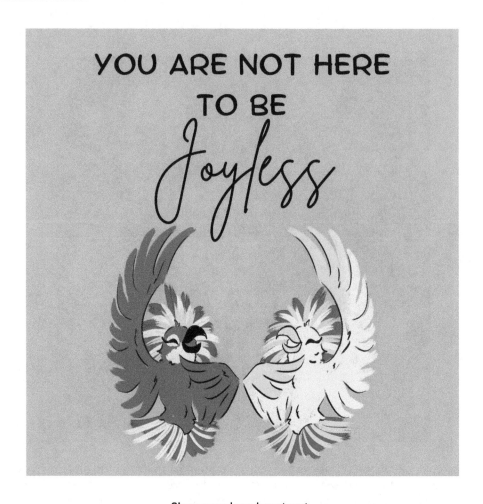

YOU ARE NOT HERE
TO BE
Joyless

Sing your dang heart out.
Dance badly.
Move your body.
Connect with the sky.
Watch clouds.
Get up for sunrise, it's worth it.
Feel molecules of sunshine bounce off your face.
Stretch your arms out in the wind.
Have a nap.
Talk to the ever-loving trees.
Breathe the forest floor.
Pet the moss.
Boop a cow's nose.
Swim naked in a lake.
Smell rain.
Let your feet linger in grass.
Listen to your heartbeat.
Rub softness on your cheek.
Brush your teeth.
Look into someone's eyes.
Be the last to release a hug.
Laugh until you cry.
Cry until you laugh.
Be ridiculous.
Love beyond reason.

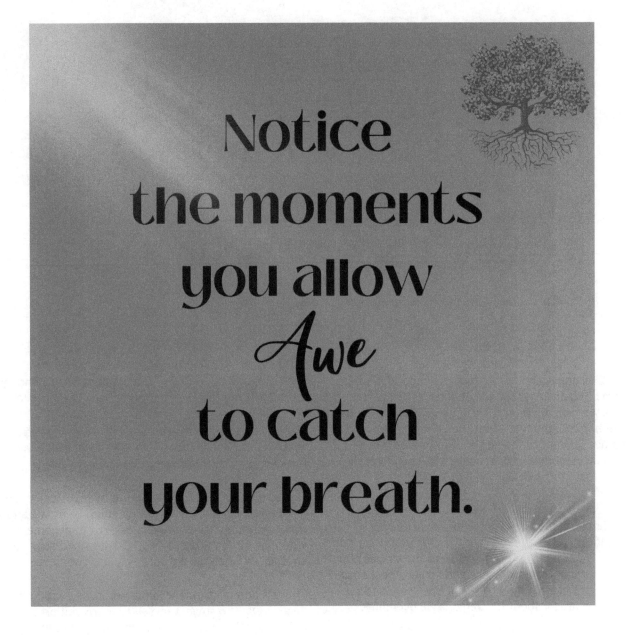

Notice
the moments
you allow
Awe
to catch
your breath.

What is your default?
Do you notice the awesome or the awful?
Do you savor the sweet juice dripping on your tongue or find an excuse to call it bitter?
We face days and nights of opportunity.
Sunshine, through the leaves, can be blinding or bonding.
Epiphany can come from looking up, even when peering inside.
Little fireworks in the brain and heart, when noticed, change who we are.
Significance is born in a moment if we dare to hold it.

> # I don't feel like the hero in my own life. I feel much more complicated, loving, and human than that.

Stories of challenges and heroic journeys abound. The symbolism of obstacles is spoken of in terms of the challenges we face on the way to something great. There are lots of books and information about archetypes such as the wounded healer or the teacher. Different archetypes describe behaviors that may resonate with you. You can read about them through Carl Jung or Dr Clarissa Pinkola Estés.

The symbolism of obstacles for me, however, is how I perceive inner challenges. Who are the demons we face and what are they asking us to do? I believe all the stories about the devil, mystical villains, dragons and slayers, witches and witch hunters, Daniel in the lion's den, Medusa, Baba Yaga, Sirens, Cthulu, are all about the demons we overcome or succumb to.

What if we accepted these characters as parts of ourselves and invited them for tea, along with the other, more "civilized" bits? Not so much as entities to kill and conquer, but to accept and love. Combining the wild and the socialized may seem a mismatch, when in truth, it's how we feel seen and loved for the whole of who we are. We've been taught to fight off the wild creatures who live inside us, further feeding our disconnection.

I might be alone in this, but I don't like watching the hero's saga. The story of a "good" guy getting pushed down over and over until he finds a way to become strong enough to overpower the forces of evil and finally have justice.

The violence of this makes me cringe, my heart aches, my eyes well up. The justice at the end is not satisfying to me, not enough to want to watch the pain.

Every one of us has a fluid mixture of angel, demon, wild and tamed, hurtful, and ignorant, compassionate, and wise flowing through us. These characteristics become prominent when the need for protection arises, when taking care of another, or when we are surprised by joy and vulnerability.

There is enough torment in the world, and within those I love, to want to subject myself to more of it on purpose. I'm happy when justice is served, though heartbroken at the debris left on the trail. I don't feel joy at the win, but discombobulation at the trauma that occurred.

I much prefer seeking consolidation within myself, accepting, and loving the Medusa inside me, as she hopes to be seen as whole and not just for her appearance, my inner Baba Yaga, who wants to impart her wisdom of the woods, and my equal parts witch and hunter, who believe in magic while still affected by fear. I don't feel like a hero. I feel much more complicated, loving, and human than that.

We....ALL of us, everybody.... deserves compassionate health care, education, housing.

We should not have to mantra the s@#! out of this statement in order to believe it.

Compassion matters from those who have taken an oath (even a hyperbolic one) to do no harm.

I saw a medical doctor yesterday.

Since covid, I don't go to the doctor unless I really need to, and as most people when seeking healthcare, I was feeling vulnerable.

I always hope that the physician I'm going to see is having a good day and will offer calming to the nervous system...and the nervousness...once I'm able to speak with them.

Counting on luck is an unsettling way to approach an appointment, but it's been this way for too long. Unfortunately, it did not go well. The doctor became unhinged and straight up yelled at me for daring to ask one too many questions, a total of three. They wanted me to make another appointment even though each of my concerns were related. When I became frustrated at the structure of this payment system, they berated me for an extra 2 minutes while typing out a requisition.

This is not compassion, nor even care.

Caring would have been offering compassionate, or even detached witnessing to my frustration.

We are human.

I understand everyone has challenges, however, being in allied healthcare I know that professionals are trained and expected to leave their baggage at the door.

If I hold myself to higher standards than physicians, we are not ok.

This encounter left me stunned and upset.

I physically felt the mistreatment flowing through the tissues of my legs, likely in the form of adrenaline and other fight or flight hormones. My body wanted to run far and fast from humiliation. For a few minutes, I sat there feeling responsible for creating the situation.

But as I reflected, I understood that I had only asked to be heard.

The doctor's reaction to that was their choice.

If we embody mistreatment, we begin to believe we deserve it, we become used to it and therefore tolerant. If we are treated like crap, we FEEL crappy. It makes sense to me why our society keeps getting sicker. Autoimmune disease is on the rise. This means the body attacks itself. Embodiment of self-blame is ironic when poor systemic treatment and lack of compassion is hurting us.

I want you to know, to feel it in your bones, that you deserve better than this.

You deserve compassionate witnessing.

You deserve dignity.

You deserve to feel heard.

Every. single. person. deserves. humanity.

I deserve compassionate care.
I deserve compassionate care.
I deserve compassionate care.
I deserve compassionate care.
I deserve compassionate care.
I deserve compassionate care.
I deserve compassionate care.
I deserve compassionate care.
I deserve compassionate care.
I deserve compassionate care.
So do you, all of the above.

> # HUG YOUR PEEPS.
> # LOVE YOUR MESSINESS.
> # IT'S ALL WE GOT
> # MY FRIENDS.

All of us are messy.

Nobody has a neat and tidy life unless they aren't living.

Even after we die, the love we leave behind blows worlds apart.

Pieces of the lost are not forgotten but remain in the form of memory and energy.

I hold both love and sadness as I write these words.

Uplifted by spirit, by people who mean the world to me, even though I feel broken by the cost that society has brought to the hearts and bodies of those who fall through the cracks of dignity.

Pressures of injustice reign, smothering the sanity of compassion.

Accepting my messiness means allowing the conflicts within, between the grief, the rage, the love, and the unlikely opening to all the diversity, fears, and hope intertwining.

Connection is the way through the terror of the inhumane.

We cannot suffer alone, we must not.

There will always be light and dark inside each of us, the doubtful and humiliated, the longing for truth and the finding of it.

We are oh so complex.

And as our inner parts flow with peace, love, fear, and grief, so does our world.

We've been ingesting contradiction in the form of bootstraps and white knights.

When disconnection blinds our senses, the feeling of community suffers, as we wait for someone to save us.

We separate from ourselves when we forget each other.

I know I'm not the only empath, the only person who feels this much, this deeply, the tumult, the great grief that humans carry.

It's so very prominent if one pays attention.

Some days are overwhelming, even for those of us who give much focus to seeing the constant stream of love in joyful moments, all around us.

This poem of discontent does not have a lighthearted ending, no soundbite to quote. We don't always get over it, come out on top, or become a hero.

We are mushy bags of feelings, and we need each other in order to stay standing or sitting...and breathing.

Love and connection really do matter.

Hug your peeps, love your messiness.

It's all we got, my friends.

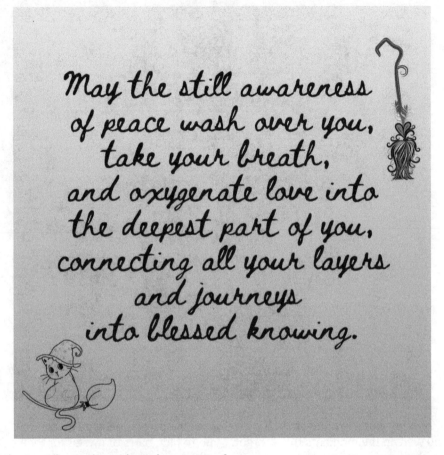

May the still awareness
of peace wash over you,
take your breath,
and oxygenate love into
the deepest part of you,
connecting all your layers
and journeys
into blessed knowing.

My story is made of all the transformations I have been part of.
Each breath an exchange of the physical and energetic.
My path of existing and allowing moved through experiences of ignorance and arrogance, trying to fit in that softened into acceptance and learning, and then understanding and love.
Each stage gaining momentum or stalling and living into the next.
As awareness and wisdom fed the capillaries of my consciousness, streams of soul blood diffused through breath to become oxygenated.
The steps creating the dance, the energy of the dance feeding ongoing movement.
Infinity, each feeding the other.
Symbiosis.

My outer existence eventually mirrored my inner journey, crossing timelines with every decision I made, like water trickling over ridges of a washboard.
I became.
I am still becoming.
Let your knowing become you.
Dare to discover what is at the root of your beliefs and fears.
Stay curious about the timelines you will visit next.
You, too, have moments of joy and passion, sorrow, and uncomfortable numbness.
You, too, have a journey, like mine, sometimes bitter, some sweet.
May the still awareness of peace wash over you, take your breath, and oxygenate love into the deepest part of you, connecting all your layers and journeys into blessed knowing.

WHEN FEAR AND CONFUSION
IS LOUD OUTSIDE,
I WISH FOR YOU A GLIMPSE OF YOUR TRUTH
AS A REMINDER THAT
INSIDE
IS WHERE YOUR CLARITY EXISTS.

It may not be true for everybody, but the times that I have felt most lost or confused were in the moments that I forgot to look inside, check in with myself, seek my center, or honor how I felt.

The noise of what's going on around us, chatter that clutters the mind and constipates the connection to our integrity, can be overwhelming when it is not balanced by our sense of self.

It's easier to be convinced to compromise values if our default is to ignore them or don't know what they are.

There are relationships and situations in my past, and I'm sure in yours, that we would not allow or would react differently to if we were to encounter them today.

The need to keep relationships stasis quo dictated some of my choices, so much so that it felt as though I didn't actually have a choice.

This is how it feels to me when my self-worth is tied up with someone else's behavior toward me.

At some point, I became aware that some people wanted me to hide parts of myself for their own comfort.

The clue appeared after I complied for fear of losing them, when I finally realized the sense of lack and sadness came from losing myself.

It may not be possible to be completely aligned and honor our whole selves 100% of the time, though it's important to seek a few relationships that value our honesty and wholeness, support all pieces of us, and how we evolve.

This is self-loving.

We do have a choice, even when we don't see it clearly.

Sometimes, all we need is a glimpse of our insides to remember how to see what's outside with more clarity.

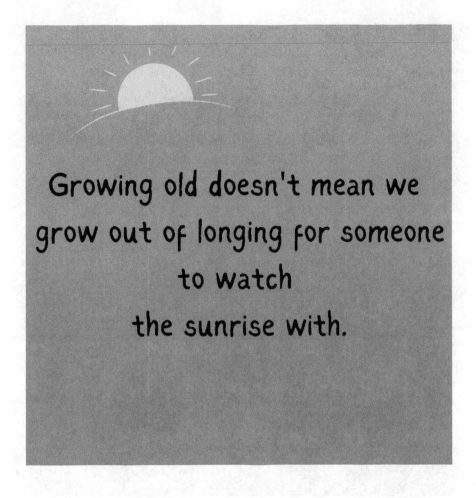

Growing old doesn't mean we
grow out of longing for someone
to watch
the sunrise with.

For many months, I spent my Thursdays with a beautiful, kind-hearted man, in the care residence that was his home.

Some days we did massage, other days we focused on rehab to strengthen his arms and legs after hip surgery.

He loved coffee, food, music, smiling, and sitting in the sunshine. What really lit him up though, was companionship, someone to talk with, to engage with in a meaningful way.

He was a teacher through his working career and knew so much about an exorbitant number of things.

We all encounter a great range of identities as we move through this precious life. Moving into a care home can help with medical needs and physical safety, though it can be difficult to honour the full lives and where each person came from before arriving here. But sometimes, I can see it in their eyes.

When I showed up a few weeks ago, he was sitting in the lounge with many others, listening to a rousing, and very loud André Rieu concert playing on the tv. He didn't want to leave, so we decided to do his treatment right where he sat.

My Mum was a huge André Rieu fan, so I knew the music well. Several of us hummed along, caught in the bliss that connects people's hearts.

We stood up with the walker a couple of times, and during the rest periods while he sat, I held both his hands and danced to the joyous music. He looked at me directly in the eyes, engaged, excited, and grinning from ear to ear while we arm danced. Connected in heart, through music, love, and joy.

We may not know everything they went through to get here, but we can honour other people's journeys by celebrating with them and giving them our time, our hearts, and our presence. Everybody wants to be seen and everyone deserves that.

This beautiful, kind-hearted, music lover passed away just two weeks after our dance.

What a privilege it was to get to know you and give you my heart. I celebrate you today and everyday, Thom. Thank you for allowing me to be part of your precious life.

I have never once healed another person.

My goal is to offer relief to a small part of the human spirit, and once relief starts to seep in....ahhh.... that's when people begin to heal themselves.

I am not the healer; I prefer instigator of intrinsic healing.

Healing isn't only one thing.

It can mean becoming free from illness, injury, or disability.

It can also mean becoming free from disabling thoughts regarding our conditions, internal or external.

Trying on different perspectives can be incredibly freeing.

Identifying with relief is a challenge when looking through the lens of suffering.

There have been oh so many times I have come across a spot on a person's body during massage therapy that they had no idea was holding tension.

Treatment of this area will often cause relief in an area they didn't realize they needed it, a lifting of an unconscious restriction.

Relief in one area can lead to shifts in the primary, more likely conscious, areas of pain or discomfort.

This happens in the mind and spirit as well.

Any number of unconscious beliefs, triggers, biases, habits, or reactions contribute to our suffering.

Myriad happenings can reveal the once unconscious restriction that kept our other pieces tied up, uncertain of their origins.

A glimpse of relief in either sense opens a metaphorical window, which allows awareness to flow in like a breeze, offering a slight lifting as the ribcage expands with a new breath.

Just a crack is all we usually need to feel hope again, that healing may be possible, in whatever form that takes.

Revealing the crack, the glimpse of relief, can spark the solo journey to discovering what healing means for each person.

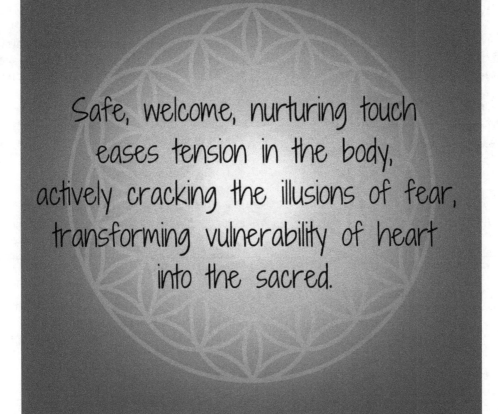

Safe, welcome, nurturing touch
eases tension in the body,
actively cracking the illusions of fear,
transforming vulnerability of heart
into the sacred.

Being held when it feels right becomes a healing space, an opportunity for opening to oneself, and to another.

Trust is critical in this environment.

In my experience, many people feel safe to speak earnestly during a calming massage therapy treatment if the therapeutic relationship has nurtured trust.

Speaking of one's pain is one of the most vulnerable subjects for people to talk about.

I've listened to the surprise that arises when someone becomes overwhelmed with pain, grief, or fear.

It could be that touch opens a portal to the emotions, or that the feeling of safety does.

Having someone in any area of life truly listen and hold you with non-judgement opens a magical cabinet to the Narnia of the heart.

This allowing creates a sacred moment between two beings, and within the one who is sharing.

I've felt this moment like a transcendence of my pain into a feeling of diffusion, like particles of pain and shame lift from my body and heart, and float into the ethers to be taken care of by the earth and spirit.

It's almost as if fear keeps us hooked, tethered to a story that has become solidified by our minds.

Noticing a shift in the body is a powerful moment because it brings doubt into awareness.

Doubt that this unshakeable fear, thoughts that have become tension over time, may not be rooted too deep for us to excavate.

When relief and ease are seen as an option, the foundation of fear becomes questionable.

And when we question our fears, sacred healing is possible.

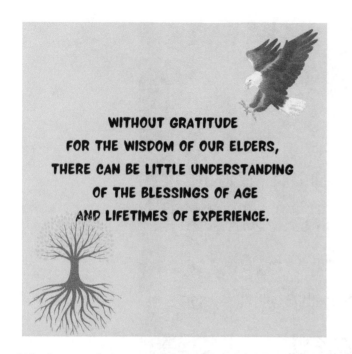

WITHOUT GRATITUDE
FOR THE WISDOM OF OUR ELDERS,
THERE CAN BE LITTLE UNDERSTANDING
OF THE BLESSINGS OF AGE
AND LIFETIMES OF EXPERIENCE.

Why is our culture so afraid of aging and dying? We have all been touched by life-altering or life- ending disease. We've been affected by the way we ourselves and our loved ones have been cared for by our healthcare systems.

In her book, if women rose rooted, Sharon Blackie wrote, the cultural narrative IS the culture. At the moment, the culture of the aged is a frightening one. During the first 3 months of the covid-19 shutdown, more than 14,000 Canadians died. More than 11,000 of those unfortunate deaths were in senior care homes. And because there were no visitors allowed, many of these folks died alone. This culture looks like isolation.

In 2021, anti-aging was a 67-billion-dollar industry and is projected to rise to 120 billion by 2030. When looking young is the ideal, western society creates a sort of youth-to-death pipeline. Media icons are expected to be young, until one day they die. No aging in between. It's a shock to the media machine when a celebrity demands to be seen without photo-shop.

This culture feels inauthentic.

Residences that house people who can no longer care for themselves, their hygiene, cook for themselves, have limited mobility, cognitive decline, and continual medical needs, are convenient for a society that relies on productive, working citizens. Families are often swamped with work in order to afford the cost of living, too busy and financially dependent to take a hiatus to be a full-time caregiver for their olders. This age group often struggles as the sandwich generation, caring for parents while still having children at home.

This culture feels like exhaustion.

The way we view what happens in our later years contributes to the aversion we have to facing these topics. If isolation, inauthenticity, and exhaustion is what we have to look forward to, it's no wonder we are scared to live into these types of scenarios.

Without gratitude for the wisdom of our elders, there can be little understanding of the blessings of age, forest, rivers, or humans, and lifetimes of experience.

It is crucial to examine the ways we have forgotten our elders and determine appropriate shifts in how we proceed as a humanity that is inextricably entwined with nature and the delicate balance between environment and humanity, oxygen, and vitality.

Someone who is able to connect with and be a compassionate witness to a whole human and their needs, or a whole planet, is necessary for integration and visibility in our communities. Healthy change requires integrity, compassion, and visibility in order to include all people in micro movements, innovative ideas to try, and possibilities for a different future for humans and the planet.

We can learn a lot from nature. When an elderly tree falls, the community comes together to keep feeding that tree nutrients, right where it landed, their offspring adjusting their root systems and the mushroom communication networks continue to provide electrical connection between the tree and its woods. The old tree has continued wisdom to share until it is eventually absorbed into the forest floor, becoming nutrients for their children, fungus, and creatures of the wood, because of their dis-integration. This is regenerative.

Thoughtful programs, once created, and even IN the creating OF them, people may not be so frightened of aging & dying, and trust community to care for them with empathy and love when their time comes. What an honor it would be to dissolve into nourishment for others.

Both areas need to be addressed, nature and human nature. It's time for love and compassion to be action words. There are many options to moving forward with integrity. Reciprocity, respect, and gratitude are values we can embody while moving toward compassionate AND regenerative goals.

> ## BEING TOUCH-DEPRIVED CAN MANIFEST AS ANXIETY. OUR CULTURE HAS FORGOTTEN WHAT A MIRACLE SAFE, KIND, CONSENSUAL TOUCH IS.

With more than 4 million touch receptors in our skin, it makes sense that we hunger for touch. Touch that feels nurturing is crucial to regulation of the nervous system. The epidemics of anxiety and depression have grown in huge numbers since covid contributed to contact starvation between people.

Self-regulation requires co-regulation in early life. This means that our bodies learn to react to our environments somewhat through the compassionate presence of a caregiver. Our bodies intuitively read the energy of the nervous system of our primary nurturer and learn to respond to it with our own.

Intentional and welcome pressure on the skin conveys care, and the body responds, often with relaxing of muscle tension and calming of the nervous system.

The miracle is the mystery of how skin receptors transform touch into safety, love, emotion, and relief.

As with all our senses, touch is communication between two beings. If someone could not see or hear, touch would be able to speak for the three senses.

Affection has always been a connection for people. We crave this connection, as it's been built into us since humans began.

To address the crisis of anxiety, adding touch therapies can be a useful shift in approach. Sterile medicine is not going to fix it alone. The most touch-starved people in our communities can feel disconnected from themselves, and I've seen how touch can bring about joy and relief for so many. However, some folks don't want to feel the feelings that arise if they were to connect. This is where other therapies may be helpful.

Personally, I feel relief from anxiety when I play in dirt, stand barefoot in grass, breathe deeply inside a forest, move my body, and receive affectionate touch from someone I trust. I feel transformed after massage therapy and melt into a long hug with a loved one. Mental health has a lot to do with our bodies as well. Though, of course, seeking out mental health professionals can be the best thing in some circumstances.

There is magic in our bodies. Our skin holds great healing potential, and our nervous systems can be taught to calm through kind touch, intention, and practice.

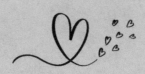

*The more we grasp how few
breaths we have in these human bodies,
the more we realize
that spreading love and kindness
is the best way to create community.*

There must be a river of love inside each of us longing to be uncovered,

With silver strands of moonlight and the glowing of a million suns,

Existing under the brush of trance and poison,

Guised by layers of overgrown confusion, fermented, throwing off the scent of truth,

Rused by falsehoods and fanatics of the psyche.

Oceans of milky sky reflecting the billions of souls on the planet,

Intertwining as we move past and through each other,

Attracting and repelling energy, some bouncing off, some bonding like hydrogen atoms to those who feel like oxygen.

This air we breathe is a gift from earth,

She has been able to give us life, nourishing each moment with her exhales,

It is senseless to use such an offering to utter hateful words into the ears of other precious beings, into the air that unironically keeps us alive,

When we are here to be infused with beauty and love.

These bodies gain much from kindness and acceptance, nurturing and presence,

Spreading love into community melts like sunrise coming over the mountain, slowly washing rays of awakening over the land, connecting us to a universe that did not exist before this moment,

Breathing in sync, in silent knowing.

As we are lost without each other, without being known, without affection and acceptance,

We are love together,

We are found, we are home.

Sharing is caring they say, a loving legacy.

Our bodies do not live forever,

But through a connected community, the love in our hearts can.

> Remembering to breathe
> during the pain,
> within the tension, through the grief,
> allows it to keep moving.
> Holding the breath builds pressure.
> Ebb and flow, inhale, exhale,
> is nature's way.

Pain, worry, grief, and sadness, all can trigger us to hold onto the breath, as if everything will fall apart if we exhale.

The truth is, we fall apart sometimes.

Tears and wails, cathartic screams, and thrashing about may look uncivilized to some, but can be profoundly healing from the inside.

Holding our breath can seem like the only kind of control we have at times, as if trying to stop the next hiccup or the next truth from escaping our lips.

Control is illusion, easy to understand in a bout of hiccups, a fit of sneezes, or as a muscle spasm.

We may not be able to stop these, but we can manage symptoms and realize that breathing through moments it feels hardest can bring relief.

As a massage therapist, I encounter a lot of folks who don't breathe. Or at least those who inhale so shallowly that it appears to create a delineation between solid rock and soft tissue. As if the breath gets stuck in the chest and makes it brittle, instead of strong and mobile. If breath only reaches a few inches, it neglects to nourish the softness of the belly, the expansion of the ribcage, the digestive forces of the gut. This neglect can be painful, even as it tries to save us from other kinds of pain.

Noticing how we breathe can help us pay attention to our oxygen-starved parts. When I ask my patients to inhale toward an area that my hands are treating them, most often, it softens more readily than just with treatment alone.

If you find it difficult or vulnerable to breathe fully and expansively, I recommend seeking someone experienced in breathwork instruction.

Breath changes our pain, our awareness, our perspective, can decrease tension, and helps us fall apart in the most necessary ways.

May you be lucky enough
to cry tears of peace,
be winded by beauty,
gutted by love,
and broken open by compassion.

When I die, I want you to be gutted.

I want the momentary catch of your breath to be filled with love.

May tears of joy flood your eyes, flow down your cheeks, and bring nourishment to your heart.

Taste more sweetness on your breath as you inhale my spirit and forever exhale only compassion for yourself and others.

Feel vibrant and warm because I have touched you with my hands or my heart.

If I have loved you and looked upon your face, allow a bit of yourself to come with me, leaving you stripped of pain and sorrow, self- love remaining, free to see yourself as I do, a being of pure love.

Remember me and dance in the moonlight while shooting stars light up your eyes and your soul.

Move into dark times with bolstered strength as I move with you.

Look at those you meet and see my eyes shining back at you.

Living becomes lighter upon the wind of another's love, embracing the memories that are pieces in your wholeness.

Let wondrous fractaled rainbows in sunlight remind you of your beauty, your impact, spreading expansively over the majesty of the land, people, creatures, the water of earth, and the water inside you.

Your tears reflect all the colors that exist, not just grief or joy but every emotion, every thought, every prayer, every piece of home, clarity, and blessed confusion.

You are an embodied miracle.

What you are, what you do, makes a difference.

Take me with you, into your lungs, your heart, and feel gutted in love, in joy, with peace guiding your inner river, and beauty catching your breath, every time.

Practice has most always been the way to increase skill level, craft, and understanding.

What I give my attention and intention to creates a cycle of return into my experience.

What we do more of, becomes deeply embedded in neural pathways, habitually requires less attention as time goes on, and develops the freedom for nuance, flair, and creative expression.

This past year, I have been intentionally focused on movement in the areas of compassion, love, and nourishment.

For myself, and also for my community, for those who would benefit from an increase in the areas of compassion, love, and nourishment.

Giving attention to the quality and meaning of life for the elderly and the dying in our communities began years ago, however,

I'm widening and deepening the reach for those who have made a great impact on my life.

People make imprints on our hearts.

Like an inverted leaf fossil embedded in a rock, the memory of our encounters accessible as stone one moment, other times fleeting and impossible to pin down.

Memories morph, slight variations change the details in our recall.

Tuning into the feelings of solitude and interactions can add layers of understanding that become wisdom.

Neural pathways play a part in what and how we reflect, but our bodies and hearts feel and know the passing moments more accurately.

Recognizing the signatures of beloved relationship within carries context to the past, present, and future.

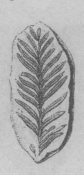

PEOPLE MAKE IMPRINTS ON US,
LIKE EMOTIONAL FOSSILS
EMBEDDED DEEPLY
IN OUR HEARTS.

Like holding a heart in front of the sun, peering through it, to determine what's inside.

I am a questioner and a lover, no doubt.

Soft, confident branches of everything these words embody, create a framework, trunk and arms to embrace the imprints in other people's hearts.

A fossil tea party, where we show each other what made us, and perhaps add some flair to our moments together.

Fossils can be stagnant brick walls, blocking love from the softness within, they can be a filter through which to view our experiences, the people around us, and they can be pieces of antiquity that show us where we've come from.

I try to appreciate history and relationships for what I may learn from them, though what I love most are the feelings my body can hold and open to upon their consideration, so that I may forever be broken open by compassion and continue to be changed by love.

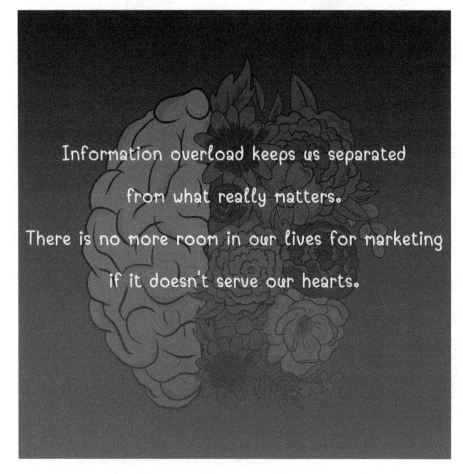

Information overload keeps us separated from what really matters.
There is no more room in our lives for marketing if it doesn't serve our hearts.

Discovering what means the most to me has been an uphill challenge.

Within the society of 'more is better' economics,

Taking in sales pitches and billboards of promises,

Landscapes littered with needless frippery that becomes refuse before tomorrow.

Economics that exist to beget wealth alone is crassitude.

In these environs, who do we serve?

Not humanity, nor creature, or planet.

Alignment with self required a severing from plastic identities of the tv screen,

No longer relating to the fears of missing the latest and greatest,

Unable to recall the insecurity that endless products filled.

Marketers turned psychologists sell their souls for profit shares,

Image creation, a vast canyon away from filling a need.

Knowing who they serve behind the scenes when not asking for money from middle earners is the classy wave of activism,

Accountability, the new judge of character.

If our hearts did the marketing, the message would be compassion,

Love would be the proceeds,

Connection, the profit,

Support, the advertiser,

Community, the network, using satellites to share solutions and spread relief,

Reciprocity and regeneration, the new economics.

Every self-help guru would advocate for social justice,

Each politician, an example of right relationship.

Humans would be as generous and creative as the earth itself.

Self-improvement is most effective when the aim is to also improve the world around us.

As Liz Gilbert says, "There's no such thing as one-way liberation."

May we always recognize and support those who speak to our hearts and follow through with action.

Soul has gravity.

There is a beautiful weightiness to an authentic moment.

It is like landing into grounding while simultaneously easing the breath and slowing down time.

The knowing of an encounter with our own pure meaning, that it will become a core memory, is the juice of life.

Joy brings us in.

Grief does too.

They effortlessly drop us into our bodies and gift us humility and vulnerability.

Emotion is vulnerable and real.

We are deeply drawn to embodied alignment in those we share space with.

These folks may spark fear, trust, compassion, happiness, or even disgust.

The point is we feel something stirring because they have a kind of magnitude.

With so much going on in the world to be drawn into, it is beneficial to listen first for the gravity of our own souls.

The silence that splits atoms.

Anabolic instead of catastrophic.

Those who want to pull us into hate and war cannot hear the voice of soul.

We do best when we avoid incite and notice insight.

In the depths, we hear creation,

The sound of creativity born,

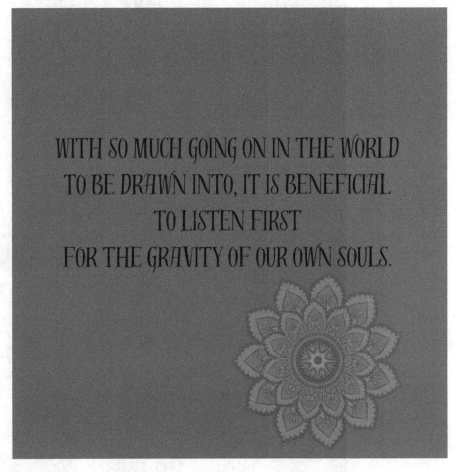

WITH SO MUCH GOING ON IN THE WORLD TO BE DRAWN INTO, IT IS BENEFICIAL TO LISTEN FIRST FOR THE GRAVITY OF OUR OWN SOULS.

The coo of the mama within,

The river that moves guts and births planets and sprouts seeds.

Every moment we swim in that river, we become the flow, the water, the force, the source.

I urge you to turn off the news today,

Be with the self you haven't allowed yourself to hear in a long while,

Sit with the gravity of the outer world interplaying with your inner world, give love to it all.

Let it reconcile within you.

You have the capacity to hold depth and meaning,

For you are the gravity.

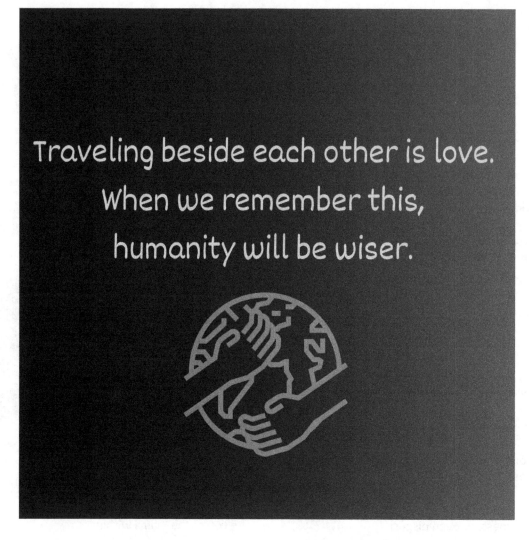

Traveling beside each other is love.
When we remember this,
humanity will be wiser.

Not everyone has the patience to rip their perspective into a thousand pieces and reassemble it as they learn new things.

We continue to hold our hurts as if they were glass, unable to put them down lest they shatter and leave us vulnerable.

Trigger finger jumpy from hypervigilance.

Love becomes a shadow hidden under thoughts of revenge, like the eclipse blocks the sun, light extinguished until further notice.

The ache one feels, unrelenting, feeding unquenchable desire for relief,

Turning pain into rocket fire.

Unable to feel humanity amongst the noise inside,

Voices that streamline blame and shift accountability outside the purview.

A land never owned, the excuse for hate,

Reciprocity foreign to power-hungry fingertips,

Devouring the very thing that would save them.

Visions of holy, drilling the holes of destruction,

Smearing the dirt from one side to the other and back again,

Until nobody is left standing.

When will this road no longer be a race to the finish, but a path to walk beside each other?

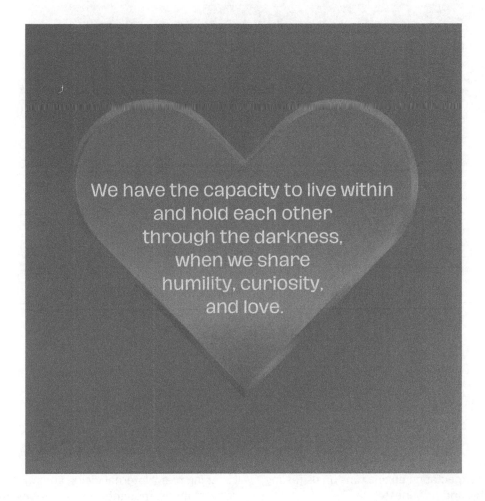

We have the capacity to live within
and hold each other
through the darkness,
when we share
humility, curiosity,
and love.

It is courageous to remember, through life and death, peace and war, suffering and joy, calm and fervor, still and tumult, that we are constants in the streams of energy, soul, and connection.

Courage is hard when we feel emotional, psychological, and physical pain. We want to ease the suffering the same way we believe it came to us, from the outside in, however, since it is most often sparked from within, learning to connect with relief is an internal endeavor.

Just like when we plug something into an electrical source and it turns on, because the energy was already there, the moment we tune into the connectedness of all beings, we light up because the stream is always there. We forget when we are overwhelmed with tasks and feelings, feel disconnected or worried.

As the moon's shadow eclipses the sun this morning, we are united in a humanity facing toward the heavens, looking for answers, for peace, for comfort, for sanity, for sustenance, mystery, and miracles.

We can be hidden by our darkness, what we think are flaws and missteps, afraid what they might do to us if we acknowledge and ask them to teach us, how we may be perceived by our communities, our societies.

We are so much more than these. We are living courage. Just being here proves that. We have the capacity to live within and through the darkness, to help others see in the dark, to hold them, and to be held when we share humility, curiosity, and love.

These heartbreaking times are enmeshed in our flesh and in our desires for a kind and just world. Allowing grief and hope to become one inside of us is a loving way to integrate our ever-changing, dichotomous nature and keep empathy in our hearts.

This, my friends, is courage.

> **When we no longer base our self-worth on the external characteristics that society deems desirable at the moment, we have more time to align with the values that rise from the inside.**

Much of the societal expectation engine runs on us feeling inadequate, unworthy, and powerless.

Marketing often sells us solutions to manufactured problems.

A conversation with a friend today reminded me that even the self-help industry is guilty of manipulation for the purpose of profit.

Being discerning is so very important when it comes to our energy, time, and relationships.

Connecting with those who resonate with what we feel deep inside is crucial to our well-being and mental health.

This doesn't mean we only talk to people if they believe what we believe. In fact, having people who feel safe challenging our beliefs and behaviors are integral to our awareness and growth.

I discover the most about myself when I ask myself powerful questions and allow others to be catalysts for reaching into what truly aligns with my soul and spirit.

Listening to my internal dialog and my body's reactions to conversations, thoughts, and situations outside of me leads to knowing more completely what I don't want in my life and what I do.

I began believing in my worthiness more as I trusted the internal whispers that felt most authentic, loving, and joyful to my body and heart.

I stopped believing in the opinions of those who aren't aligned with themselves, those who don't know my path, and those who do not serve others in this world.

The relationships we have with ourselves evolve when we use and grow and trust our innate intuition.

This is also what changes the relationships we have with others and with the world.

I believe a universe is born with every new friendship; with every person we spend time with.

Our worthiness is a foundation for the worlds we want to create in our lifetimes.

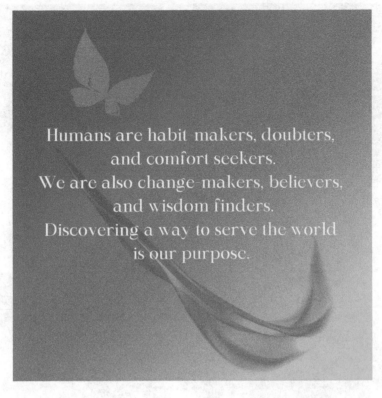

Humans are habit-makers, doubters,
and comfort seekers.
We are also change-makers, believers,
and wisdom finders.
Discovering a way to serve the world
is our purpose.

We cannot run away from this.

There are millions of ways to distract,

Whiling away days, months, years,

Scrolling, "reality shows," acquisition, desiring money, freedom, comfort, as people die, as the planet suffers, as creatures become extinct because of us.

Disconnection allows us to hide from our shadows and the deep and blatant suffering of our people, all people.

The world is filled with our people,

The earth houses our non-human relations, those who feed us, shelter us, give us meaning, give us life.

And yet, we fail to acknowledge, to reciprocate.

Complacency arises from fear, from disconnection, and from believing we are powerless.

We go to great lengths to not see, to not hear.

And then complain about being stuck in a rut, about being purposeless, about boredom.

It has become habitual.

We are afraid to explore the things that are heartbreaking and nonsensical, the joyful and the limitless.

We are scared to grow old, to see our loved ones suffer, to die,

And yet, we don't live.

Humans are habit-makers, doubters, and comfort seekers,

We are also change-makers, believers, and wisdom finders.

There are causes for everything under the sun, and change happens literally every second.

If you have not started an initiative to serve the world, find one, join one that speaks to your soul,

Be a questioner of systems, a seeker of truth, a lover of life, a designer of your daring destiny, a singer of hopeful songs, even while people and planet suffer.

We cannot run away from this,

We cannot hide from the change that is coming,

And so, we must find a way to join.

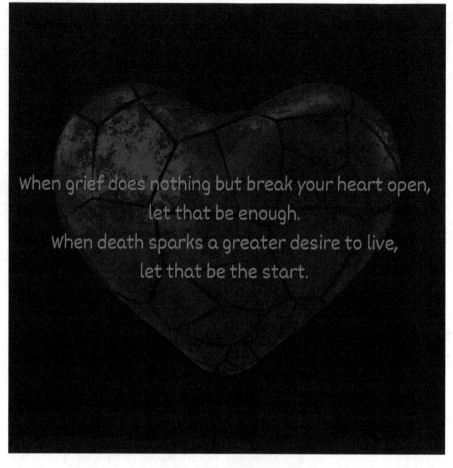

When grief does nothing but break your heart open,
let that be enough.
When death sparks a greater desire to live,
let that be the start.

Death is too intimate and finite for some people to hold,
Others mourn with candles lit,
Peace elusive, prayers, and birthday wishes unfulfilled,
Why must we die to find it?
Mountaintop wisdom up so high,
Bears and scorpions in the sky,
Walking together as below the earth quakes,
Love and monsters make hearts break.
The destroyers have forgotten,
To themselves will be begotten,
What they do to one or many,
No more illusions, only unity.
Lonely and destitute, attacker and attacked,
Lost and hurt, no going back,
Senseless pain because of words,
From belief in sides, we must be cured.
The world is watching, but will we act,
Flourishing life needs a new pact,
Unjust horrors burn our eyes, burn the lands,
I pray for compassion to guide our hands.
Grief is such an internal experience that we can often feel alone,
Talk to your friends, talk to your government.
If war does nothing but light a fire in your raging heart, let that be enough.
If destruction does nothing but fill you with heart-opening compassion, let that be enough.
If death brings you the desire to live, let that be a start.

Remaining above water can be drying, dehydrating.
Dip your toes in the coolness underneath, slowly submerge into discovery.
Especially when you don't know what to expect.
Your soul is buoyant in uncertain spaces.

Float beneath the surface,
Linger in the depths.
Distortion in the dry air becomes clearer as you sink down.
The first drought of cold water makes you choke... and then awaken.
The sun feels different down here,
It's not dehydrating like the desert sand.
It looks like moving rainbows,
And tastes like heaven with a side of bittersweet.
Brackish layers of home, comfort in the liminal.
A nourishing bog with all manner of creature and insecurity,
The scent of renewal and calm bubbling under the greenish skin.
Illuminating the love within the fear.
Storms way above do not shake,
Shadows do not shade,
Mere ripples form from crashes of thunder.
For underneath, you are held in the mandala of molecules unified.
Vibrating as one.
Surfing the tide alone is not sustainable,
Without the pull of the ocean floor and the movement of the inverse curl as it hugs every ragged rock and smooth pebble.
Grounded, supported, while surfacing anew.
In the depths, you are buoyant.
Floating on the wisdom of the well-traveled water.

My darling child, it is okay
to take care of yourself
while the world does not rest.
Otherwise, the war inside
becomes too loud.

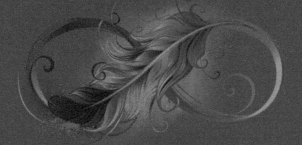

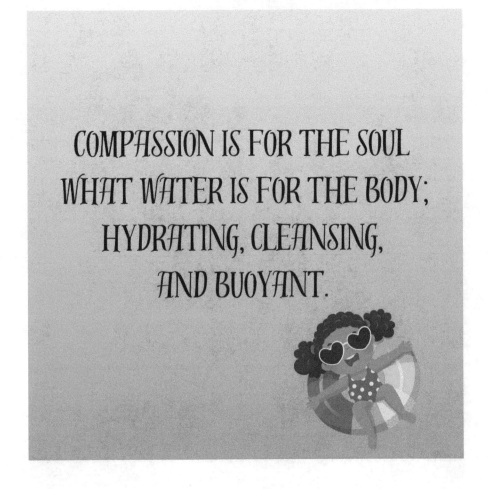

COMPASSION IS FOR THE SOUL
WHAT WATER IS FOR THE BODY;
HYDRATING, CLEANSING,
AND BUOYANT.

When we are lonely, miserable, longing, disconnected, suffering, seeking, mildly grumpy, or even hangry, being heard frees us.

Our minds, hearts, and nervous systems need to be known in order to thrive.

Compassion is a loving path to give others the gift of nourishment.

And it doesn't only go one way.

The moment we think a compassionate thought or feel it opening our heart, we are also being fed.

The lack of empathy, when directed toward us, can be extremely painful individually.

Without compassion for our humanity, we feel like a number, devalued, unimportant, invisible, less than.

This feeds frustration, anger, and sometimes the desire to retaliate.

On a larger scale, this can catalyze war.

When we are hydrated, our energy and vitality flow smoothly.

When we are seen, we are refreshed, clean.

Resentment can melt away when we are held in our pain.

Our spirit lifts and connection grows when we are valued and given space to be honest and to share what we hold inside.

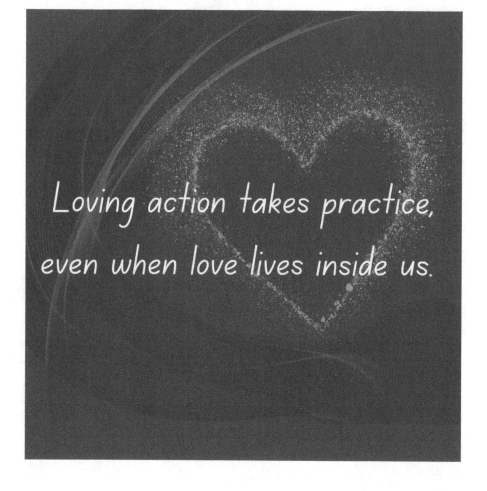

Loving action takes practice, even when love lives inside us.

If you forget who you are or how much you are worth, if you get distracted while listening to someone you care for, if something drives you into fear and away from love, or if your touch doesn't land with as much purpose and intention as you meant it to, try to remember that you are practicing, in this moment.
Remember who you are striving to be.
Remember to practice alignment with your integrity when you notice you are not.
Practice holding yourself with compassion.
Practice is ongoing, your evolution is ongoing.
Check in with yourself.
Connect with the hearts of others.
Vulnerability is a practice.
Hearing the whispers of soul is a practice.
Letting go is a practice.
Death and rebirth are inevitable.
Daily.
Reopen your mind.
Re-break your heart.
Hold it until it heals... again.
Daily.
Loving action takes practice, even when love lives inside us.
Just because it's inside doesn't always mean it's easy to express.
Practice who you want to be every time you are reborn, in a new moment, a new day, or a new life.

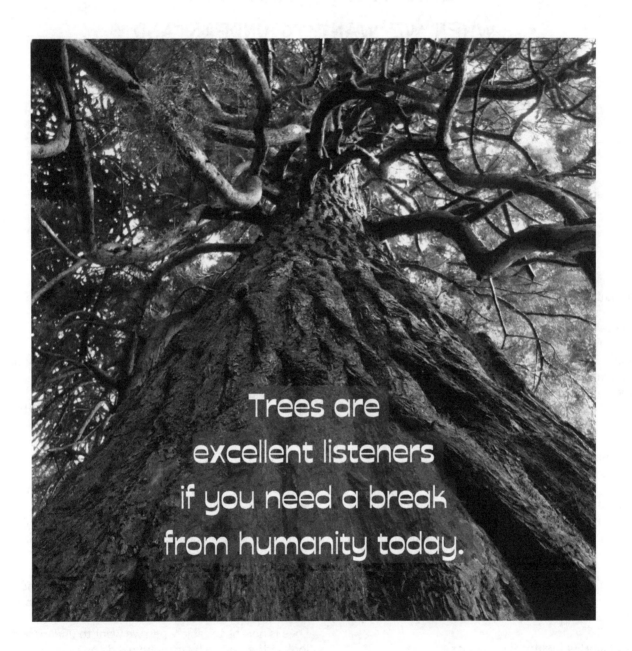

Trees are
excellent listeners
if you need a break
from humanity today.

LOVE IS NON-NEGOTIABLE WHEN WE WANT TO UNDERSTAND HOW TO LOOK AT THE HUMAN HEARTS WHO NEED COMMUNITY.

Out of sight doesn't mean they don't exist.

Do you see me?
I am a lonely woman living in a care home.
I don't get many visitors.
My children and grandchildren have busy lives.
They feed me well here and my room has a nice view.
I just wish I had someone to talk to and hold my hand.

Do you see me?
I have dementia.
Sometimes I can't see myself.
It's scary in my head, so confusing.
I try to hold on to the good memories I have, because they are what has meant the most to me in my life.
I just wish I had someone to reassure me and hold my hand in the dark.

Do you see me?
I'm became a mother too young.
I was abused in my relationship, so I did drugs to escape my pain.
Now my baby lives with someone else.
I just wish I had someone to help me heal so I can be a good mama.

Do you see me?
I left home when I was 12.
I went through my teens on the street.
Now I'm in jail because I stole things so I could eat and feed my friends.
We all had to look out for each other.
I just wish I had someone to see me for my strengths and my sacrifices.

Do you see me?
I have so much pain.
The doctors I've seen can't find anything wrong in my body, so they say it is all in my head.
It's been so long; I don't remember what life was like before.
I just wish I had someone that could make sense of all this and help me find relief.

Visibility is important when we want to understand systems.
Compassion is crucial when we want to understand humanity.
Love is non-negotiable when we want to understand how to look at the human hearts who need community.

The next revolution,
from the inside, from the deep,
must be of right relationship and reciprocity.

Sometimes, I feel that we have landed in the wrong timeline on earth. It was supposed to be more beautiful than this, more just, more loving, more conscious. Humanity is so often inhumane.

My heart aches so badly for people and animals and rivers and trees for all that they suffer because of choices made by people who are disconnected and out of balance. You see it. We all have our own versions of hell that present themselves in cycles.
We carry versions of violence within us, parts of us ingrained oppressive colonizer, other parts open and vulnerable, longing for liberation and healing.

I want to change so many things for so many people. I have a weak stomach for violence and a thin skin for indignity. To witness injustice is painful, but to experience it is unthinkable. So settlers, we must look.

There are countless violations of humanity. Unending wars against people and the planet, injustice is rampant. Billionaires exist. The lack of affordable housing is violence. There are constant attacks on children in schools, attacks on the LGBTQ+ community, and continued ignorance and violence toward our Indigenous peoples.
It's easy to get lost in pain and fear when there is so much of it.

The gospels of love don't travel far enough, awaken everybody, or embed into the hearts of all. The profound words of revolutionaries don't sink in through every ear, the songs of community don't echo in the heartbeats of the whole. The rhythms of nature do not reach the politicians of corruption.

Who cares and dares to face the pain of others when so muddled with our own?
Scars deep enough to hold oceans of tears torment us in dreams, in movies, in the dark, in the faces of others and the faces of our addictions and anxieties.

The dread must have its opposite wave, the undercurrent that peels back the layers of decay, bringing with it a sheer force, a mobility of desire, a new, collective breath. The reckoning must be of right relationship and reciprocity. Where else can we go from here?

Our instinctual nature
can be heard more easily
when we are close to the ground,
can smell the dirt,
are able to witness birth and death
in front of our eyes,
and the feeling of warmth waning
as we move
further from the sun.

My house is cold this morning, and it feels like the beginnings of winter. The sun in the distance is bright but noncommittal with its warmth.

Two crows sit upon the fence, looking at me. I ask them if they're cold, and they reply, of course not!

It's only the threshold of autumn, but the remnants of summer that lingered on the air last week are gone. My bones are chilled, and my blankets are warm. This makes it hard to jump out of bed with the same fervor as in spring or summer. My sloth days are coming.

I always feel a twinge of sadness when the season changes, except from winter to spring when the light returns. My body senses that it's time to harvest, make soup, and rest. I don't, however, have the luxury of honouring my instincts alone. The restful spirit in me must forgive my busyness each year, the restless anxiety that rises from going against my nature. Awareness of this melancholy helps me understand my feelings, but it does nothing to solve the economics of this world, at least yet.

I guess balance is what it's all about.

Hibernation and rebirth.

Cycles of growth, change, and sleep.

We have internal seasons, though they can be hard to access due to the unstoppable energy of lights, media, corporations, and billionaires, forever pointing toward constant growth, as if that was ever a natural thing.

A cycle goes round, not only up.

Our instinctual nature can be heard more easily when we are close to the ground, can smell the dirt, are able to witness birth and death in front of our eyes, and the feeling of warmth waning as we become further from the sun.

So today I am sad for untouchable reasons.

Though I still feel love and peace in the melancholy.

I wish the world would hibernate for 3 months every year to let everyone and everything rest and reset, so we could catch up on living and reconnect with the wild nature within.

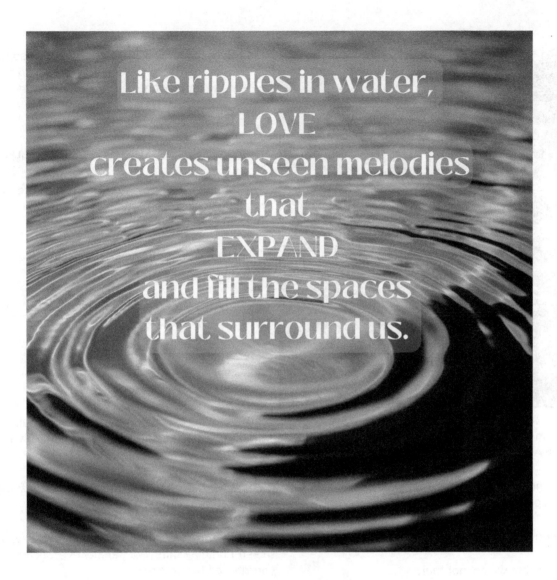

Like ripples in water,
LOVE
creates unseen melodies
that
EXPAND
and fill the spaces
that surround us.

From inside the rings of ripples
I feel the never-ending longing for the shore
From inside the wings of wild birds
I am cradled, free, and sure
Discovery is an eternity
Horizons stretch beyond the sea
I am the ripple, blessed by whispers of the wind, savoring the warmth of sunshine infusing through my fluid skin
I am the moth playing on the breeze
I speak without words, entice the bees
Hear love songs flowing softly from the trees
Currents guide my ebb and shimmer
Seeing above and beneath the glowing glimmer
With senses that don't need a body
One with the outer One with the inner
Portals to the otherworld iridescent and alive
Morphing unseen melodies, molecules revive
Dimensions of the deep, shadows overcome
Rhythms of the ocean wide
From ripples I become

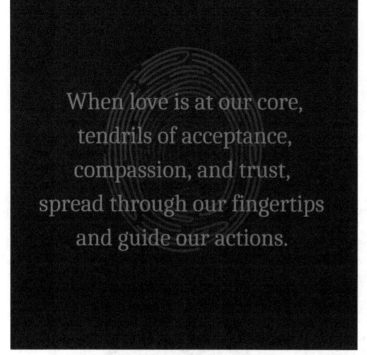

When love is at our core, tendrils of acceptance, compassion, and trust, spread through our fingertips and guide our actions.

We, in North America, are witnessing devastation in the form of wars in Africa, the Middle East, and Eastern Europe.

They are by far not the only places with atrocities and destruction happening in the world.

They break our hearts, nonetheless.

We are watching, but we are not there.

Some of us may have escaped areas of war, some of us may have family in these areas, some of us can only imagine what people are being faced with at this very moment.

As difficult as it is to hear about, it is much much worse for people losing their lives and families, communities, and countries.

This may be obvious, though our nervous systems get involved anyway.

The fight or flight response is commonly known, but there are two others, fawn, and freeze.

The freeze response can create a sense of helplessness.

Watching from afar is fear-inducing and may cause folks to feel helpless.

On top of our responsibilities, economic needs, drug crises, and hardships here at home, it's hard to pile more worry and anxiety onto our plates.

I feel helpless sometimes too.

I encourage you to take care of your mental health, first.

Put your hand on your chest and feel the sensation of your hand on your skin as you breathe or notice the support of the surface you're sitting on.

Take a break from the news, connect with a friend, or talk to a therapist.

Remember your joy, because only focusing on grief and anxiety is exhausting.

If you feel angry and want to see something change, take one small action to help move the energy and reach out to someone outside of yourself.

Search online for one organization you could contact if or when you feel ready to connect with others who are helping a cause you deeply value.

Meet a few friends for tea and discuss an action you could take together that would feel meaningful.

Even just donating a few dollars to people saving lives on the ground may shift your perspective, because you have contributed to some relief.

When we contribute to another's relief, compassion grows in our hearts, making it easier to breathe, and to continue toward meaningful action.

If we are scared to move an injured joint once there is healing and then still after, the ability to use its full range decreases or remains stagnant, in a sense.

Similarly, if we remain stuck in our fear, disgust, and helplessness, we can become immobilized.

If we remember to listen for the love underneath our shock and sadness, it can be comforting to realize that without this love, we wouldn't be devastated in the first place. Let this love drive our action and compassion and allow us to hope for change.

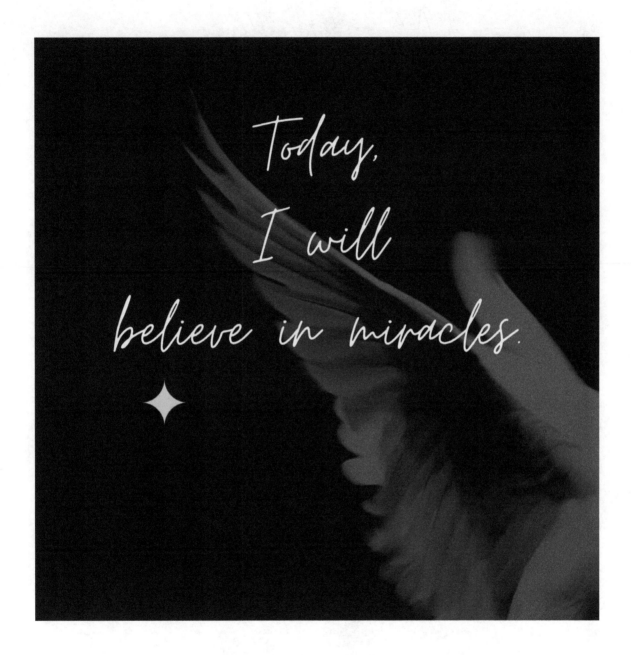

Today, I will believe in miracles.

Pay attention. They are everywhere.
Tell your miraculous story.

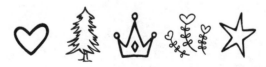

Notes and Reflections

Notes and Reflections

Notes and Reflections

Notes and Reflections

Notes and Reflections

Notes and Reflections

References

The Benefits of Play for Adults – Helpguide.org, https://www.helpguide.org/articles/mental-health/benefits-of-pla-for-adults.htm

What to do when you feel like you can't do anything right, https://www.verywellmind.com/what-to-do-when-you-feel-like-you-cant-do-anything-right-5218204

Understanding Motivation, https://developingchild.harvard.edu/resources/understanding-motivation-building-the-brain-architecture-that-supports-learning-health-and-community-participation/

https://www.healthline.com/health/mental-health/tend-and-befriend#theories

Somatic Experiencing, https://www.frontiersin.org/articles/10.3389/fpsyg.2015.00093/full#

Therapeutic Intention: Into the Next Generation, https://www.researchgate.net/publication/314196423_therapeutic_intention_into_the_next_generation

Developing and training intuition:

https://positivepsychology.com/intuition-training/

https://www.takingcharge.csh.umn.edu/activities/exercising-developing-your-intuition

Six habits of highly compassionate people, https://greatergood.berkeley.edu/article/item/six_habits_of_highly_compassionate_people

The Compassionate Instinct, https://greatergood.berkeley.edu/article/item/the_compassionate_instinct

Defining your list of values and beliefs, https://soulsalt.com/list-of-values-and-beliefs/

What to do if you or a loved one lack empathy, https://www.verywellmind.com/what-to-do-if-you-or-a-loved-one-lack-empathy-5199257

Compassion Fatigue, https://www.stress.org/military/for-practitionersleaders/compassion-fatigue

Nerve injury and repair, https://pubmed.ncbi.nlm.nih.gov/14641646/

Neuropathic pain, https://pubmed.ncbi.nlm.nih.gov/18003941/

Massage Therapy improved symptoms of MS, https://pubmed.ncbi.nlm.nih.gov/34338108/

What is gaslighting, https://www.wholeheartedworkshops.com/what-is-gaslighting-could-it-be-happening-to-you/

The ability to listen, https://cooalliance.com/blog/why-the-ability-to-listen-is-the-ultimate-soft-skill/

Active listening, MindTools.com, https://www.mindtools.com/commskll/activelistening.htm

How to improve listening skills, Indeed.com, https://www.indeed.com/career-advice/career-development/how-to-improve-listening-skills

Daring Leadership Assessment, Brenebrown.com, https://daretolead.brenebrown.com/assessment/

Community: Activities that build interdependence: Rollins teaching resources, https://rollins.instructure.com/courses/6578/pages/community-activities-that-build-interdependence

Health promotion and illness prevention, https://pubmed.ncbi.nlm.nih.gov/2707681/

Embodiment of Emotion throughout the Lifespan, https://www.frontiersin.org/research-topics/8911/embodiment-of-emotion-throughout-the-lifespan-the-role-of-multi-modal-processing-in-perception-cogni

The power of touch in senior care,

https://plushcare.com/blog/advantages-of-human-touch-hugs/

https://www.goldencarers.com/the-power-of-touch-in-senior-care/5505/

Measuring what counts in life, https://www.frontiersin.org/articles/10.3389/fpsyg.2021.795931/full

What is an Oriki, https://awesomelyluvvie.com/2021/03/oriki-challenge.html

Hugging study, https://link.springer.com/article/10.1007/s10919-022-00411-8

What is regenerative capitalism? https://www.weforum.org/agenda/2022/01/regenerative-capitalism-industry-explainer/

Sense of Self: What it is and how to build it, https://www.healthline.com/health/sense-of-self

The power of labels, https://turnersyndromefoundation.org/2021/07/13/the-power-of-labels/

Living through loss, https://livingthroughloss.ca/grief-and-loss-training/

The Power of Human Connection,

https://www.betterup.com/blog/human-connection#:~:text=Human%20connection%20is%20a%20deep,you%20a%20sense%20of%20belonging.

https://www.mindbodygreen.com/articles/how-to-know-if-you-have-emotional-connection-with-someone

Healwell.org https://www.healwell.org/flawed-research

https://www.familycaregiversbc.ca

Elder care resources, https://hr.ubc.ca/health-and-wellbeing/mental-health/elder-care-resources

Compassion in Caregiving, https://www.compassionincaregiving.com

Jung archetype, https://jungplatform.com/store/the-archetype-of-the-wounded-healer

Healing definitions, https://www.ncbi.nlm.nih.gov/pmc/articles/PMC1466870/

Continuity of care importance, https://www.ncbi.nlm.nih.gov/pmc/articles/PMC2083711/

Continuity of care study, https://www.ncbi.nlm.nih.gov/pmc/articles/PMC4979943/

Healthy reasons to walk in the rain/nature,

https://m.footfiles.com/wellness/relaxation/article/8-healthy-reasons-to-walk-in-the-rain

https://www.psychologies.co.uk/walking-in-the-rain-benefits/

https://www.researchgate.net/publication/327946184_health_benefits_of_walking_in_nature_a_randomized_controlled_study_under_condtions_of_real-life_stress

The effect of deep and slow breathing on pain perception, autonomic activity, and mood processing – an experimental study, https://pubmed.ncbi.nlm.nih.gov/21939499/

Neuroscience of gratitude, https://positivepsychology.com/neuroscience-of-gratitude

The importance of patient dignity in care at the end of life, https://www.ncbi.nlm/nih.gov/pmc/articles/PMC4847835/

The heart vs. the mind (scientific explanation), https://cognitiontoday.com/the-heart-vs-mind-battle-that-need-not/

The importance of developing curiosity,

https://psychcentral.com/blog/the-importance-of-developing-curiosity

https://andersonuniversity.edu/sites/default/files/student-success/importance-of-being-curious.pdf

https://communityedition.ca/buliding-resilience-curiosity-is-key/#:~:text=A%20continuously%20curious%20adult%20will,compelling%2C%20confident%20and%20resilient%20life.

https://psychologytoday.com/blog/resilient-leadership/201604/are-you-curious-person-why-you-may-also-be-more-resilient

Human connection,

https://www.discovermagazine.com/health/how-human-connection-affects-our-hearts-and-hormones

https://www.psychologytoday.com/us/blog/wired-love/201909/commitment-connection-in-culture-fear

Forest bathing, https://greatergood.berkeley.edu/article/item/why_forest_bathing_is_good_for_your_health

Touch reduces pain,

https://www.ncbi.nlm.nih.gov/pmc/articles/PMC/3988987/

https://www.frontiersin.org/articles/10.3389/fnint.2022.956510/full

Nested vulnerability, https://www.ncbi.nlm.nih.gov/pmc/articles/PMC7163976/

How learning affects evolution, https://journals.plos.org/plosone/article?id=10.1371/journal.pone.0219502

https://www.scienceofpeople.com/core-values/

"The effects of therapeutic touch on spiritual care and sleep quality in patients receiving palliative care." (Aslan, Cetinkaya, Perspectives in Psychiatric Care, Wiley Online, April 2021) https://doi.org/10.1111/ppc.12801 https://onlinelibrary.wiley.com/doi/ftr/10.1111/ppc.12801

"Massage Therapy for symptom reduction and improved quality of life in children with cancer in palliative care: A pilot study." (Genik, et al. Complement Ther Med, National Library of Medicine, PubMed, January 2020) https://pubmed.ncbi.nlm.nih.gov/31987232

How many thoughts do we have per day, https://healthline.com/health/how-many-thoughts-per-day#thought-origins

How does consciousness evolve, https://www.frontiersin.org/articles/10.3389/fpsyg.2018.01537/full

"Six weeks of massage therapy produces changes in balance, neurological and cardiovascular measures in older persons." (Sefton, Yarar, Berry, National Library of Medicine, PubMed Central, September 2012) https://www.ncbi.nlm.nih.gov/pmc/articles/PMC3457720/

Benefits of massage therapy on elderly two times per week, "A randomised study of the effects of massage therapy compared to guided relaxation on well-being and stress perception among older adults." (Sharpe, Williams, et al. Science Direct, Complementary Therapies in Medicine, September 2007) https://www.sciencedirect.com/science/article/abs/pii/S0965229907000064

"Massage Therapy for hospitalized patients receiving palliative care." (Groginger, Nemati, Cates, et al. Journal of Pain and Symptom Management, May 2023) https://www.jpsmjournal.com/article/S0885-3924(23)00046-5/fulltext

https://rehabs.com/pro-talk/how-relationships-regulate-our-nervous-system/

"The 2030 Problem: Caring for aging baby boomers." (Knickman, Snell, Health Services Research, National Library of Medicine, PubMed central, August 2002) https://www.ncbi.nlm.nih.gov/pmc/articles/PMC1464018/

https://census.gov/library/stories/2019/12/by-2030-all-baby-boomers-will-be-age-65-or-older.html

"Violence against seniors and their perception of safety in Canada." (Conroy, Sutton, Canadian Centre for Justice and Community Safety Statistics, July 2022) https://www.150.statcan.gc.ca/n1/pub/85-002-x/2022001/article/00011-eng.htm

9.6 million Canadians will die by 2050, https://nnpcn.com/the-baby-boomer-bulge/

Japan in-home care program, https://www.oecd.org/g20/topics/global-health/

"How lack of love in childhood robs us of love in adulthood." (Cikanavicius, PsychCentral, September 2019) https://psychcentral.com/blog/psychology-self/2019/09/trauma-lack-of-love

https://www.lifehack.org/868295/relationship-values

Scarcity mentality, https://www.wedmd.com/mental-health/signs-sociopath

Empathic listening, https://www.berkeleywellbeing.com/empathic-listening.html

"Cheering enhances inter-brain synchronization between sensorimotor areas of player and observer." Mirror neurons and brain connectivity with cheering, (Koide, Shimada, Japanese Psychological Research, Wiley Online Library, July 2018) https://onlinelibrary.wiley.com/doi/full/10.1111/jpr.12202

"How nature nurtures: Amygdala activity decreases as the result of a one-hour walk in nature." (Sudimac, Sale, Kuhn, Molecular Psychiatry, September 2022) https://www.nature.com/articles/s41380-022-01720-6

https://www.linguajunkie.com/japanese/beautiful-japanese-words

"Medical center researcher explores what happens when we touch." https://news.columbia.edu/news/medical-center-researcher-explores-what-happens-when-we-touch

Printed in the USA
CPSIA information can be obtained
at www.ICGtesting.com
LVHW070554221223
767101LV00009B/511